Nursing Diagnosis in Clinical Practice:

Guides for Care Planning

Dedication

We dedicate this book to those frontline nurses who continue to struggle for an independent realm of nursing practice.

NURSING DIAGNOSIS IN CLINICAL PRACTICE:

Guides for Care Planning

Kathy V. Gettrust, R.N., B.S.N.
Case Manager
Midwest Medical Home Care
Milwaukee, Wisconsin

Paula D. Brabec, R.N., M.S.N.
Nurse Consultant
Wheaton, Illinois

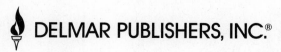

DELMAR PUBLISHERS, INC.®

Notice to the reader

Publisher does not warrant or guarantee any of the products described herein or perform any independent analysis in connection with any of the product information contained herein. Publisher does not assume, and expressly disclaims, any obligation to obtain and include information other than that provided to it by the manufacturer.

The reader is expressly warned to consider and adopt all safety precautions that might be indicated by the activities described herein and to avoid all potential hazards. By following the instructions contained herein, the reader willingly assumes all risks in connection with such instructions.

The publisher makes no representations or warranties of any kind, including but not limited to, the warranties of fitness for particular purpose or merchantability, nor are any such representations implied with respect to the material set forth herein, and the publisher takes no responsibility with respect to such material. The publisher shall not be liable for any special, consequential or exemplary damages resulting, in whole or in part, from readers' use of, or reliance upon, this material.

Delmar Staff:
Executive Editor: David Gordon
Project Editor: Christopher Chien
Production Coordinator: Sandra Woods
Art Supervisor: John Lent
Design Coordinator: Karen Kunz Kemp

COPYRIGHT © 1992
BY DELMAR PUBLISHERS, INC.

Printed in the United States of America
Published simultaneously in Canada
by Nelson Canada,
a division of The Thomson Corporation

10 9 8 7 6 5 4 3 2

Library of Congress Cataloging-in-Publication Data

Nursing diagnosis in clinical practice: guides for care planning/ Kathy V. Gettrust, Paula D. Brabec.
    p. cm.
  Includes bibliographical reference and index.
  ISBN 0–8273–4852–5 (textbook)
  1. Nursing diagnosis. 2. Nursing care plans.   I. Gettrust, Kathy V. II. Brabec, Paula D.
  (DNLM: 1. Nursing Diagnosis. 2. Patient Care Planning.   WY 100 N975143)
RT48.6.N87 1992
610.73—dc20
DNLM/DLC
for Library of Congress
    91-25195
    CIP

Contributors

We are fortunate to have found a nationally diverse group of contributors. Each possesses quality credentials and expertise in specific nursing diagnoses. Their knowledge has been invaluable to this book.

Linda S. Baas, R.N., M.S.N., C.C.R.N.
Visiting Assistant Professor —
Miami University,
Oxford, Ohio.
- Activity Intolerance
- Activity Intolerance: Risk
- Infection: Risk

Colleen Creamer-Bauer, R.N., M.S., C.C.R.N.
Cardiovascular Clinical Nurse Specialist—
Merritt Hospital,
Oakland, California.
- Cardiac Output, Altered
- Tissue Perfusion, Altered Peripheral

Kathleen Beyerman, R.N., Ed.D.
Director of Education and
Staff Development—
Winchester Hospital,
Winchester, Massachusetts.
- Sleep Pattern Disturbance

Christine Brugler, R.N., M.S.N.
Gerontological Nurse Consultant—
Warren, Ohio.
- Relocation Stress

Phyllis Cerone, R.N., B.S.N., C.C.R.N.
Critical Care Educator—
Northwest Community Hospital
Arlington Heights, Illinois.
- Swallowing, Impaired

Marga S. Coler, R.N., C.S., CTN, Ed.D.
Professor, School of Nursing—
University of Connecticut,
Storrs, Connecticut.
- Fear

Carol Lewis Cullinan, R.N., C., M.S.N., F.N.P.
Clinical Nurse Coordinator—
Rhode Island Hospital,
Providence, Rhode Island.
and Janice K. Janken, R.N., Ph.D.
Associate Professor—
University of North Carolina at Charlotte,
Charlotte, North Carolina.
and Clinical Nurse Researcher—
Presbyterian Hospital, Charlotte,
North Carolina.
- Sensory Perception, Altered: Auditory

Patricia Danaher-Dunn, R.N., M.S.
Community Consultation Liaison Program—
Milwaukee County Mental Health Complex,
Wauwatosa, Wisconsin.
- Family Processes, Altered
- Social Interaction, Impaired
- Social Isolation

M. Kathleen Eilers, R.N., M.S.N.
Associate Administrator, Programs—
Milwaukee County Mental Health Complex,
Wauwatosa, Wisconsin.
- Adjustment, Impaired
- Denial, Impaired
- Role Performance, Altered

Julia D. Emblen, R.N., Ph.D.
Dean, Department of Nursing—
Trinity Christian College,
Palos Heights, Illinois.
- Fatigue
- Grieving, Anticipatory
- Grieving, Dysfunctional

Kathleen Fitzgerald, R.N., M.S., C.E.T.N.
Clinical Nurse Specialist, Nutritional
Support—
Northwestern Memorial Hospital,
Chicago, Illinois.
- Bowel Incontinence
- Diarrhea

Marilyn Frenn, R.N., Ph.D.
Assistant Professor—
Marquette University,
Milwaukee, Wisconsin.
Assistance from Helena Lee, R.N., M.S.N.
Clinical Nurse Specialist—
Milwaukee County Mental Health Complex,
Milwaukee, Wisconsin.
and Sharon Willadsen, R.N., B.S.N.
Graduate Student—
Marquette University,
Milwaukee, Wisconsin.
- Health Maintenance, Altered
- Health Seeking Behaviors (Specify)
- Nutrition, Less than Body
  Requirement
- Nutrition, Less than Body
  Requirement: Risk
- Nutrition, More than Body
  Requirement
- Nutrition, More than Body
  Requirement: Risk

Laina M. Gerace, R.N., Ph.D.
Assistant Professor of Psychiatric Nursing,
College of Nursing—
University of Illinois at Chicago,
Chicago, Illinois.
and Jill Anderson, R.N., M.S.N.
Clinical Specialist in Psychiatric Nursing,
University of Illinois Hospitals and Clinics,
Chicago, Illinois.
- Thought Processes, Altered

Joan T. Harkulich, R.N., M.S.N.
Director of Research and Professional
Services—
Care Services,
Beachwood, Ohio.
- Communication, Impaired Verbal
- Protection, Altered
- Relocation Stress

Elizabeth Hiltunen, R.N., M.S., C.S.
Medical-Surgical Clinical Nurse Specialist—
WalthamWeston Hospital and Medical
Center,
Waltham, Massachusetts.
- Conflict: Decisional (Specify)

Kay Koneazny, R.N., M.S.N.
Psychiatric Case Manager,
Milwaukee, Wisconsin.
- Coping: Defensive
- Coping, Impaired Individual

S. Jill Ley, R.N., M.S., C.C.R.N.
Clinical Nurse Specialist—
Pacific Presbyterian Medical Center,
San Francisco, California.
- Fluid Volume Deficit
- Fluid Volume Deficit: Risk
- Fluid Volume Excess

Colleen Lucas, R.N., M.N., C.S.
Medical-Surgical Clinical Nurse Specialist—
Good Samaritan Hospital and Medical
Center,
Portland, Oregon.
• Injury: Risk

• Poisoning: Risk

• Trauma: Risk

Vicki E. McClurg, R.N., M.N.
Assistant Professor, School of Health
Science—
Seattle Pacific University,
Seattle, Washington.
Assistance from Ginna R. Wall, R.N., M.N.,
Dona J. Lethbridge, R.N., Ph.D.
and Mary Henrikson, R.N., C., M.N.,
A.R.N.P.
• Breastfeeding, Effective

• Breastfeeding, Impaired

Marilyn A. McCubbin, R.N., Ph.D.
Assistant Professor, School of Nursing—
University of Wisconsin-Madison,
Madison, Wisconsin.
• Coping, Family: Compromised

• Coping, Family: Disabled

• Coping, Family: Potential for Growth

Peg A. Mehmert, R.N., C., M.S.N.
Associate Director of Nursing—
Assistance from Carol Dickel, R.N.
Clinical Research Assistant,
Suellyn Ellerbe, R.N., M.N.
Vice President of Nursing,
and Diane C. Kolb, R.N., B.A.
Director, Mercy Continuing Care—
Mercy Hospital,
Davenport, Iowa,
and Rosemary J. McKeighen, R.N., Ph.D.,
F.A.A.N.
Professor Emeritus, College of Nursing—
University of Iowa,
Iowa City, Iowa.
• Bathing/Hygiene Deficit

• Dressing/Grooming Deficit

• Feeding Deficit

• Toileting Deficit

Ann Moore, R.N., M.Ed.
Staff Development/QA Coordinator—
Milwaukee County Mental Health Complex,
Wauwatosa, Wisconsin.
• Parental Role Conflict

• Parenting, Altered

• Parenting, Altered: Risk

Brenda S. Nichols, R.N., D.N.Sc.
Associate Professor, School of Nursing—
Old Dominion University,
Norfolk, Virginia.
- Disuse Syndrome: Risk
- Physical Mobility, Impaired

Joan Norris, R.N., Ph.D.
Professor and Associate Dean, School
of Nursing—
Creighton University,
Omaha, Nebraska.
- Self-Esteem Disturbance: Chronic Low
- Self-Esteem Disturbance: Situational

Joan Randall, R.N., M.S.
Vice President, Clinical Services—
VNA of Orange County,
Anaheim, California.
- Home Maintenance Management,
  Impaired
- Knowledge Deficit (Specify)
- Oral Mucous Membrane, Impaired

Marilyn J. Rantz, R.N., M.S.N., N.H.A.
Administrator, Lakeland Nursing Home,
Elkhorn, Wisconsin.
- Diversional Activity Deficit

Polly Ryan, R.N., M.S.N.
Doctoral Candidate, University of Wisconsin—
Milwaukee,
Milwaukee, Wisconsin.
- Noncompliance: Dietary
- Noncompliance: Prescribed Medications
- Noncompliance: Smoking

Judith K. Sands, R.N., Ed.D.
Associate Professor, School of Nursing—
University of Virginia,
Charlottesville, Virginia.
- Dysreflexia
- Pain, Acute
- Pain, Chronic

Kathleen Herman Scanlon, R.N., M.S.N.
Assistant Professor, Department of Nursing—
Elmhurst College,
Elmhurst, Illinois.
- Constipation
- Constipation: Colonic
- Constipation: Perceived

Jan A. Sheldon, R.N., M.S., C.R.R.N.
Nurse Manager, Spinal Cord Injury Program.
Assistance from Mary A. Gollinger, R.N., M.S.,
C.R.R.N.
Administrative Director of Nursing—
Marianjoy Rehabilitation Center,
Wheaton, Illinois.
- Body Image Disturbance
- Unilateral Neglect

Anne Marie Voith Sherman, R.N., M.S.N.
Quality Assurance Coordinator—
Blue Cross/Blue Shield,
Milwaukee, Wisconsin.
- Incontinence: Functional
- Incontinence: Reflex
- Incontinence: Stress
- Incontinence: Urge
- Incontinence: Total
- Urinary Retention: Acute
- Urinary Retention: Chronic

Georgene C. Siemsen, R.N., C.S., M.S.
Clinical Nurse Specialist, Gerontology,
Good Samaritan Hospital and Medical Center,
Portland, Oregon.
- Aspiration: Risk
- Suffocation: Risk

Gladys Simandl, R.N., Ph.D.
Assistant Professor
and Leona VandeVusse, R.N., C.N.M., M.S.
Adjunct Assistant Professor,
College of Nursing—
Marquette University,
Milwaukee, Wisconsin.
- Sensory Perception, Altered
- Sensory Perception, Altered: Touch
- Sexuality Patterns, Altered
- Spiritual Distress

Linda Slimmer, R.N., Ph.D.
Professor, Department of Nursing—
Elmhurst College,
Elmhurst, Illinois.
- Hopelessness
- Powerlessness

Carrol A. M. Smith, R.N., M.S.
Assistant Professor,
Department of Nursing
Elmhurst College,
Elmhurst, Illinois.
- Rape-Trauma Syndrome
- Rape-Trauma Syndrome: Compound Reaction
- Rape-Trauma Syndrome: Silent Reaction

Nancy A. Stotts, R.N., Ed.D.
Associate Professor, Department of Physiological Nursing—
University of California,
San Francisco, California.
- Skin Integrity, Impaired
- Skin Integrity, Impaired: Risk
- Tissue Integrity, Altered

Sharon Summers, R.N., Ph.D.
Associate Professor, School of Nursing—
University of Kansas Medical Center,
Kansas City, Kansas.
- Body Temperature, Altered: Risk
- Hyperthermia
- Hypothermia

Cynthia C. Valentin, R.N., Ph.D.
Consulting Psychologist
Ancillary Home Health Care,
Wauwatosa, Wisconsin.
- Personal Identity Disturbance

Karen Goyette Vincent, R.N., M.S., C.S.
Psychiatric Clinical Nurse Specialist—
Brockton/West Roxbury V.A. Medical Center,
Brockton, Massachusetts.
- Anxiety

Claudia M. West, R.N., M.S.
Assistant Clinical Professor, School of Nursing—
University of California, San Francisco,
San Francisco, California.
- Airway Clearance, Impaired
- Breathing Pattern, Impaired
- Gas Exchange, Impaired

Von Best Whitaker, R.N., Ph.D.
Assistant Professor, School of Nursing—
University of Texas–Health Science Center at San Antonio,
San Antonio, Texas.
- Sexual Dysfunction
- Violence: Risk

Marcia Williams, R.N., M.S.N.
Clinical Nurse Specialist.
Assistance from Alice Kramer, R.N., B.S.N.
Nurse Clinician—
St. Luke's Medical Center,
Milwaukee, Wisconsin.
- Post-Trauma Response

Jenny A. Zaker, R.N., M.Ed., C.C.R.N.
Critical Care Educator—
Northwest Community Hospital,
Arlington Heights, Illinois.
- Thermoregulation, Impaired

Contents

SECTION I: NURSING DIAGNOSIS: HISTORY AND PRACTICE

SECTION II: NURSING DIAGNOSIS CARE PLANNING GUIDES

Titles set with asterisk and boldface are newly developed nursing diagnoses not on NANDA list.

Foreword

Much of what we collectively experience as a species presents itself as a spiral growth process, a coming full circle to a new place which is at the same time a familiar place, one reframed by fresh insights or greater depth. This book exemplifies this spiral growth process. For several years now, the efforts begun in 1973 in St. Louis to organize nursing's phenomena of concern, i.e., nursing diagnoses, have been manifested in increasingly sophisticated reflections of that first effort. Such reflections have focused on improving patient care in nursing terms, institutionalizing these improvements, and making them tangible. Now, spiraling forth, new manifestations emerge with fresh insights and greater depth. This book exemplifies that emergence. It is good news for all of us.

This book reflects the explosive growth of nursing practice in the intervening years. We understand our practice better; we describe it more clearly. We have delineated and accepted responsibility for our roles in health care in a way that has expanded both the scope and depth of that practice. We reflect a growing sense of confidence and pride in these developments. Using this book creatively thus enables you, as the reader, to observe these changes and become a participant in and continue this growth.

Nursing care delivery always confronts the practicing nurse with the delicate balance between the intelligent use of generalizable knowledge and the innovative response to the unique needs of each individual client. One way to optimize quality care is to increase the efficiency of our use of generalizable knowledge. We can then more deliberately focus on innovative individualizations and the human and humane expressions of care.

To achieve this balance, we need continuously improved resources. This book is such a resource. It enables the practicing nurse to hone discriminating powers in both dimensions of care. It can increase efficiency; it can further the process of describing the generalizable aspects of care; it can provide indicators of opportunities for individualization of care.

Years of working in the North American Nursing Diagnosis Association (NANDA) taught me many things about our capacity for creative collaboration. Often it seemed that people would explain to me in painful detail the deficiencies of NANDA's efforts and assure me that they elected to either utilize or create an alternate system for one reason or another. I would point out to them that, because NANDA enabled consensus and collective ownership and development, they could make the difference, create the solution; they could improve the NANDA system rather than merely criticizing or competing. I would note that common language is a worthy goal, and requires a common ground. People would demur; it seemed that having a language they personally embraced was for them a greater good than the goal of a common language for the common good. This always struck me as moderately benighted.

This book manifests for me the obverse of that experience. All of what I consider the best in struggling for both the common ground and the common language are reflected here. The capacity for growth, development, continued dialogue, and ongoing growth are the "stuff" of this book. The emergence of this book reminds us that this approach works. Joining a common effort, improving and expanding it, making it work for all of us: These goals are possible and this book makes that evident. Diversity of voices is indeed enriching when joined in a common effort.

Thus it is a pleasure to welcome you to our journey through this book. We have all grown since our first cycles on this spiral. It is my hope that you will enjoy, benefit from, use, and value this cycle of the spiral as much as I have.

It is a wonderful exemplar of our collective and continuous growth.

Phyllis B. Kritek, R.N., Ph.D., F.A.A.N.
Dean and Professor, College of Nursing
Marquette University
Milwaukee, Wisconsin

Preface

Contemporary nurses play a key role in the delivery of health care. The body of knowledge required to practice nursing with expertise is growing rapidly as the nursing profession continues to evolve. Current facts, principles, and concepts of health and illness coupled with the knowledge of individual differences, situational variances, and environmental influences must be readily known in order to meet this demand.

While the nursing role is expanding, the health care environment is struggling with contracting time and financial resources. To meet these challenges, nurses must practice more knowledgeably and efficiently than ever before. In order to provide quality patient care, it must be planned and coordinated. Care plans, written and utilized properly, provide direction and continuity of care by facilitating communications among care givers.

The purpose of this book is:

1. To provide an easy-to-use, comprehensive, and well-organized information source for care plan construction. It has application for both the novice and the experienced diagnostician practicing in a variety of settings.

2. To enhance the understanding of all currently accepted nursing diagnoses developed by the North American Nursing Diagnosis Association (NANDA).

3. To use the nursing process model, as opposed to medical model or systems/disease classification, as an efficient method of organizing thought processes to plan and implement nursing care.

4. To equip the nurse with a prototype for care plan construction with an understanding that critical thinking be applied to each individual situation.

5. To assist the educator by incorporating theory and research-based data into the practice setting.

This book has two important and unique features: First, each nursing intervention is supported by a scientific rationale; every practicing nurse needs to have a strong theoretical base. Unfortunately, all too often, nurses intervene without a clear understanding of the reasons for their actions. When the purpose for care is understood, the nurse can practice more intelligently and tailor actions to each individual's needs.

Second, this book reflects both the changing role of nursing toward a more independent practice and the changing focus of nursing toward community-based health care by including interventions for clients in both inpatient and community settings. With the current trend of nursing practice moving from inpatient to community settings, communication and documentation must be consistent to assure continuity of care as the client moves from one area of the health care system to another.

Experts from a wide geographical area who represent the state of the art of nursing practice have contributed to this undertaking. We have utilized nurses in the area of service and education so as to incorporate both the practical realism of the staff nurse and the theoretical idealism of the nurse scholar.

It is difficult to comprehend the progress nurses have made in developing their nursing taxonomy and theory, adapting to their expanding roles, and reaching for more independent practice. The 1990s will see nurses armed with the tools of a unified language and a scientific base confidently going on to demonstrate excellence in nursing through carefully planned and implemented interventions. We are pleased to be sharing a part in this endeavor.

Kathy V. Gettrust
Paula D. Brabec

Acknowledgements

We would like to thank Debi Folkerts, Executive Director, NANDA, for attending to our many questions and concerns. Appreciation is also given to David Gordon and Barbara Norwitz, Executive Editors; Christopher Chien, Project Editor; Debra Flis, Editorial Assistant; and other staff at Delmar Publishers who so capably guided us through the publishing process. A big "thank you" is extended to all of our dear family and friends who supported us with encouraging cards, phone calls, and the like through these past months. Gratitude is also extended to Dad and Mom Groves for their capable child care, home maintenance, taxi service, typing, and moral support that only parents can give to their children. We would especially like to thank our husbands—John Gettrust and Tom Brabec—for being "Mr. Mom" during the long hours of preparing this book. Also, thanks and hugs to Katrina and Allison Gettrust; and to Hannah, Martha, Gabriela, and Jesse Brabec for taking on additional responsibilities, respecting our work spaces, and following the house rules more carefully than usual.

Introduction

The importance of well-written and individualized care plans is known to most nurses. Quality nursing care occurs when a course of action is scientifically based and carefully developed. This takes precious time and expertise to accomplish. NURSING DIAGNOSIS IN CLINICAL PRACTICE: GUIDES FOR CARE PLANNING has been written to aid the nurse in care plan construction. Each nursing care planning guide is built around a nursing diagnosis, and includes all elements of a care plan (see Table i.1). It is well organized for easy use, and comprehensive, and selectable for individualizing care.

EXPLANATION OF FRAMEWORK AND TAXONOMY

NANDA has several classification systems in various stages of development. They are Taxonomy I-Revised, ICD coding of Taxonomy I-Revised, and (as of 1990), Taxonomy II-Draft 1 (see Chapter 1 for more information regarding the classification systems). All of the classification systems have some minor language differences. Some of the labels are different and some of the structure of the classification systems is different. Tolerance with the ambiguity and involvement in refining the classification systems need to occur during this developmental phase. The importance of having an organizing structure within which the nursing diagnoses are placed cannot be underestimated. A conceptual structure has direct relevance to the scientific understandings of nursing diagnoses but a more limited relevance to nursing practice. Given this limited relevance to nursing practice and the current state of ambiguity in the classification of nursing diagnoses, we have chosen to arrange the nursing diagnoses alphabetically.

Table i.1: Elements of a Care Plan

> Nursing Diagnosis
> Defining Characteristics
> Contributing Factors
> Expected Outcomes
> Interventions

ELEMENTS OF THE NURSING CARE PLANNING GUIDES
Nursing Diagnosis

An officially accepted working definition of nursing diagnosis was approved by the membership of NANDA at its Ninth National Conference. It states:

Nursing diagnosis is a clinical judgment about individual, family, or community responses to actual and potential health problems/life processes. Nursing diagnoses provide the basis for selection of nursing interventions to achieve outcomes for which the nurse is accountable (NANDA, 1990, p. 5).

All but three of the 100 diagnostic labels identified by NANDA through the Ninth National Conference in March 1990 are being used in this book. The exceptions are: "Altered Growth and Development," which has not been included, since the care planning guides are limited for use with the adult client; and "Altered Urinary Elimination" and "Self-Esteem Disturbance," both of which were excluded because they are viewed by us as broad, abstract categories. All specific, concrete nursing diagnoses within these categories, however, have been included.

We have also identified new diagnoses not yet on the official NANDA list; these are denoted in the table of contents by an asterisk and boldface. We endorse NANDA's recommendation for nurses to develop new nursing diagnoses as the need arises and we encourage nurses using this book to do so. For the most part, we have presented NANDA's recommendations as formulated by their national conferences. An example of this is that we have changed the terminology of the nursing diagnoses slightly to be consistent with the NANDA Taxonomy Committee's recommendations. These recommended changes in terminology were made for two reasons: First, some of the nursing diagnostic qualifying terms included in Taxonomy I-Revised, such as "potential," "ineffective," and "decreased" were viewed by the Committee as ambiguous or value-laden (Fitzpatrick, J.J., in Carroll-Johnson, R.M., 1, p. 21, 1990); they were replaced with the more measureable and less value-laden terminology of "risk," "impaired," or "altered." Second, the changes were made to increase consistency with the World Health Organization's "International Classification of Diseases" (ICD) format. (See Chapter 1 for more information about ICD).

NANDA solicits newly proposed nursing diagnoses for review by the Association. The NANDA Diagnosis Review Committee has prepared a set of guidelines. They are designed to promote the consistency, clarity, and quality of submissions. Nurses are encouraged to send new diagnoses or refinements of accepted diagnoses to the North American Nursing Diagnosis Association, St. Louis University School of Nursing, 3525 Caroline St., St. Louis, MO 63104.

Definition

Each care planning guide has a definition included after the nursing diagnosis. The definition provides a clear, precise description of the nursing diagnosis that differentiates it from related diagnoses. It is used along with the defining characteristics to aid the nurse in verifying a particular diagnosis. Some of the definitions used were developed by NANDA, while others were the product of the individual contributor who developed the care planning guide. NANDA definitions, when used, are cited. If no citation appears at the end of the definition, it can be assumed that it was the work of the original contributor.

Defining Characteristics

Data collection is frequently the source for identifying defining characteristics, sometimes called signs and symptoms. These data, once gathered, are then organized into meaningful patterns and used along with the definition to verify the diagnosis. They are the behaviors, either subjective or objective, exhibited by the client. Subjective information stems from the client's perception and includes physical feelings, such as, achiness, and expressions of emotions or thoughts, for example, panic. Objective information is observable by others. Some examples are physical findings, chart information such as x-ray and laboratory results, and nonverbal manifestations of the client or family. Both subjective and objective data are important in substantiating the diagnosis. The diagnosis must be precise and reflect substantiated data from the client, family, and other health care professionals. In most instances, multiple defining characteristics are required to verify a diagnosis. Because some of the same defining characteristics may apply to related nursing diagnoses as well, it is important to obtain enough information to identify the correct nursing diagnosis. For example, the nursing diagnoses "Stress Incontinence" and "Urinary Retention" both list dribbling and small volume of urination (less than 50 cc) as defining characteristics. Additional data need to be obtained to clearly focus on which of these problems the client is experiencing. Some authors have differentiated defining characteristics that are critical for formulating a given nursing diagnosis from those that are supporting but not critical. Critical defining characteristics are viewed by Gordon (1982) as "the major criteria for diagnostic judgment. They are found nearly always when the diagnosis is present and are absent when the diagnosis is absent" (p. 17). Although we value the work which has been done in this area, we have chosen not to distinguish between critical and supporting defining characteristics, since the research on which to base such differentiation is limited.

Contributing Factors

Contributing factors suggest a link or connection to the nursing diagnosis. These have sometimes been termed etiologies, causes, or related factors. In the absence of substantial research in the area of contributing factors, it is highly speculative to assign a single cause for a nursing diagnosis. There is frequently more than one contributing factor for a given diagnosis. For example, immobility, muscle spasms, and tissue damage may all be contributing factors for the client with the nursing diagnosis of "Pain." Contributing factors provide direction for identifying appropriate nursing interventions. If there are numerous unrelated contributing factors such as contractures, lack of knowledge and confusion, for example, for the nursing diagnosis "Bathing/Hygiene Deficit", it becomes difficult to include interventions to address each of them in one diagnosis. In that instance, the nurse needs to question whether the correct contributing factor(s) has been chosen or if there is a need to look deeper. If satisfied that the unrelated contributing factors are correct, it may be more workable to list the nursing diagnosis on the care plan more than once, accompanied by each contributing factor and corresponding interventions. There may be times when the contributing factors are questionable or unknown. In those cases, a question mark or "unknown" should be indicated on the care plan and revised as additional information becomes available. Many times nursing care needs to be given despite this unknown. For example, if the contributing factors for the nursing diagnosis of "Fear" were unknown, we would try to allay the fear and make educated guesses as to the reason(s) for it until more information became available.

There is disagreement at present regarding inclusion of pathophysiological/medical diagnoses in the list of contributing factors. Frequently, a medical diagnosis does not provide adequate direction for nursing care. For example, the nursing diagnosis of "Constipation" related to a cerebrovascular accident does not suggest specific nursing interventions. It is more useful for the nurse to identify specific causes of the constipation such as weak abdominal musculature, impaired mobility, or a diet low in roughage. This, in turn, suggests more specific interventions. However, there are times when the medical diagnosis provides the best available information. This tends to occur with the more medically oriented diagnoses such as "Altered Cardiac Output" or "Impaired Gas Exchange." Because it is necessary to acknowledge the interrelatedness of nursing and medicine when determining contributing factors, we have decided to include medical terminology when it seems appropriate.

Risk Factors

A nursing diagnosis designated as potential, which is now termed high risk, "is a clinical judgment that an individual, family or community is more vulnerable to develop the problem than others in the same or similar situation" (North American Nursing Diagnosis Association, 1990, p. 116). These nursing diagnoses are supported by risk factors that direct nursing actions to reduce or prevent the problem from developing. Since these nursing diagnoses have not yet occurred, risk factors replace the listing of actual defining characteristics and contributing factors. Most nursing diagnoses can be considered as actual or high risk; for example, "Impaired Skin Integrity" or "High Risk for Impaired Skin Integrity." Prevention of problems is within the scope of nursing practice and, therefore, high-risk nursing diagnoses need to be identified. The nurse needs to ascertain whether the risk is sufficiently high to warrant intervention. If so, a high-risk nursing diagnosis should be assigned.

Expected Outcomes

Expected outcomes, sometimes termed patient goals, are observable behaviors or data which measure changes in the condition of the client after nursing treatment. They are objective indicators of progress toward prevention of the development of high-risk nursing diagnoses or resolution/modification of actual diagnoses. The expected outcomes are arranged into long-term outcomes with short-term outcomes indented below them. For example, in the nursing diagnosis "Impaired Skin Integrity," "Client will have completely healed skin" might be the long-term outcome, while "Epithelial cells on surface of the wound are replaced" and "Dermal repair is characterized by healthy granulation tissue" would be short-term. Like other elements of the care plan, expected outcome statements are dynamic. Some outcomes are readily attained, while others may take longer to achieve. The nurse must review the outcomes periodically and modify them as the client progresses. Assigning specific "target or evaluation dates" or "time frames" for evaluation of progress toward outcome achievement is crucial. These evaluation dates must be realistic and reflect the realities of the client situation. Since there are so many considerations involved in when the outcome could be achieved (for example, varying lengths of stay, individual client condition), these care planning guides do not include evaluation dates. The date needs to be individualized and assigned, using the professional judgment and discretion of the nurse caring for the client.

Nursing Interventions

Nursing interventions are the treatment options/actions the nurse employs to prevent, modify, or resolve the nursing diagnosis. They are driven by the contributing factors and selected based on the expected outcomes to be achieved. Treatment options should only be chosen if they apply realistically to a specific client condition. For example, it would probably not be realistic for a client with a diagnosis of "Impaired Physical Mobility" related to contractures to perform active range of motion to all joints.

We have included independent, interdependent, and dependent nursing interventions as they reflect current practice. We have not made a distinction between these kinds of interventions because of institutional differences and increasing independence in nursing practice. The interventions that are interdependent or dependent will require collaboration with other professionals. The nurse will need to determine when this is necessary and take appropriate action.

The severe problems created by escalating health care costs culminated with a prospective payment scheme for reimbursement of health care services. The Diagnosis Related Group (DRG) classification system was developed, which assigned a relative cost weight to all medical diagnoses. The federal government used these cost weights to determine the actual payment made to a hospital for a client's care. This has resulted in "rationing of hospital and physician resources through its mechanism of predetermined payments" (Halloran, Kiley, & England, 1988, p. 22). As a result, early discharge has become more common, and the client population is continuing to shift from long inpatient stays to home care options for health care. With that shift, a growing number of nurses are employed in community health. Since there are differences in nursing care based on the setting, we have attempted to address both environments by separating the nursing interventions into three major divisions: The first major division is UNIVERSAL interventions, which we are defining as nursing actions appropriate to all clients in all settings; the second major division is INPATIENT interventions, which are nursing actions appropriate to clients confined to a hospital, nursing home, rehabilitation facility, or other inpatient setting; the third major division is COMMUNITY HEALTH/HOME CARE interventions, which are nursing actions appropriate to clients being cared for in their homes by themselves or family members, but which require periodic nursing visits. For nurses practicing in an inpatient setting, interventions would be selected from the UNIVERSAL and INPATIENT divisions. For nurses practicing in a community health/home care setting, interventions would be selected from that and the UNIVERSAL divisions. In some care planning guides, all interventions are listed under the UNIVERSAL division. In those instances it can be assumed that intervention options are the same regardless of setting.

Each of these major divisions has been separated into three logical parts: assessment, therapeutic, and teaching actions. The assessment actions are those actions designed to evaluate the client's day-to-day condition and the effectiveness of the therapeutic and teaching actions. These interventions start with verbs such as assess, monitor, or test—for example, "monitor daily dietary pattern." These assessment actions should not be confused with the data collection done *prior to* the determination of the nursing diagnosis. These assessment actions are appropriate *after* the identification of the diagnosis. The therapeutic and teaching interventions are the specific activities used to aid in problem resolution, for example, "initiate seizure precautions," or "teach how to irrigate or change catheter utilizing sterile technique." There are some care planning guides that do not have assessment, therapeutic, and teaching actions in all three major divisions. They are only included when appropriate, but when included are to be considered and implied in the previously stated order.

By necessity, we and our contributors are limited in providing information for nurses developing community care plans, since the current taxonomy of diagnostic labels focuses on individuals. There are few diagnoses which address families or groups as clients. As the taxonomy evolves, we look forward to inclusion of those diagnoses as well.

Each intervention requires a frequency. Since there are so many variables that determine the frequency of an intervention, the decision needs to be individualized and assigned, using professional judgment and discretion of the nurse caring for the client.

Rationale

The rationale provides a scientific explanation or purpose for the intervention. Every practicing nurse needs to have a strong theoretical base. Unfortunately, all too often, nurses intervene without a clear understanding of the reasons for their actions. An anecdote that illustrates this point concerns the young woman who routinely cut off both ends of a roast before baking. When asked why she did that, her response was "because that's the way my mother did it." Out of curiosity, the woman asked her mother her purpose in removing both ends. With a smile the mother replied, "I never had a pan large enough for the whole roast to fit in!" When understanding the purpose, interventions can be selected more intelligently and actions can be tailored to each individual's needs.

The rationales provided may be used as a quick reference for the nurse unfamiliar with the reason for a given intervention and as a tool for client education. These rationales may include principles, theory, and/or research findings from current literature. The rationales are intended as reference information for the nurse and, as such, should not be transcribed onto the care plan. A rationale is not provided when the intervention is self-explanatory.

Reference/Bibliography

A reference/bibliography appears at the conclusion of each care planning guide or related group of guides. The purpose of our reference/bibliography is to cite specific work used and to specify background information or suggestions for further reading. Citings provided represent the most current theory and/or research bases for inclusion in the care planning guides. We have highlighted all nursing research articles with an asterisk to emphasize their special significance to our profession.

REFERENCES/BIBLIOGRAPHY

Fitzpatrick, J.J. (1991). The translation of NANDA's taxonomy I-revised into ICD code. In R. Carroll-Johnson. (Ed.). **Classification of nursing diagnoses: Proceedings of the ninth conference.** (pp. 19–22). Philadelphia: Lippincott.

Gordon, M. (1987). **Nursing diagnosis: Process and application.** New York: McGraw Hill.

Halloran, E. J., Kiley, M., & England, M. (1988). Nursing diagnosis, DRG's, and length of stay. **Applied Nursing Research. 1** (1), 22–26.

North American Nursing Diagnosis Association. (1990). **Taxonomy I (rev. ed.).** St. Louis: Author.

SECTION ONE

CHAPTER 1

Nursing Diagnosis: A Historical Review

Nurses have been identifying specific client problems since the beginning of the profession. Movement from data collection and interpretation to intervention occurred after determining the problem. It provided the impetus for planning and was intended to identify the areas of concern for nursing intervention. Lacking any consistent language, these areas of concern were frequently described in terms of nursing problems, patient needs, clinical judgments, goals to be accomplished, or interventions to be implemented. As the profession of nursing evolved, it began to search for professional identity, to define the practice of nursing, and to distinguish itself as a separate and unique contributor to the wellness of the client. Nursing diagnosis is another step in this process. Using a consistent language, nurses can focus on problems that require intervention. The practice becomes diagnosis-based, rather than driven by the routine tasks and procedures that consume so much of the nurse's time and energy. Diagnosis-based nursing practice provides nursing that is professional, accountable, and visible (Gebbie, 1984).

The term "Nursing Diagnosis" was first used in the 1950s. McManus (1950) was a pioneer in recognizing that the identification and diagnosis of nursing problems were functions of the professional nurse. Fry (1953) described the first major function in developing a creative approach to nursing as the formulation of a nursing diagnosis and the development of an individualized care plan. The American Nurses' Association (ANA) Model Practice Act of 1955 rejected this suggestion by stating: "The foregoing shall not be deemed to include acts of diagnosis or prescription of therapeutic or corrective measures." Nurses and other health care professionals in the 1960s remained uncomfortable with the term Nursing Diagnosis, although the efforts supporting inclusion of it in nursing terminology were apparent. Chambers (1962) refuted arguments that only physicians should diagnose and even offered a working definition of nursing diagnosis: "A careful investigation of the facts to determine the nature of a nursing problem." The 1970s ushered in an increasing interest in the concept of nursing diagnosis with its addition—as a formal step into the profession's recognized thinking model—of the nursing process. Originally, the nursing process was described as a four-step model: 1) assessment, 2) planning, 3) implementation of the plan, and 4) evaluation of the plan's effectiveness. The revised nursing process model included nursing diagnosis as a separate and distinct step following the assessment phase.

Another strong influence was the publication of the Generic Standards of Nursing Practice in 1973 by the American Nurses' Association (ANA). This document presented eight mandated standards of nursing practice, based on the nursing process. The second of these stated that "nursing diagnoses are derived from health status data" (ANA, 1973, p. 2). That same year, a national task force comprising 100 nurse professionals from the United States and Canada, representing the areas of practice of education and research, convened in St. Louis, Missouri, for the First

National Conference Group for Classification of Nursing Diagnosis, later renamed the North American Nursing Diagnosis Association (NANDA). Co-directed by Kristine M. Gebbie and Mary Ann Lavin, the participants drew on their recall of client situations to generate nursing diagnoses individually and then validated them in small groups. Diagnoses were accepted by a majority vote of the conference participants (1975). The interest and support for nursing diagnoses continued to build in the 1980s. The ANA's Social Policy Statement (1980) included the term Nursing Diagnosis. It defined nursing as "the diagnosis and treatment of human responses to actual or potential health problems" (p. 9). Other professional groups and regulating agencies began to endorse the concept of nursing diagnoses. Nurse practice acts in the majority of states supported its use as a key part of the practice of nursing, and many schools of nursing began to include nursing diagnosis in their curricula. Nursing diagnosis appeared in the national board examination for registered nurses, and the Joint Commission for the Accreditation of Healthcare Organizations recognized nursing diagnosis as an effective means of documentation. In 1982, the NANDA conferences were opened to the nursing community at large. The group now convenes every two years to consider additions and revisions to the list of nursing diagnoses and to discuss taxonomic issues and methodologies for validation. The process of accepting diagnoses was, initially, by conference participants only; however, it now requires a positive vote of the NANDA membership. Publication of the proceedings of these meetings and the nursing diagnoses generated there has been augmented by books, articles, and programs. The current NANDA-approved list of nursing diagnoses following the 1990 Conference is composed of about 100 diagnostic labels that have been approved for clinical use and testing (see Table 1.2).

CLASSIFICATION SYSTEM

Although great advances have been made in the development and implementation of nursing diagnosis, nurses continue to wrestle with a taxonomic system that will provide a frame of reference for the diagnoses. NANDA defines taxonomy as "the theoretical study of systematic classifications including their bases, principles, procedures, and rules. The science of how to classify and identify." (1990, p. 5). Participants at the First National Conference Group for Classification of Nursing Diagnosis attempted "to initiate the process of preparing an organized, logical, comprehensive system for classifying those health problems or health states diagnosed by nurses and treated by means of nursing intervention" (Gebbie & Lavin, 1975, p. l). To do so, Gebbie and Lavin stated that "the first step in developing a classification is to identify all those things which nurses locate or diagnose in patients. This means nothing less than describing the entire domain of nursing" (p. 250). Although several classification systems were discussed, participants realized the enormity of the task. At the conclusion of the conference, the decision was made to list the diagnoses alphabetically and to continue the classification efforts at subsequent conferences.

As the list of diagnoses grew, NANDA realized that the alphabetized method of listing them was cumbersome and difficult to use. A group of 14 nurse theorists, chaired by Sr. Callista Roy, was asked to develop a conceptual framework for the classification of nursing diagnoses. It was developed by them during the Third and Fourth National Conferences. Their final work proposed the nine patterns of unitary man as the conceptual framework for the diagnostic classification system (Kim & Moritz, 1982, p. 235). These patterns, later renamed "Human Response Patterns"—a more familiar term—are shown in Table 1.1. At the Fifth National Conference, a taxonomy special interest group, chaired by Phyllis Kritek, was given the task of generating an initial taxonomy for the diagnostic labels. The purposes of the taxonomy were to provide a language for classifying and identifying phenomena within the realm of nursing, to provide new and different ways of looking at nursing, and to play a part in concept derivation (Kim, McFarland & McLane, 1984). The group drew upon the existing list of diagnoses and the theorists' human response patterns. The labels were separated into four levels of abstraction, with level 1 being the most abstract and level 4 being the least abstract.

Table 1.1: Human Response Patterns

Exchanging—mutual giving and receiving
Communicating—sending messages
Relating—establishing bonds
Valuing—assigning relative worth
Choosing—selection of alternatives
Moving—activity
Perceiving—reception of information
Knowing—meaning associated with information
Feeling—subjective awareness of information

At the Seventh National Conference, a classification system, Taxonomy I, was formally endorsed for development and testing. It was revised at the eighth and ninth national conferences (see Table 1.2).

Other individuals and groups interested in the further development of nursing diagnosis have formulated useful classification systems as well. To name a few, Gordon (1987) proposed a system for categorization called the "Functional Health Patterns." In 1980, the Roy Adaptation Model was devised (Reihl & Roy), and the Visiting Nurse Association of Omaha developed the Omaha System in 1986. The ANA has recognized the NANDA taxonomy as the profession's classification system (*Nursing Diagnosis Newsletter*, 1989, p. 3).

The impact of nursing diagnosis on nursing practice has been felt in many corners of the world. In 1987, Calgary, Canada, hosted the First International Nursing Conference on "Clinical Judgment and Decision Making: The Future with Nursing Diagnosis," in which 600 nurses from 36 countries participated.

The evolution of nursing diagnosis continues into the last decade of this century. NANDA carries on the work of developing and refining the taxonomy. The initial version of Taxonomy II was presented at the 1990 National Conference. This classification scheme uses axes—defined as dimensions of human condition considered in the diagnostic process. These axes will provide a means for the classification system to include diagnoses of three types of clients (individuals, families and communities); to provide wellness aspects of diagnostic concepts; and to designate the appropriate developmental stage of the client. The level of abstraction determines the level of placement of a diagnosis; i.e., level 2 or level 3. The work on Taxonomy II is in the early stage of development. (see Table 1.3). Concurrently, the Taxonomy Committee of NANDA and representatives from ANA decided to develop a translation of nursing diagnosis into the World

Table 1.2: Taxonomy I—Revised 1990

PATTERN 1: EXCHANGING	
1.1.2.1	Altered Nutrition: More than body requirement
1.1.2.2	Altered Nutrition: Less than body requirement
1.1.2.3	Altered Nutrition: Potential for more than body requirement
1.2.1.1	Potential for Infection

1.2.2.1	Potential Altered Body Temperature
1.2.2.2	Hypothermia
1.2.2.3	Hyperthermia
1.2.2.4	Ineffective Thermoregulation
1.2.3.1	Dysreflexia
*1.3.1.1	Constipation
1.3.1.1.1	Perceived Constipation
1.3.1.1.2	Colonic Constipation
*1.3.1.2	Diarrhea
*1.3.1.3	Bowel Incontinence
1.3.2	Altered Urinary Elimination
1.3.2.1.1	Stress Incontinence
1.3.2.1.2	Reflex Incontinence
1.3.2.1.3	Urge Incontinence
1.3.2.1.4	Functional Incontinence
1.3.2.1.5	Total Incontinence
1.3.2.2	Urinary Retention
*1.4.1.1	Altered (Specify Type) Tissue Perfusion (Renal, cerebral, cardiopulmonary, gastrointestinal, peripheral)
1.4.1.2.1	Fluid Volume Excess
1.4.1.2.2.1	Fluid Volume Deficit
1.4.1.2.2.2	Potential Fluid Volume Deficit
*1.4.2.1	Decreased Cardiac Output
1.5.1.1	Impaired Gas Exchange
1.5.1.2	Ineffective Airway Clearance
1.5.1.3	Ineffective Breathing Pattern
1.6.1	Potential for Injury
1.6.1.1	Potential for Suffocation
1.6.1.2	Potential for Poisoning
1.6.1.3	Potential for Trauma
1.6.1.4	Potential for Aspiration
1.6.1.5	Potential for Disuse Syndrome
#1.6.2	Altered Protection
1.6.2.1	Impaired Tissue Integrity
*1.6.2.1.1	Altered Oral Mucous Membrane
1.6.2.1.2.1	Impaired Skin Integrity
1.6.2.1.2.2	Potential Impaired Skin Integrity

PATTERN 2: COMMUNICATING

2.1.1.1	Impaired Verbal Communication

PATTERN 3: RELATING

3.1.1	Impaired Social Interaction
3.1.2	Social Isolation
*3.2.1	Altered Role Performance
3.2.1.1.1	Altered Parenting
3.2.1.1.2	Potential Altered Parenting
3.2.1.2.1	Sexual Dysfunction
3.2.2	Altered Family Processes
3.2.3.1	Parental Role Conflict
3.3	Altered Sexuality Patterns

PATTERN 4: VALUING

4.1.1	Spiritual Distress (distress of the human spirit)

PATTERN 5: CHOOSING

5.1.1.1	Ineffective Individual Coping
5.1.1.1.1	Impaired Adjustment
5.1.1.1.2	Defensive Coping
5.1.1.1.3	Ineffective Denial
5.1.2.1.1	Ineffective Family Coping: Disabling
5.1.2.1.2	Ineffective Family Coping: Compromised
5.1.2.2	Family Coping: Potential for Growth
5.2.1.1	Noncompliance (Specify)
5.3.1.1	Decisional Conflict (Specify)
5.4	Health Seeking Behaviors (Specify)

PATTERN 6: MOVING

6.1.1.1	Impaired Physical Mobility
6.1.1.2	Activity Intolerance
6.1.1.2.1	Fatigue
6.1.1.3	Potential Activity Intolerance
6.2.1	Sleep Pattern Disturbance
6.3.1.1	Diversional Activity Deficit
6.4.1.1	Impaired Home Maintenance Management
6.4.2	Altered Health Maintenance
*6.5.1	Feeding Self Care Deficit
6.5.1.1	Impaired Swallowing
6.5.1.2	Ineffective Breastfeeding
#6.5.1.3	Effective Breastfeeding
*6.5.2	Bathing/Hygiene Self Care Deficit
*6.5.3	Dressing/Grooming Self Care Deficit
*6.5.4	Toileting Self Care Deficit
6.6	Altered Growth and Development

PATTERN 7: PERCEIVING

*7.1.1	Body Image Disturbance
*7.1.2	Self Esteem Disturbance
7.1.2.1	Chronic Low Self Esteem
7.1.2.2	Situational Low Self Esteem
*7.1.3	Personal Identity Disturbance
7.2	Sensory/Perceptual Alterations (Specify) (Visual, auditory, kinesthetic, gustatory, tactile, olfactory)
7.2.1.1	Unilateral Neglect
7.3.1	Hopelessness
7.3.2	Powerlessness

PATTERN 8: KNOWING

8.1.1	Knowledge Deficit (Specify)
8.3	Altered Thought Processes

PATTERN 9: FEELING

*9.1.1	Pain
9.1.1.1	Chronic Pain
9.2.1.1	Dysfunctional Grieving
9.2.1.2	Anticipatory Grieving
9.2.2	Potential for Violence: Self-directed or directed at others
9.2.3	Post-Trauma Response
9.2.3.1	Rape-Trauma Syndrome
9.2.3.1.1	Rape-Trauma Syndrome: Compound Reaction
9.2.3.1.2	Rape-Trauma Syndrome: Silent Reaction
9.3.1	Anxiety
9.3.2	Fear

#New diagnostic categories approved 1990
*Categories with NANDA-modified label terminology

Table 1.3: Taxonomy II Draft #1

HUMAN RESPONSE PATTERN: CHOOSING

Level 2
Coping, Impaired
Decisional Conflict
Health Management
Health Seeking Behaviors
Level 3
Coping, Compromised
Coping, Defensive
Coping, Dysfunctional
Denial, Impaired
Noncompliance

HUMAN RESPONSE PATTERN: COMMUNICATING

Level 2
Verbal Communication, Impaired
Violence: Risk Self Directed or Directed at Others
Level 3
Dysreflexia

HUMAN RESPONSE PATTERN: EXCHANGING

Level 2
Body Temperature, Altered: Risk
Breastfeeding, Impaired
Gas Exchange, Impaired
Infection: Risk
Injury: Risk
Sleep Pattern Disturbance
Tissue Integrity, Altered
Level 3
Airway Clearance, Impaired

Aspiration: Risk
Breathing Pattern, Impaired
Developmental Delay
Hyperthermia
Hypothermia
Nutrition, Altered, Less than Body Requirements
Nutrition, Altered, More than Body Requirements
Nutrition, Altered, More than Body Requirements: Risk
Oral Mucous Membrane, Impaired
Poisoning: Risk
Skin Integrity, Impaired
Skin Integrity, Impaired: Risk
Suffocation: Risk
Thermoregulation, Impaired
Trauma: Risk

HUMAN RESPONSE PATTERN: FEELING

Level 2
Anxiety
Fear
Post-Trauma Response
Level 3
Fatigue
Grieving: Anticipatory
Grieving: Dysfunctional
Pain: Acute
Pain: Chronic
Rape-Trauma: Compound
Rape-Trauma: Silent
Rape-Trauma: Syndrome

HUMAN RESPONSE PATTERN: KNOWING

Level 2
Level 3

HUMAN RESPONSE PATTERN: MOVING

Level 2
Home Maintenance Management, Impaired
Urinary Elimination, Altered
Level 3
Activity Intolerance
Activity Intolerance: Risk
Bathing/Hygiene Deficit
Bowel Incontinence
Constipation: Colonic
Constipation: Rectal
Diarrhea
Disuse Syndrome: Risk
Diversional Activity Deficit
Dressing Deficit
Feeding Deficit

Incontinence: Functional
Incontinence: Reflex
Incontinence: Stress
Incontinence: Urge
Incontinence: Total
Physical Mobility, Impaired
Swallowing, Impaired
Toileting Deficit
Urinary Retention

HUMAN RESPONSE PATTERN: PERCEIVING
Level 2
Sensory Perception, Altered
Sexuality, Altered
Social Isolation
Thought Process, Altered
Level 3
Body Image Disturbance
Constipation: Perceived
Hopelessness
Personal Identity Disturbance
Powerlessness
Self-Esteem Disturbance: Chronic Low
Self-Esteem Disturbance: Situational
Social Isolation
Unilateral Neglect

HUMAN RESPONSE PATTERN: RELATING
Level 2
Role Performance, Altered
Social Interaction, Impaired
Level 3
Parental Role Conflict
Parenting, Altered
Parenting, Altered: Risk

HUMAN RESPONSE PATTERN: VALUING
Level 2
Sexual Function, Altered
Spiritual Distress
Level 3

Health Organization's (WHO) International Classification of Diseases (ICD) coding format. The ICD organizes an international data base for health care and is used to standardize the reporting of mortality and morbidity rates. WHO publishes a revised ICD every 10 years. Currently, work is being done on the 10th edition (ICD-10). Nursing's translation of nursing diagnoses into ICD was based on Taxonomy I-Revised. The nine human response patterns were retained as the overall classification structure and were placed in alphabetical order, for example, choosing, communicating, and exchanging. The diagnoses under the appropriate patterns were also placed in alphabetical order (see Table 1.4, p. 9). The translation of nursing diagnoses into ICD code was viewed by the Committee as a first step in efforts to include nursing language in the broader

Table 1.4: The Proposed ICD-10 Version of NANDA's Taxonomy I Revised: "Conditions that Necessitate Nursing Care." Prepared by NANDA Board of Directors, Taxonomy Committee and ANA Liaison, January 28, 1989.

HUMAN RESPONSE PATTERN: CHOOSING		
*Y00	Family Coping, Impaired	
	Y00.0	Compromised
	Y00.1	Disabled
Y0l	[Health Seeking Behavior]	
	Y0l.0-9	Health Seeking Behaviors, (Specify)
*Y02	Individual Coping, Impaired	
	Y02.0	Adjustment, Impaired
	Y02.1	Conflict: Decisional
	Y02.2	Coping: Defensive
	*Y02.3	Denial, Impaired
	Y02.4	Noncompliance
HUMAN RESPONSE PATTERN: COMMUNICATING		
Y10	[Communication, Impaired]	
	Y10.0	Verbal
HUMAN RESPONSE PATTERN: EXCHANGING		
Y20	[Bowel Elimination, Altered]	
	Y20.0	Bowel Incontinence
	Y20.1	Constipation: Colonic
	Y20.2	Constipation: Perceived
	Y20.3	Diarrhea
*Y21	[Cardiac Output, Altered]	
Y22	[Fluid Volume, Altered]	
	Y22.0	Deficit
	Y22.1	Deficit: Risk
	Y22.2	Excess
*Y23	Injury: Risk	
	*Y23.0	Aspiration
	*Y23.1	Disuse Syndrome
	*Y23.2	Poisoning
	*Y23.3	Suffocation
	*Y23.4	Trauma
Y24	[Nutrition, Altered]	
	Y24.0	Less than Body Requirement
	Y24.1	More than Body Requirement
	*Y24.2	More than Body Requirement: Risk
Y25	[Physical Regulation, Altered]	
	Y25.0	Dysreflexia
	Y25.1	Hyperthermia
	Y25.2	Hypothermia
	*Y25.3	Infection: Risk
	*Y25.4	Thermoregulation, Impaired
Y26	[Respiration, Altered]	
	*Y26.0	Airway Clearance, Impaired
	*Y26.1	Breathing Pattern, Impaired

	Y26.2	Gas Exchange, Impaired
Y27		Tissue Integrity, Altered
	*Y27.0	Oral Mucous Membrane, Impaired
	Y27.1	Skin Integrity, Impaired
	Y27.2	Skin Integrity, Impaired: Risk
Y28		[Tissue Perfusion, Altered]
	Y28.0	Cardiopulmonary
	Y28.1	Cerebral
	Y28.2	Gastrointestinal
	Y28.3	Peripheral
	Y28.4	Renal
Y29		Urinary Elimination, Altered
	Y29.0	Incontinence: Functional
	Y29.1	Incontinence: Reflex
	Y29.2	Incontinence: Stress
	Y29.3	Incontinence: Urge
	Y29.4	Incontinence: Total
	*Y29.5	Retention

HUMAN RESPONSE PATTERN: FEELING

Y30		Anxiety
Y31		[Comfort, Altered]
	Y31.0	Pain, [Acute]
	Y31.1	Pain, Chronic
Y32		Fear
Y33		[Grieving]
	Y33.0	Anticipatory
	Y33.1	Dysfunctional
Y34		Post-Trauma Response
	Y34.0	Rape Trauma Syndrome
	Y34.1	Rape Trauma Syndrome: Compound Reaction
	Y34.2	Rape Trauma Syndrome: Silent Reaction
*Y35		Violence: Risk

HUMAN RESPONSE PATTERN: KNOWING

Y40		[Knowledge Deficit]
	Y40.0-9	Knowledge Deficit (Specify)
Y41		Thought Processes, Altered

HUMAN RESPONSE PATTERN: MOVING

Y50		[Activity, Altered]
	Y50.0	Activity Intolerance
	Y50.1	Activity Intolerance: Risk
	Y50.2	Diversional Activity Deficit
	Y50.3	Fatigue
	Y50.4	Physical Mobility, Impaired
	Y50.5	Sleep Pattern Disturbance
*Y51		Bathing/Hygiene Deficit
*Y52		Dressing/Grooming Deficit
*Y53		Feeding Deficit
	*Y53.0	Breastfeeding, Impaired

	Y53.1	Swallowing, Impaired
Y54		Growth and Development, Altered
Y55		Health Maintenance, Altered
Y56		Home Maintenance Management, Impaired
*Y57		Toileting Deficit

HUMAN RESPONSE PATTERN: PERCEIVING

Y60		[Meaningfulness, Altered]
	Y60.0	Hopelessness
	Y60.1	Powerlessness
Y61		[Self Concept, Altered]
	Y61.0	Body Image Disturbance
	Y61.1	Personal Identity Disturbance
	Y61.2	Self-Esteem Disturbance: Chronic Low
	Y61.3	Self-Esteem Disturbance: Situational
*Y62		[Sensory Perception, Altered]
	Y62.0	Auditory
	Y62.1	Gustatory
	Y62.2	Kinesthetic
	Y62.3	Olfactory
	Y62.4	Tactile
	Y62.5	Visual
	Y62.6	Unilateral Neglect

HUMAN RESPONSE PATTERN: RELATING

Y70		Family Processes, Altered
Y71		Role Performance, Altered
	Y71.0	Parental Role Conflict
	Y71.1	Parenting, Altered
	Y71.2	Parenting, Altered: Risk
	Y71.3	Sexual Dysfunction
Y72		Sexuality Patterns, Altered
Y73		[Socialization, Altered]
	Y73.0	Social Interaction, Impaired
	Y73.1	Social Isolation

HUMAN RESPONSE PATTERN: VALUING

Y80		[Spiritual State, Altered]
	Y80.0	Spiritual Distress

NOTES:
Items in brackets are not NANDA accepted diagnoses.
Items with an asterisk (*) are changes in terminology from NANDA diagnostic labels.
NANDA diagnoses not specifically identified are embedded in the coding system.

scientific community as well as the broader health care community (Fitzpatrick in Carroll-Johnson, in press). Following NANDA board approval, a new draft was submitted to ANA for endorsement and submission to WHO. The list of nursing diagnoses was also submitted to the publishers of the ICD-CM (clinical modification). The ICD-CM is the United States' adaptation of the ICD coding system and includes reasons for patient services and interventions. "The ICD-CM provides the major coding schema used by most third-party payors and reporters of health care resource utilization—a function of the data base that is unique in the United States. Inclusion of nursing diagnoses in the ICD-10CM would document patient conditions requiring nursing care" (Warren & Hoskins, 1990, p. 167). At this time, WHO has not decided to include the NANDA Taxonomy in ICD-10; however, work and discussion will continue between ANA and the International Council of Nursing (ICN) toward its possible inclusion in future revisions of both ICD and ICD-CM. If accepted for the 1993 publication of the ICD-10 or for the American adaptation of this coding system, nursing will then be in a position to have health statistics compiled on nursing diagnoses through an international nursing data base within the ICD framework.

Interest in nursing diagnosis and its application in clinical practice continues to grow. Its contribution to the identity of nursing as a profession, facilitation of nurses' autonomy in judgments about client care, and use in promoting the knowledge base of nursing as a science are just a sampling of its usefulness. The process of identifying and classifying nursing diagnoses is far from over. Many questions and controversies about it exist. It will be through the use of nursing diagnoses in clinical practice, the collaboration between professionals and the systematic testing and validation of the nursing diagnoses, that the answers will be found.

REFERENCES/BIBLIOGRAPHY

American Nurses' Association. (1973). **Standards of Nursing Practice.** Kansas City, MO: Author.
American Nurses Association. (1980). **Nursing: A Social Policy Statement.** Kansas City, MO: Author.
Chambers, W. (1962). Nursing diagnosis. **American Journal of Nursing, 62**(11), 102–104.
Fitzpatrick, J.J. (in press). The translation of NANDA's Taxonomy I—revised into ICD code. In R. Carroll-Johnson. (Ed.). **Classification of nursing diagnoses: Proceedings of the ninth conference.** Philadelphia: Lippincott.
Fry, V.S. (1953). The creative approach to nursing. **American Journal of Nursing, 53,** 301–302.
Gebbie, K.M. (1984). Nursing diagnosis: What is it and why does it exist? **Topics in Clinical Nursing, 5**(4), 1–9.
Gebbie, K.M., & Lavin, M.A. (Eds.). (1975). **Classification of nursing diagnoses: Proceedings of the first national conference.** St. Louis: Mosby.
Gordon, M. (1987). **Nursing diagnosis: Process and application.** New York: McGraw-Hill.
Kelly, L.Y. (1974). Nurse practice acts. **American Journal of Nursing, 74,** 1310–1319.
Kim, M.J., McFarland, G.K., & McLane, A.M. (Eds.). (1984). **Classification of nursing diagnoses: Proceedings of the fifth national conference.** St. Louis: Mosby.
Kim, M.J., & Moritz, D.A. (Eds.). (1982). **Classification of nursing diagnoses: Proceedings of the third and fourth conferences.** New York: McGraw-Hill.
McManus, R.L. (1950). Assumptions of the functions of nursing. **Regional Planning for Nursing and Nursing Education.** New York: Bureau of Publications, Teachers College, Columbia University, p. 54.
North American Nursing Diagnosis Association. **Taxonomy I** (Rev. 1990). St. Louis: NANDA.
North American Nursing Diagnosis Association. (Spring, 1989). President's message. **Nursing Diagnosis Newsletter.** NANDA, **15,** 3.
Reihl, J.P., & Roy, C., Sr. (1980). **Conceptual models for nursing practice** (2nd ed.). New York: Appleton-Century-Crofts.
Simmon, D.A. (1986). Implementation of nursing diagnosis in a community health setting. In M.E. Hurley (Ed.). **Classification of nursing diagnoses: Proceedings of the sixth national conference.** St. Louis: Mosby.

CHAPTER 2

Nursing Diagnosis: An Integral Part of the Nursing Process

Nursing diagnosis is an important part of the nursing process and practice, but it cannot be taken out of context. For the entire process to function, all five steps—data collection, diagnosis, planning, intervention or implementation, and evaluation—must be completely, accurately, and professionally utilized. This chapter contains information on how to function within the nursing process, and Chapter 3 provides a case study as an example of how the process works in practice.

DATA COLLECTION

Data collection, the first phase of the nursing process, is the systematic, comprehensive gathering and analysis of relevant information about the client in order to obtain a baseline, or database. Its purpose is to gain knowledge about the present health status and risk for potential health problems; historical, physical, spiritual, social, and mental data; present needs; and past coping mechanisms. This process begins when there is a felt need for change.

Data collection is a multifaceted and complicated process which, when broken down into its individual components, can be more readily understood. For this reason the ensuing discussion is divided into the following sections: sources of information; kinds of information; verification of the data; cues and inferences; diagnostic reasoning; information gathering through data collection and assessment; timing of data collection; and data and defining characteristics and contributing factors.

Sources of Information

The data may be obtained from several sources. The client provides the best source of information, but significant others may also be helpful, especially when the client is too ill or confused to communicate appropriately. Data may also come from medical records, laboratory and diagnostic reports, and from health care personnel involved in care.

Kinds of Information

Data are of two kinds: subjective and objective. Subjective data are obtained primarily through interaction or interview. These data include those things that are reported by the client or others and involve feelings or perceptions. The historical information surrounding the illness, reports of body sensations such as pain or numbness, and feelings about the illness experience are subjective data.

13

Objective data are obtained through the physical examination, observation, and review of laboratory, x-ray, and other records. Affect, mood, and expressive abilities, while occurring during the interview, are objective data since *how* the client communicates is relevant to this data, not what is being said.

In a nutshell, subjective data primarily include what the client says while objective data are what the nurse observes.

Verification of the Data

It is important to understand the distinction between objective and subjective data so that it is verifiable and communicated appropriately as stated by the ANA Standards for Nursing Practice (1973), which are the basis for today's guidelines for data collection.

One way to verify the data is to compare what is being said (the subjective information) with what is being observed (the objective information). For example, a client in a substance abuse treatment unit who had just returned from a weekend pass stated, "I didn't go near any drugs while I was out." Observation of the client, however, indicated dilated pupils, slurred speech, and belligerent behavior. In this case, the subjective and objective data do not coincide, further investigation is necessary, and the discrepancy needs to be communicated appropriately in the chart and to other members of the health care team.

When verifying the data, caution is advised since what is being heard can be influenced by the nurse's personal perceptions or interpretations of events, values and beliefs, past experiences, and knowledge base. Care needs to be exercised to control the entrance of these components into the data.

On occasion the data cannot be verified totally, but there remains a strong suspicion that a problem exists. In this case, one or two of the defining characteristics may be present, but there is not enough evidence to corroborate existence of the problem. This likely diagnosis is prefaced with the word "possible." The possible diagnosis is different from NANDA's risk diagnoses in the following way: The selection of a risk diagnosis is made after matching client signs and symptoms with diagnosis risk factors, and interventions are aimed at prevention of problem occurrence. The selection of a possible diagnosis is based on a suspicion that a problem exists, and interventions are aimed at determining whether or not the problem really exists by collecting more information.

Cues and Inferences

Little and Carnevali (1976) have identified a process for validating data accurately. They suggest information be separated into *cues* and *inferences*. Information acquired through the senses— sight, smell, hearing, taste, and touch—falls into the cue category. This information includes the subjective reports of the client and significant others, and all the observable or objective data. Inferences include the conclusions or judgements about those cues. Again, the distinction is important so that inferences are not regarded as fact, but rather are considered as a point for further investigation.

For example, the defining characteristics of the Rape Trauma Syndrome care planning guides in this book point out the wide variety of emotional reactions displayed. One victim may appear calm and subdued while another victim may be fearful, anxious, and crying. Both reactions are genuine and based in the client's emotional make-up. In this example the nurse could infer that the victim who appeared calm and subdued had not been raped; however, it is the nurse's moral and legal responsibility to report the cues accurately and to avoid making incorrect inferences.

The nurse walks a fine line during the data-collection phase of the nursing process. The determination of nursing diagnoses is dependent upon the application of critical thinking to determine what data are necessary for collection, to organize them, and to determine the significance of symptoms, while at the same time using caution to avoid making unverifiable judgments or inferences about the data.

Diagnostic Reasoning

In order to utilize this critical thinking the nurse needs to utilize the process of diagnostic reasoning, which has received recent increased attention in nursing literature.

Radwin (1990) discusses several theories about the thinking processes essential to diagnostic reasoning. One of those theories, the Information Processing Model, is similar to the ideas of Little and Carnevali (previously discussed) in that the practitioner obtains cues or characteristics, infers relationships among cues, and then groups or clusters the cues for the formation of diagnostic hypotheses, which are then tested until the most likely diagnosis is chosen.

For example, if during the interview, the client continually coughs, the practitioner looks for contributing historical information about the cough, adventitious or absent lung sounds, fever, and other pertinent data in order to obtain cues. After all the data have been collected, the information is studied and clustered so that the signs and symptoms seen in this client can be compared to the defining characteristics of possible respiratory-related problems. At this point all the possible problems should be considered, and in this instance the problems of Risk of Infection, Suffocation, or Aspiration; Impaired Gas Exchange; Ineffective Airway Clearance; and Ineffective Breathing Pattern are plausible diagnoses. When the signs and symptoms most closely match the defining characteristics of a diagnosis or diagnoses, those hypotheses have been tested, and the diagnoses are chosen.

An interesting point about the Information Processing Model is that the diagnostic decision made are influenced by experience. That is, the novice or student will have more difficulty generating accurate and complex diagnoses, but with nursing experience, the determination of diagnoses improves. Also, like the Little and Carnevali ideas, inferences cannot be regarded as fact because if they are inaccurate, they will yield faulty diagnoses.

Radwin goes on to point out, however, that intuitive reasoning does play a part in clinical judgment, but that, again, experience is important. In other words, sometimes the experienced nurse senses or intuitively knows that there is a problem, and this enables the competent handling of the situation.

And finally this reasoning process is useful for not only determining problems, but also identifying client strengths and assets which will be of assistance in balancing the focus on both problem areas and strengths, as well as for defining those innate qualities which will fortify the client throughout the illness.

Information Gathering through Data Collection and Assessment

There can be confusion among beginning practitioners about data collection and assessment, probably because the terms are used interchangeably. The action of obtaining information about clients does occur throughout the nursing process, and both data collection and assessment have many features in common. But they occur at two different points in the nursing process and have slightly different purposes.

As previously stated the data collection is done to obtain a database. The database includes information about the client before treatment begins and usually is obtained during the initial contact with the client. Therefore, the database is static, and it serves as a point of comparison for changes in the client condition after treatment is rendered.

The confusion about data collection and assessment can be avoided by labeling the first phase of the nursing process "data collection" and avoiding the use of the word "assessment" during this phase.

The term "assessment," then, need only be applied during the intervention phase of the nursing process. For the purpose of this book, assessment is defined as the function of gathering *ongoing* information about the client's dynamic condition in response to treatment. The purpose of assessment is to gather information to evaluate and change care, and reorder diagnostic priorities. Words such as "monitor" or "assess" can be used to describe the actions during this phase of the nursing process.

Timing of Data Collection

On occasion it is not possible to collect all the pertinent data on the initial contact with the client because of life-threatening conditions, fatigue, or essential hospital procedures that interfere with the interview. In this case the time frames of data collection and assessment overlap, but the purpose does not change. When information for the database needs to be collected at a later time, it involves discussion about the client's condition before treatment began, and the database expands to include this new information. All interactions to monitor changes in the client's condition after treatment are part of the implementation or intervention phase of the nursing process.

Data and Defining Characteristics and Contributing Factors

As previously stated, after the data collection is complete, and the data have been verified as much as possible, they are clustered into groups of information for identification of patterns. Most schools of nursing and hospitals have a preferred method for data organization, such as Maslow's Hierarchy of Needs, Gordon's Functional Health Patterns, or NANDA's Human Response Patterns. Whatever method is used, the information obtained through the data collection is organized or clustered to provide clues for patterns.

These patterns then point the way to a specific diagnosis by fitting into the defining characteristics of that diagnosis. Defining characterisics are those signs and symptoms that are frequently seen with a particular diagnosis. Not all the defining characteristics need to be present for a diagnosis to be selected, and this determination depends upon the practitioner's expertise.

Many other authors list risk factors as part of the defining characteristics, but for the purposes of this text we have listed risk factors under the heading of "risk factors" for all the risk-related diagnoses, and for the actual problems we have listed the signs and symptoms under the heading of "defining characteristics."

After the diagnosis is determined, the practitioner needs to identify the contributing factors or causes. Contributing factors are extremely important because they drive the interventions or treatment. For example, once it has been determined that the diagnosis of Unilateral Neglect in a particular client is related to unilateral blindness, the interventions can be aimed at compensating for the blindness in an effort to relieve the neglect. Or in the case of Risk of Suffocation related to a lack of awareness of hazards in the environment, intervention should be aimed at education to reduce the risk.

It may seem difficult to put all these components together to determine the link between the data collection, the defining characteristics, the diagnostic label, and the contributing factors, but the educated, competent practitioner can find the link by applying organized, critical thinking to the process.

NURSING DIAGNOSIS

The most recent definition approved by NANDA at its ninth national conference states,

> *"Nursing diagnosis is a clinical judgment about individual, family, or community responses to actual or potential health problems/life processes. Nursing diagnoses provide the basis for selection of nursing interventions to achieve outcomes for which the nurse is accountable" (NANDA, 1990, p. 5).*

Key components of this definition are:

1. The diagnoses are made by nurses who, by virtue of their education and experience, are professional and licensed, and are competent and accountable for their nursing judgments.

2. Nursing clinical judgments are made about a variety of client populations—individual, family, or community.

3. Nursing diagnoses can be actual or potential, and result because of a careful, systematic data collection performed during the initial contact and as a feedback mechanism resulting from ongoing assessments.

Nursing diagnosis is probably the most important and pivotal part of the nursing process. It depends entirely on the complete and accurate collection of data and is in turn responsible for the success of the care plan.

The importance of the nursing diagnosis is further demonstrated by its complexity. While being a discrete component of the nursing process, it necessitates continuous re-evaluation through feedback of the other parts. While being an independent province of nursing, it is also a cooperative action in that the diagnosis selection process is enhanced by the input of the client, other health care professionals, and the use of reference material.

The nursing diagnosis statement consists of two or three components. In both statements, the first part is the diagnostic label. The labels used in this book are—for the most part—taken from those developed by NANDA, and although there are other classification systems, those designated by NANDA are the most widely used.

In the two-part statement, only the diagnostic label and the contributing factors are used. The label is supplemented with a "related" or "due to" clause that identifies the contributing factors. These are sometimes called causes, etiologies, or related factors. The two-part statement is more commonly used by practicing nurses.

In the three-part statement, the diagnostic label, the defining characteristics, and the contributing factors are used. This format is sometimes used by students because it provides in writing the basis for the diagnostic label selection. An example of a three-part statement is "Impaired

Adjustment related to lack of future-oriented thinking as evidenced by impaired cognition and inadequate support systems."

In this book, those diagnoses that involve risk labels have only a two-part statement because there are no contributing factors or defining characteristics. The statement contains the diagnostic label and the risk factors. An example of a risk statement is "Risk of Altered Body Temperature due to burn injuries." (See figure 2.1)

Nursing diagnoses are distinct from medical diagnoses. In general, nursing diagnoses are more holistic then are medical diagnoses. For example, the medical diagnosis of diabetes mellitus describes the inadequate metabolism of carbohydrate, fat and protein, and intervention would be aimed at the balance of diet, exercise, and insulin. Nursing diagnoses, however, would center on the ability to complete activities of daily living and to function in the face of the signs and symptoms presented by this illness. The interventions include teaching to administer insulin, to eat properly, and to exercise as prescribed in the medical treatment plan, but they might also address the nursing problems of fear, fatigue, potential for infection, and altered peripheral tissue perfusion that are the responses to actual or potential health problems.

Furthermore, medical diagnoses tend to be static: That is, the diagnosis of diabetes mellitus would probably remain throughout the time of the hospitalization and home care. The nursing problems, however, are dynamic and multiple.

The physician collects data about signs and symptoms to define problems about structure and function of the human body, while the nurse collects data about signs and symptoms to define or diagnose human responses to health problems.

Once the diagnosis and contributing factors are determined, planning begins.

Figure 2.1: Nursing Diagnosis Statements

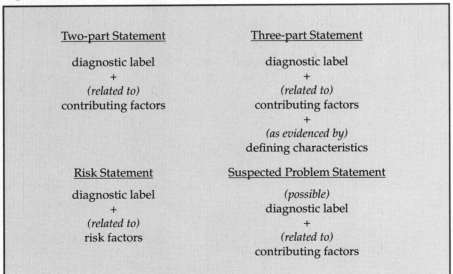

Two-part Statement	Three-part Statement
diagnostic label	diagnostic label
+	+
(related to)	*(related to)*
contributing factors	contributing factors
	+
	(as evidenced by)
	defining characteristics
Risk Statement	Suspected Problem Statement
diagnostic label	*(possible)*
+	diagnostic label
(related to)	+
risk factors	*(related to)*
	contributing factors

PLANNING

During the planning phase the nurse ordinarily organizes diagnoses according to priority guidelines, establishes outcome criteria, and writes the nursing care plan.

Priority Setting

Although the client should be involved in every part of the nursing process, the importance of the client's input in setting priorities cannot be overemphasized. The entire care plan is destined to fail if the client does not believe that a problem exists and if there is no commitment to intervention. The process of setting priorities begins in the diagnosis phase and continues into the planning phase when deciding on interventions. This process decides to some extent which interventions are most important and need to come first; mostly, however, the setting of priorities determines which diagnoses or problems warrant intervention—a decision based on client-felt needs and compliance.

Christensen and Kenney (1990) provide the following guidelines for establishing priorities:

1. Actual or imminent life-threatening concerns are considered before actual or health threatening concerns.

    Life-threatening problems are Risk for Violence, Impaired Airway Clearance, or Altered Tissue Perfusion; these diagnoses must often be made quickly based on nursing judgment. Life-threatening concerns are one of the few conditions in which client input may be bypassed. If there is a Risk for Violence related to drug abuse, for example, the client will probably fail to believe that a problem exists and will not be committed to intervention, and yet intervention must occur; or, if there is Impaired Airway Clearance related to foreign body ingestion, the client is probably incapable of input, and intervention is necessary immediately.

2. Temporal, human, and material resources are examined deliberately.

    Priority should be assigned based on the time it will take to resolve the problem versus the time the nurse has with the client. The hospital nurse will probably have three or four days with a surgical client. The home care nurse may see a client once a week for a month or so; then longer periods of time will elapse between visits. Noncompliance, for example, is more commonly dealt with in the home care setting because it involves longer periods of time for resolution; Acute Pain related to a back injury, however, needs high-priority attention in the hospital setting.

    Human and material resources should also be considered when setting priorities. An elderly client living on a fixed income in a high-crime area of the inner city is likely to experience social isolation. In this setting it is also likely that there will be inadequate people and money to provide assistance toward more socialization. However heartbreaking it may be, this diagnosis might receive low priority because it has little chance of resolution.

3. The client is involved in determining the priority of concerns.

    As previously stated, the client must be involved whenever possible in the setting of priorities so that understanding of the problems, as well as values and beliefs, can be taken into account. If there is no belief that smoking is the cause of Impaired Gas Exchange, for example, then this concern needs to receive low priority so that efforts can be aimed toward diagnoses and interventions that can be accomplished.

4. Scientific and practice principles provide rationale for decisions.

    The professional nurse, by virtue of education, is equipped with theories, models, and principles to judge priorities. For example, using Maslow's (1968) hierarchy of needs, the unmet basic and growth needs must be given highest priority. Knowledge about physiologic principles leads the nurse to give higher priority to altered cardiopulmonary tissue perfusion than to knowledge deficit.

An in-depth discussion of prioritizing diagnoses is given here, despite the fact that the contributors to the Care Planning Guides in this book were not asked to assign priority to diagnoses. This planning step is so highly individualized to each specific situation, nurse, and client that it cannot be done in these hypothetical situations; but it is an essential component in the actual delivery of care.

Establishment of Outcome Criteria

The expected outcome, or goal, is a statement that describes the desired or favorable client condition that can be achieved through nursing interventions. They are the standard or criteria by which the effectiveness of the interventions is measured.

Outcomes should be stated in terms of expected or desired client behavior, they should be specific and measurable in time, and they should contain long- and short-term components.

Having a time component is one of the ways in which an outcome is measurable. The time component was not included in the Care Planning Guides in this book since it is very specific to the individual situation. For example, the outcome of "the client walks one block per day within X number of weeks" is variable depending on the medical diagnosis, age, and exercise tolerance.

The short-term components are designed as vehicles to achieve the long-term components, and are necessary so that progress can be sensed and used as impetus to attain the next step. Using the example above, the long-term outcome might be "The client will walk one block per day within two weeks." The short-term outcomes would then be: "Endurance allows walking outside and sitting for thirty to sixty minutes daily for the next three days;" "The pulse rate does not go over 100;" and "There are no feelings of shortness of breath or exhaustion after walking one-half block during the next week."

Writing the Care Plan

Once the diagnoses are established and the outcomes are defined, interventions are designated and written into the care plan. Interventions or nursing strategies can be determined by the use of Care Planning Guides contained in this book or other nursing literature, by brainstorming with others as in a nursing conference, by making inferences about possible alternatives, by utilizing pertinent nursing research, and by using scientific rationales.

Interventions are primarily of three types: assessment, therapeutic, and educational. There are also evaluative interventions. But just as we have advised against using the word "assessment" in the data collection phase, it also seems appropriate to use the word "evaluate" only in that phase, as the overall nursing process is clearer if we avoid overlapping term usage.

Assessment interventions are designed to monitor the client's dynamic condition in order to compare the information received through assessment with that in the database and other data obtained during intervention. This provides a feedback mechanism for the determination of the overall effectiveness of care.

Therapeutic interventions are designed to provide comfort or alleviate symptoms, perform specific treatments, diminish or eliminate high risk factors, maintain status quo, and provide for consultation with other professionals.

Teaching interventions assist the client to gain knowledge about disease processes, health practices, and treatment actions. They encompass both counseling and teaching.

The most important point here is that determining interventions is a highly individualized process. The practicing nurse must never be lulled into thinking that writing a care plan can be accomplished by merely opening a book and copying complete care plans. The Care Planning Guides contained in this book are education- and experience-based suggestions for care as it relates to specific nursing diagnoses. The intention is that the guides should be applied to specific situations based on sound nursing judgment.

IMPLEMENTATION (INTERVENTION)

Implementation is the process of putting the nursing care plan, which includes both medically and nursing determined interventions, into action so as to attain the desired outcomes.

The goal of nursing intervention is to achieve client independence. In some instances the goal may also be to make the client as comfortable as possible—as in terminal illness—but independence on the part of the family and client is still important. As evidence of the benefit of client independence, for the past few years, clients have been assisted to self-administer IV pain medication (PCA, or patient-controlled analgesia), and it has been found that when the client feels in control of pain relief, far less medication is used.

At the onset of illness or immediately after surgery the client may be unable to participate in care, and interventions may be aimed at things done *to* or *for* the client (e.g., turning, changing dressings, or monitoring body temperature). But even these nursing actions are aimed at upgrading the client's condition to a point of participating in care. Later the interventions should be primarily of a teaching nature so that the nurse is preparing the client for functioning without the assistance of health care personnel.

EVALUATION

This final phase of the nursing process is defined as the ongoing comparison or appraisal of the degree to which the outcomes have been accomplished.

The evaluation phase is probably the most neglected part of the nursing process, and yet it provides important feedback for changing priorities and revising the care plan.

When evaluation demonstrates that outcomes have been accomplished, the nurse can remove the related diagnoses and interventions from the care plan and proceed to focus attention on other problems. When outcomes have not been accomplished, the nurse needs to ask why. Was the data collection flawed? Was the etiology assigned to the diagnosis incorrectly? Has too little time elapsed for the outcome to occur? Did the client lack belief in the plan? Were the interventions inadequate to resolve the problem? When these questions are answered, the nurse will know where the plan needs revision. (See figure 2.2 for an overall picture of the nursing process and its products. See also figure 2.3 for a diagram of the nursing process and its feedback mechanism).

CONCLUSION

Expert, professional nursing care depends on the systematic and continuous use of the five phases of the nursing process. At each step, scientific or theoretical information provides the basis for nursing action, while the practicing nurse provides the critical thinking and judgment for appropriate application.

Figure 2.2: The Nursing Process: Actions involved and products of the actions

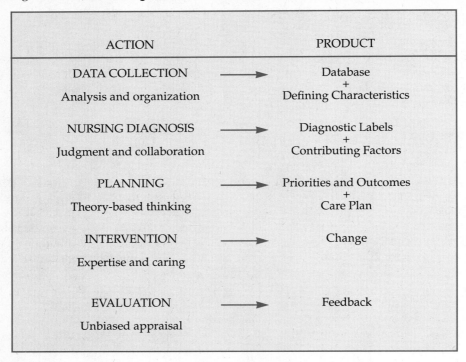

Figure 2.3: The Nursing Process: Interrelatedness of parts and feedback mechanism (Note: The database is static and the information contained does not change, but through ongoing collection of data the database may expand. This is essential so that there is a genesis or point of beginning for comparison during the evaluation phase.)

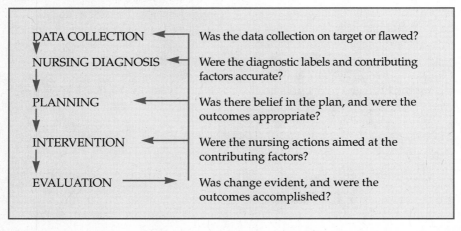

REFERENCES/BIBLIOGRAPHY

Alfaro, Rosalinda. (1990). **Applying nursing diagnosis and nursing process: A step-by-step guide** (2nd ed.). Philadelphia: Lippincott.

American Nurses' Association. (1973). **Standards of nursing practice**. Kansas City, MO: ANA.

Carpenito, L.J. (1989–1990). **Nursing diagnosis: Application to clinical practice.** Philadelphia: Lippincott.

Christensen, P.J., & Kenney, J.W. (1990). **Nursing process: Application of conceptual models.** St. Louis: Mosby.

Kozier, Barbara, & Erb, Glenora. (1987). **Fundamentals of nursing: Concepts and procedures.** Menlo Park, CA: Addison-Wesley.

Little, D., & Carnevali, D. (1976). **Nursing care planning.** Philadelphia: Lippincott.

Maslow, A.H. (1968). **Toward a psychology of being** (2nd ed.). New York: Van Nostrand Reinhold Co.

North American Nursing Diagnosis Association. **Taxonomy I** (Rev. 1990). St. Louis: NANDA.

Phipps, W.J., Long, B.C., & Woods, N.F. (1987). **Medical-surgical nursing: Concepts and clinical practice.** St. Louis: Mosby.

Radwin, L.E. (1990). Research on diagnostic reasoning in nursing. **Nursing Diagnosis, 1**(2), 70–77.

CHAPTER 3

The Nursing Process in Action

Mr. Rhyner, a 60-year-old, slightly obese male, entered the Emergency Department on the evening of January 6. He was accompanied by his wife, who was anxious and tearful but controlled. She reported that Mr. Rhyner had been watching TV when he stated he had a headache. Within minutes he became confused and then "fell asleep;" when Mrs. Rhyner could not wake him, she summoned an ambulance.

The Emergency Department record stated the following significant history and physical findings:

- Mrs. Rhyner reported that Mr. Rhyner is a heavy smoker with a history of hypertension who, for the past two months, has been having periods of headache with difficulty speaking, which passes within an hour. Mr. Rhyner had refused to see a doctor because he said, "They'd lecture about smoking and eating, and you've got to die of something."
- Lethargic but arousable state with slurred verbal response to stimulation of left side
- Pupils equal and react to light and accommodation (PERLA), full visual field assessment not possible, but suspicious right homonymous hemianopsia as no response to right stimuli
- Face flushed
- Right face, arm, and leg flaccid
- Vitals: Temperature 100; Pulse 88; Resp 14; BP (rt) 168/100; (lt) 180/110
- No nuchal rigidity, no bruits over carotids
- Cardiovascular unremarkable
- Lungs clear except for expiratory rales at bases bilaterally
- Abdomen soft, no distention, bowel sounds normal, urinary incontinence
- Integument shows no evidence of bruising or trauma, right arm and leg cool to touch, left extremities warm
- Reflexes (within normal limits) (WNL) except right Babinski positive
- CT scan, skull x-ray, and EKG WNL
- CBC and arterial gases WNL
- Lumbar puncture revealed clear, colorless fluid, negative for red and white cells with protein and glucose WNL; pressure 190 mm H_2O

Mr. Rhyner's medical diagnosis was TIA or possible CVA, probably of embolitic origin. He was admitted to a medical unit with the following:

- Keep open IV of 5% dextrose in Ringer's lactate
- Indwelling urinary catheter
- Oxygen per nasal cannula at 4L/min
- Aldomet (Methyldopa HCl) 250 mg IV q 6 h given over 60 min
- BP q 30 min during IV infusion of Aldomet, then q 2 h
- MRI and cerebral angiography when stable
- NPO until speech therapy evaluation, and then oral intake per therapist
- Bed rest with HOB flat, turn q 1 hour, being certain respiratory passages are open in all positions

Mrs. Kemper, a gerontology nurse practitioner, admitted Mr. Rhyner to the medical unit and became his primary nurse. She carefully read the Emergency Department report, collected her admission forms and data collection tools, and went to greet Mr. and Mrs. Rhyner. While helping to put Mr. Rhyner to bed, Mrs. Kemper used her observational skills to note the following:

- Level of consciousness (LOC) and mood
- Communication abilities
- Skin condition for color and injury
- IV rate, solution, and infusion site
- Oxygen flow rate and cannula position
- Indwelling urinary catheter drainage and attachment

Mrs. Kemper greeted Mr. and Mrs. Rhyner and attempted to involve both of them in the data collection and in decisions regarding care. She explained each step of these processes and collected only data that was essential for Mr. Rhyner's safety and well-being, did not stress or overtax him, was relevant to his hospital stay, and ruled out possible complicating factors. She deferred items that were unimportant at this time and could either be assessed later or deemed not applicable at all. She collected the following data:

- Brief past medical history with careful attention to hypertension and cardiovascular and kidney disease
- Current medication usage
- Allergies
- General health habits, i.e. smoking, alcohol use, appetite, sleep
- Elimination patterns with last bowel movement (LBM)
- Conceptual patterns of sight and hearing in addition to the usual use of eyeglasses or a hearing aid
- Handedness
- Social history with emphasis on family, spiritual, and other support systems for past coping
- Vital signs with careful attention to BP in both arms in sitting and supine positions
- Pupil reaction, eye movement, and vision
- LOC, mentation, mood and ability to communicate

- Ability to swallow
- Heart and lung sounds
- Bowel sounds
- Extremity control, strength, awareness of body parts
- Felt needs

Mrs. Kemper now had the subjective and objective signs that made up the defining characteristics, and she had obtained clues for the contributing factors. For example, Mrs. Rhyner stated Mr. Rhyner was right-handed, wore glasses for reading, smoked one pack of cigarettes per day, had a bowel movement every three to four days, and would only eat "real food" like butter, whole milk, and eggs. Objectively, Mrs. Kemper observed that Mr. Rhyner's right extremities were flaccid, he was lethargic but arouseable, and he became angry when he was unable to recall words or speak clearly.

Mrs. Kemper's admission form asked for additional information which she deferred because Mr. Rhyner seemed tired. For example, she did not delve into Mr. Rhyner's activities of daily living (ADL) or his usual nutritional patterns. She knew he would be on bed rest for the next several days and NPO until swallowing could be evaluated, making these data unimportant at this time.

Care at this time was guided by the use of critical thinking, diagnostic reasoning, knowledgeable decision making, and the use of science-based rationales. Some of the rationales utilized in this situation were:

- The careful and appropriate collection of data determines the selection of nursing diagnoses that lead to effective intervention and treatment.
- Compliance is enhanced when decisions about care and ADLs are shared by the nurse and the client.
- Careful and continual assessment of the client experiencing cerebral perfusion deficit during the first hours after onset is essential, as the condition can change and worsen quickly.
- Cerebral emboli are frequently caused by cardiomegaly-generated clots.
- The use of eyeglasses, a hearing aid, or any other device that sharpens the senses can assist in the compensation of unilateral neglect.
- Cerebral perfusion after stroke is assisted by rest and quiet with the HOB flat.
- Hypertension is a major cause of heart and kidney failure and stroke, and is associated with aneurysm formation and congestive heart failure.
- Circulatory load is assessed through the monitoring of IV fluid administration, indwelling urinary catheter drainage, and blood pressure. The safe administration of Aldomet is dependent upon the frequent updating of this information.
- Coping with present stressors is enhanced when past coping mechanisms and support systems are recalled and utilized.

Mrs. Kemper oriented Mr. and Mrs. Rhyner to the hospital and room and suggested that Mrs. Rhyner get some sleep. He explained that Mr. Rhyner would need to stay in bed with the HOB flat, and that he would not be allowed to eat or drink anything until it was certain he could swallow adequately. She stated she would be back every half hour or so, and she apologized for having to interrupt Mr. Rhyner's sleep. She then explained why it was necessary, and Mr. Rhyner did not seem upset about the procedures. The Rhyners had no questions, and they both appeared to be in control. Mrs. Kemper left to begin work on the care plan.

Mrs. Kemper's first task was to go over the data and to check her admission forms to be certain that they were as complete as possible, and that she was attempting to understand the clients' point of view rather than imposing her own values on the Rhyner's responses. For example, she disliked smoking and overeating because of the associated health problems, and she had an obligation to investigate further; but she had to be careful not to lecture or to waste energy if these problems seemed unresolvable.

Her next task was to organize the data into clusters for problem definition and then to prioritize the problems. Data had been collected on felt needs, and these would be validated throughout the nursing process.

Mrs. Kemper relied on her own expertise, consulted with colleagues, very carefully considered felt needs, and used books on care planning to select the following diagnoses and contributing factors:

- Impaired Health Seeking Behaviors, possibly related to lack of knowledge about consequences or lack of motivation
- Impaired Verbal Communication related to a decrease in circulation to the brain
- Possible Colonic Constipation, probably related to less than adequate levels of fluid and fiber intake, and physical activity
- Risk for Aspiration related to reduced level of consciousness and impaired swallowing
- Risk for Altered Nutrition: Less than Body Requirement related to impaired swallowing and risk for aspiration
- Risk for Impaired Skin Integrity related to immobility and altered sensation
- Altered Cerebral Tissue Perfusion related to interruption of arterial flow
- Total Incontinence related to sensory motor impairment
- Anxiety related to a change in health status
- Possible Unilateral Neglect related to hemianopsia and sensory motor impairment

The next task at hand was to define long- and short-term expected outcomes for each diagnosis. Some examples of outcomes are:
Client will evacuate soft formed stool at least every third day.
Physical activity as tolerated to enhance peristalsis is performed daily.
2000–3000 cc fluid is ingested daily.
Client will attend to neglected side of body with minimal cues within one week.
All body parts are kept free of injury daily.
Scanning techniques to enhance body awareness are learned within four days.
Face, neck, chest, and affected arm washing are completed independently within three days.

And finally, Mrs. Kemper planned interventions specific to this set of problems or diagnoses and to this client. They were:

- Monitor vital signs q 1/2 h while Aldomet is running, then q 1 h through the night
- Assess LOC and pupil response q 1 h
- Assess for reasons for impaired health seeking behaviors of smoking and incorrect eating; assess for knowledge in these areas

- Monitor bowel movements
- I/O
- Keep open IV of 5% dextrose in Ringer's lactate
- Aldomet 250 mg IV q 6 h over 60 min
- Oxygen per nasal cannula at 4 L/min
- Side lying position with HOB flat, turn q 1 h
- Rotating water pressure mattress in place at all times
- When communicating use questions that require simple responses; speak and stand toward unaffected side
- Referral to speech therapy to assess swallowing in A.M.
- Referral to ophthalmology to assess for hemianopsia in A.M.
- Referral to PT and OT when stable
- Referral to respiratory therapy for evaluation
- MRI in A.M.
- Keep side rails up
- Indwelling urinary catheter care
- Provide reassurance and teaching about all procedures
- Continually orient to right side of body, i.e., during bath time say, "I'm going to wash your right arm now."

(See figure 3.1 for example of partial care plan.)

Mrs. Kemper carried out these interventions until her shift ended, and whenever she found Mr. Rhyner awake she used that time to teach him about the MRI he would be having in the morning, to briefly explain the procedures she was doing, and to assess for fears and anxiety. She said good night and introduced Mr. Rhyner's night nurse during her last visit that evening.

During the next few days, Mr. Rhyner stabilized and his speech improved. Although his urinary catheter was removed, he was still incontinent, so a condom-type drainage system was used. His right paralysis remained, but his ability to swallow was normal, and he began PT and OT. Through interaction with Mr. Rhyner, the nursing staff learned that he was not a compliant person, and was often angry and impatient. He had two sons who lived some distance away and had only his wife to care for him, since the couple did not have many friends or other support systems.

Utilizing evaluation, the final step of the nursing process, the nurses determined that some of the problems resolved and new problems developed. Therefore, the diagnoses, expected outcomes, and interventions changed continually.

After two weeks in the hospital, it was determined that Mr. Rhyner was ready for discharge. Based on the existing resources, and the Rhyner's needs, it was decided that Mr. Rhyner would be discharged home with a referral to a community nursing service for skilled nursing care, a home health aide, PT, OT, and a social work evaluation.

At this point the nursing process began anew as Mr. Rhyner entered another phase of the health care system. His community health nurse collected data relating to strengths, resources, and problems, assigned nursing diagnoses, planned care, intervened, and evaluated for change.

Figure 3.1: Example of Partial Patient Care Plan

Medical Diagnosis:
Transcient Ischemic Attack (TIA)   Mr. William Rhyner
Possible Cerebral Vascular   Age – 60
Accident (CVA)
Primary Nurse: Mrs. Kemper, R.N.

Date	Nurse Diagnosis	Expected Outcome	Evaluate by	Interventions/Frequency
01/06	Impaired verbal communication	Long-term: Client will send understandable messages through congruent verbal/ nonverbal means.	01/09	1. Monitor for nonverbal indicators of problems, e.g., facial grimacing, rubbing of body part-q contact.
	Related to: Decreased cerebral perfusion	Short-term: Needs are communicated with minimal frustration.	01/07	2. Listen for vocalizations such as moaning or groaning. 3. Provide continuity in care giving assignments—daily. 4. Communicate while facing unaffected side-q contact.
		Alternative methods of communication are used.	01/07	5. Use questions requiring simple responses. 6. Explain exactly what is being done in the process of providing all care.
01/06	Risk for impaired skin integrity	Long-term: Client's skin will remain intact.	01/10	1. Evaluate skin condition and integrity-q shift. 2. Reposition q 1 h. (Refer to turning schedule at HOB).
	Risk factors: Altered sensation Lack of mobility	Short-term: No symptoms of skin trauma are experienced.	01/07	3. Rotating water pressure mattress on bed at all times. 4. Keep skin clean—daily/PRN.
		All skin surfaces are intact, warm, and pink.	01/07	5. Apply moisturizer to skin following bath and PRN. 6. Use pull sheet to mitigate shearing of skin-q contact.

After two months, Mr. Rhyner continued to smoke half a pack of cigarettes per day, but he had improved his eating habits, and had complied with his medication regime; he was ambulatory with a cane, had regained bladder control, and was using his right arm and hand with bracing assistance. After three months, he was discharged from the community nursing service.

Mr. Rhyner had come through a difficult illness, and he remained not without problems. But because of nursing intervention that was compassionately, scientifically, and individually applied, he was practicing better health habits, was independent despite being physically challenged, and had learned a great deal about resources available to him in the event of a future change in his health status.

REFERENCES/BIBLIOGRAPHY

Carpenito, L.J. (1989–1990). **Nursing diagnosis: Application to clinical practice.** Philadelphia: Lippincott.

North American Nursing Diagnosis Association. (1990). **Taxonomy I** (Rev. 1990). St. Louis: NANDA.

Phipps, W.J., Long, B.C., & Woods, N.F. (1987). **Medical surgical nursing: Concepts and clinical practice.** St. Louis: Mosby.

Welsh, Brady. (1990). **Outline for patient study: Rush medical college.** Chicago: Rush-Presbyterian-St. Luke's Medical Center.

SECTION TWO

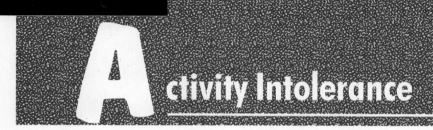

Activity Intolerance

A state in which an individual has insufficient physiological or psychological energy to endure or complete required or desired daily activities (NANDA, 1990, p. 72).

Linda S. Baas, R.N., M.S.N., C.C.R.N.

. . . .

DEFINING CHARACTERISTICS

Abnormal blood pressure response:
> Diastolic pressure increase of 15 mm Hg or more during activity or exercise
> Drop in systolic pressure of 15 mm Hg or more during activity or exercise
> Excessive increase in systolic blood pressure response when performing a specific task
> Failure of the systolic pressure to rise with increasing intensity of activity or exercise
> Failure of the systolic pressure to return to baseline within five to ten minutes of the end of the bout of activity or exercise
> Postural hypotension

Abnormal heart rate response:
> Chronotropic incompetence (failure of the heart rate to rise with activity)
> Excessive increase in heart rate to low-level activity, e.g., greater than 125% of resting heart rate with less than three metabolic equivalents (METs) intensity (See Table 1 to determine the energy equivalents (in METs) for various activities)
> Failure of heart rate to return to resting level within five to ten minutes of the end of the bout of activity or exercise

Confusion during activity

Cooling of skin temperature during exercise or activity

Crackles auscultated in lung fields

Diaphoresis

Dizziness while performing an activity

Dyspnea on exertion

Dysrhythmias, e.g., heart block, premature ventricular contractions, rate-dependent bundle branch block, or ventricular tachycardia or fibrillation

Electrocardiographic changes of myocardial ischemia—exacerbated or occurring during activity, exercise, or recovery, e.g., T wave inversion or ST-segment depression, elevation, or normalization

Table 1: Estimated Energy Requirements of Selected Activities

MILD	(METs)	VIGOROUS	(METs)
Baking	2.0	Badminton	5.5
Billiards	2.4	Chopping wood	4.9
Bookbinding	2.2	Climbing hills:	
Canoeing (leisurely)	2.5	No load	6.9
Conducting an orchestra	2.2	With 5-kg load	7.4
Dancing, ballroom (slow)	2.9	Cycling (moderately)	5.7
Golf (with cart)	2.5	Dancing:	
Horseback riding (walking)	2.3	Aerobic or ballet	6.0
Playing a musical		Ballroom (fast)	
instrument:		or square	5.5
Accordion	1.8	Field hockey	7.7
Cello	2.3	Ice skating	5.5
Flute	2.0	Jogging (10-minute mile)	10.2
Horn	1.7	Karate or judo	6.5
Piano	2.3	Roller skating	6.5
Trumpet	1.8	Rope skipping	12.0
Violin	2.6	Skiing (water or downhill)	6.8
Woodwind	1.8	Squash	12.1
Volleyball		Surfing	6.0
(noncompetitive)	2.9	Swimming (fast)	7.0
Walking (2 mph)	2.5	Tennis (doubles)	6.0
Writing	1.7		

MODERATE			
Calisthenics (no weights)	4.0
Croquet	3.0
Cycling (leisurely)	3.5
Gardening (no lifting)	4.4
Golf (without cart)	4.9
Mowing lawn	
(power mower)	3.0
Playing drums	3.8
Sailing	3.0
Swimming (slowly)	4.5
Walking (3 mph)	3.3
Walking (4 mph)	4.5

*These activities can often be done at variable intensities, assuming that the intensity is not excessive and that the courses are flat (no hills) unless so specified. Categories are based on experience of tolerance; if an activity is perceived to be more than indicated, it should be judged accordingly.
MET, metabolic equivalent (3.5 ml • kg^{-1} • min^{-1} oxygen uptake).

Hypoglycemia following activity
Increased fatigue or weakness during activity
Increased fatigue or weakness following activity
Increased perception of exertion while performing a specific task
Increased perception of dyspnea while performing a specific task
Left ventricular wall motion abnormality detected with nuclear angiography or echo-cardiography, reflecting myocardial ischemia during resting or exercise
Loss of muscle mass
Loss of muscle strength
Murmur auscultated in any cardiac listening area that is heard only during exercise or increases in intensity with exercise
Pain or discomfort, e.g., claudication, angina, skeletal-muscular, or joint
Pallor during activity or exercise
Postural hypotension
Syncope
Third or fourth heart sound (extra heart sound or gallop), auscultated in the tricuspid or mitral listening areas, that occurs only with activity
Tremors

CONTRIBUTING FACTORS

Pathophysiological

Anemia
Cardiac disorders, e.g., chronotropic incompetence, cardiac denervation, decreased cardiac output, decreased contractility, decreased or increased afterload, decreased or increased preload, heart block, non-rate responsive permanent pacemaker, or resting sinus tachycardia
Fluid or electrolyte imbalance
Illness therapies:
    Activity limitations or prescribed bedrest
    Medications, e.g., beta blockers, calcium channel blockers, nitrates, diuretics, catabolic steroids
Imbalance between myocardial oxygen supply and demand
Infection
Metabolic disorders, e.g., decreased basal metabolic rate, hyperglycemia, hypoglycemia, malnutrition, obesity
Respiratory disorders, e.g., impaired gas exchange, impaired ventilation, ineffective airway clearance
Skeletal-muscular disorders, e.g., decrease in bone density, decrease in muscle strength or mass, joint stiffness or inflammation

Psychosociobehavioral

Anxiety	Depression	Pain
Bedrest/immobility	Environmental changes	Sedentary life-style
Circadian rhythm disturbance	Fear	Sleep pattern disturbance

EXPECTED OUTCOMES

Client will report an increase in activity level.

> There is an increase in the frequency of activities or exercise bouts.
>
> There is an increase in the duration of activity or exercise periods.
>
> There is an increase in the intensity level of the activity or exercise performed.

Client will report an improvement in the ability to tolerate an activity or exercise.

> There is a decrease in perceived effort or exertion during the performance of an activity.
>
> There is a decrease in the amount of fatigue or weakness experienced one hour after the activity or exercise.
>
> There is a normal heart rate and blood pressure response to activity or exercise and recovery.

INTERVENTIONS	RATIONALE
Universal	
Assess usual/maximal MET level and the fitness classification.	Fitness classification is based on the maximal oxygen uptake and age as delineated in Table 2. One MET is equal to 3.5 ml/kg/min. Assessment of either MET level or maximal oxygen uptake will yield the other parameter.
Identify the causes of the activity intolerance.	Therapeutic guidelines for advancing activity can be individualized when the interventions consider etiology. The primary intervention is aimed at decreasing or eliminating the cause of activity intolerance.
Monitor response to activity.	Heart rate and systolic blood pressure rise with activity but return to the baseline, pre-exercise level within five to seven minutes of recovery post exercise.
Provide an exercise prescription that includes the mode, duration, frequency, and intensity of the activity.	Levels of tolerated activity are highly individualized, and interventions are aimed at tailoring the plan in any of the four areas of the exercise prescription.
Provide gradual modifications in the exercise prescription to increase activity level.	A gradual increase in one component of the exercise prescription is better tolerated and results in fewer complications and less problems with adherence. Thus an increase in intensity, duration, or frequency is advised at any point in time.

INTERVENTIONS	RATIONALE
	After adjustment to one change, an advance in another component of the exercise prescription can be attempted. This allows for reconditioning to occur within a safe range while monitoring response to the increase. Use the MET chart for gradually increasing the intensity of effort.
Refer to a supervised and/or monitored exercise program if more specific guidelines are needed due to existing pathophysiology.	Supervision or monitoring is warranted if the person is unable to perform self-monitored exercise or if the severity of cardiac or respiratory problems warrants more specific assessment of physiological parameters.
Teach self-monitoring skills for activity or exercise progression and attempt to replicate the level of exertion at a prescribed intensity.	The heart rate or perceived exertion at peak effort can be used to monitor the intensity of activity or exercise. A reconditioning heart rate is generally 60% to 80% of the maximum heart rate. Table 3 provides a general guideline for exercise heart rate levels. Perceived exertion can be rated on a scale of one to 10. Table 4 provides the Borg Scale for rating perceived exertion.
Teach guidelines for advancing the intensity of activity or exercise level.	With the training effect, heart rate and perceived exertion for a specific intensity or MET level will decrease. When this occurs, an increase in the intensity is needed to achieve the same heart rate or level of perceived exertion and allow for further increases in conditioning.
Teach guidelines for increasing frequency or duration of activity or exercise level.	A change in either duration or frequency should be attempted first. After adjustment to one change, the other parameter can be increased.
Teach guidelines for including a five-minute warm-up prior to the prescribed exercise and concluding with a five minute cooldown.	A warm-up gradually increases the cardiorespiratory response to activity and provides gradual stretching of the muscle fibers. The cooldown allows for a gradual return to baseline. In addition, cooldown provides for the removal of lactic acid from the working muscle which reduces the potential for muscle soreness post-exercise.

Table 2: Normal Values of Maximum Oxygen Uptake at Different Ages*

AGE	MEN	WOMEN
20–29	43 (± 22) [12 METs]	36 (± 21) [10 METs]
30–39	42 (± 22) [12 METs]	34 (± 21) [10 METs]
40–49	40 (± 22) [11 METs]	32 (± 21) [9 METs]
50–59	36 (± 22) [10 METs]	29 (± 22) [8 METs]
60–69	33 (± 22) [9 METs]	27 (± 22) [8 METs]
70–79	29 (± 22) [8 METs]	27 (± 22) [8 METs]

*(ml kg^{-1} • min^{-1})
MET, metabolic equivalent; 1 MET = 3.5 ml • kg^{-1} • min^{-1} oxygen uptake.
Reproduced with permission.
© "Exercise Standards, A Statement for Health Professionals," 1991, p. 2287.
Copyright American Heart Association

INTERVENTIONS

RATIONALE

Inpatient	
Monitor heart rate and blood pressure response before, during, and after ambulation, range of motion exercise, or performance of an activity.	In the presence of cardiopulmonary disorders, peak response should be limited to 20 beats per minute and a 20 mm Hg over resting level or an increase of 125%.
Monitor heart and lung sounds with activity.	Presence of an abnormal response warrants a decrease in the intensity or cessation of activity.
Monitor oxygen saturation with activity.	An arterial oxygen saturation drop of more than 10% with activity warrants the use of supplemental oxygen with activity if a cardiopulmonary disorder is present.
Ambulate for increasing distances and/or increasing frequency.	Increase tolerance of activity to prepare for the three MET level required for most activities of daily living.
Encourage chair rest rather than bedrest unless contraindicated due to pathophysiology.	Chair rest reduces the risk of postural hypotension and thromboembolism. Furthermore, chair rest can improve respiratory function.

Table 3: Normal response to progressive treadmill protocol
in healthy subjects

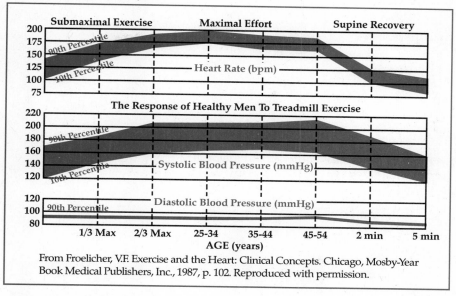

From Froelicher, V.F. Exercise and the Heart: Clinical Concepts. Chicago, Mosby-Year
Book Medical Publishers, Inc., 1987, p. 102. Reproduced with permission.

Table 4: Borg Scale for Rating of Perceived Exertion (RPE)

REVISED BORG RPE SCALE (1985)

0	nothing at all
0.5	extremely weak (just noticeable)
1	very weak
2	weak (light)
3	moderate
4	somewhat strong
5	strong
6	
7	very strong
8	
9	
10	extremely strong (almost max)
*	maximal exertion

Reproduced with permission from Borg, G. & Ottoson, D., **The perception of
exertion in physical work**, © 1986 by the Macmillan Publishing Company,
London & Basingstoke, U.K.

INTERVENTIONS	**R**ATIONALE
Encourage participation in care.	Gradually increase tolerance of the activities needed for self care. These activities are at an intensity of one to three METs.
Perform passive, active assisted, or active range of motion exercises one to four times per day.	Range of motion activity reduces the risk of immobility hazards.
Teach ways to balance activity and rest during hospitalization and after discharge.	Adequate rest is required to provide the strength to increase activity tolerance.
Community Health/ Home Care Encourage participation in a self-monitored, supervised, or monitored exercise reconditioning program.	Reconditioning requires 12 weeks of gradual increase in the activity prescription.
Increase level of intensity of social, recreational, or occupational activity.	Moderate reconditioning occurs with increases in activity other than a specific exercise prescription.
Maintain conditioning through participation in an ongoing exercise/activity program.	Maintenance is achieved when exercise entails an isotonic activity three times per week, for thirty minutes duration at an intensity of 60% to 80% of the maximum heart rate response. Lower intensity may be recommended if the duration or frequency of the activity are increased.
Teach self-monitoring skills for exercise and/or activity.	Self-care knowledge increases control, satisfaction, and adherence.
Teach ways to modify the activity/exercise during environmental changes.	Wind resistance, extremes in temperature, or increased humidity increase the effort of a specific activity. Under these conditions, reduce the intensity of the activity. Maintain the same target heart rate or level of perceived exertion.

REFERENCES/BIBLIOGRAPHY

American College of Sports Medicine. (1986). **Guidelines for exercise testing & prescription.** Philadelphia: Lea & Febiger.

American Heart Association Special Report. (1990). Exercise standards: A statement for health professionals from the American Heart Association. **Circulation, 82,** 2286–2332.

Baas, L.S. (1991). Assessment and prescription of activity for the person with cardiovascular disease. In L.S. Baas. (Ed.). **Essentials of cardiovascular nursing** (pp. 171–187). Rockville, MD: Aspen.

Baas, L.S. (1988). Caring for the person on prolonged bedrest. In P.L. Swearingen, M.S. Sommers, & K. Miller. (Eds.). **Manual of critical care: Applying nursing diagnoses to adult critical illnesses** (pp. 506–511). St. Louis: Mosby.

Borg, G., & Ottoson, D. (1986). **The perception of exertion in physical work.** Houndsmills, U.K.: MacMillan.

Dishman, R.K., Patton, R.W., & Smith, J. (1987). Using perceived exertion to prescribe and monitor exercise training heart rate. **International Journal of Sports Medicine, 8,** 208–213.

Fardy, P.S., Yanowitz, F.G., & Wilson, P.K. (1988). **Cardiac rehabilitation, adult fitness, and exercise testing (**2nd ed.). Philadelphia: Lea & Febiger.

*Fletcher, B.J., Thiel, J., & Fletcher, G.F. (1986). Phase II intensive monitored cardiac rehabilitation for coronary artery disease and coronary risk factors: A six session protocol. **American Journal of Cardiology, 57,** 751–756.

Kim, M.J., McFarland, G.K., & McLane, A.M. (1989). **Pocket guide to nursing diagnosis** (3rd ed.). St. Louis: Mosby.

*Lane, L.D., & Winslow, E.H. (1987). Oxygen consumption, cardiovascular response, and perceived exertion in healthy adults during rest, occupied bedmaking, and unoccupied bedmaking activity. **Cardiovascular Nursing, 23,** (31–36).

*Lindskog, B.D., & Sivarajan, E.S. (1982). A method of evaluation of activity and exercise in a controlled study of early cardiac rehabilitation. **Journal of Cardiac Rehabilitation, 2,** 156–165.

*Miller, N.H., Haskell, W.L., Berra, K., & DeBusk, R.F. (1984). Home versus group exercise training for increasing functional capacity after myocardial infarction. **Circulation, 70,** 645–649.

Moore, R.L., et al. (1987). Effects of training/detraining on submaximal exercise responses in humans. **Journal of Applied Physiology, 61,** 1719–1724.

North American Nursing Diagnosis Association. (1990). **Taxonomy I** (Rev. 1990). St. Louis: NANDA.

Olson, E.V. (1990). The hazards of immobility. **American Journal of Nursing, 90,** 43–46.

Wenger, N.K., & Hellerstein, H.K. (1984). **Rehabilitation of the coronary patient** (2nd ed.). New York: Wiley.

Winslow, E.H. (1985). Cardiovascular consequences of bedrest. **Heart and Lung, 14,** 236–246.

Activity Intolerance: Risk

A state in which an individual is at risk of developing insufficient physiological or psychological energy to endure or complete required or desired daily activities (NANDA, 1990, p. 74).

Linda S. Baas, R.N., M.S.N., C.C.R.N

RISK FACTORS

Pathophysiological

Bedrest or immobility

Cardiac disorders (e.g., chronotropic incompetence, cardiac denervation, decreased cardiac output, decreased contractility, decreased or increased afterload, decreased or increased preload, heart block, non-rate responsive permanent pacemaker, or resting sinus tachycardia)

Fluid or electrolyte imbalance

Illness therapies:
  Activity limitations or prescribed bedrest
  Medications (e.g., beta blockers, calcium channel blockers, nitrates, diuretics, catabolic steroids)

Imbalance between myocardial oxygen supply and demand

Infection

Metabolic disorders (e.g., decreased basal metabolic rate, hyperglycemia, hypoglycemia, malnutrition, obesity)

Pain or discomfort

Respiratory disorders (e.g., dyspnea at rest or with activity, impaired gas exchange, impaired ventilation, ineffective airway clearance)

Skeletal-muscular disorders (e.g., decrease in bone density, decrease in muscle strength or mass, joint stiffness, or inflammation)

Psychosociobehavioral

Anxiety   Environmental changes   Sleep pattern disturbance
Circadian rhythm disturbance   Fear
Depression   Sedentary life-style

Expected Outcomes

Client will report the ability to maintain usual activities.
> There is maintenance or an increase in the frequency of activities or exercise bouts.
> There is maintenance or an increase in the duration of activity or exercise periods.
> There is maintenance or an increase in the intensity level of activity or exercise performed.

Client will report the ability to tolerate an activity or exercise.
> There is maintenance or a decrease in perceived effort or exertion during performance of an activity.
> There is maintenance or a decrease in the amount of fatigue or weakness experienced one hour after the activity or exercise.
> There is a normal heart rate and blood pressure response to activity or exercise and recovery.
> There are no defining characteristics of activity intolerance.

Interventions	Rationale
Universal	
Assess usual and/or maximal metabolic equivalent (MET) level and the fitness classification.	The activity level is quantified in terms of METs. Table 1, p. 34, provides this information for common activities and exercises. Fitness classification is based on the maximal oxygen uptake and age as delineated in Table 2, p. 38. One MET is equal to 3.5 ml/kg/min. Assessment of either MET level or maximal oxygen uptake will yield the other parameter.
Identify the factor that is increasing the risk of activity intolerance and minimize the impact on functional status.	Therapeutic guidelines for preventing activity reduction can be individualized based on the risk factor profile. The primary intervention is aimed at decreasing or eliminating the factor(s) that can lead to activity intolerance.
Monitor response to activity.	Heart rate and systolic blood pressure rise with activity but return to the baseline, pre-exercise level within five to seven minutes of recovery post exercise.

INTERVENTIONS	RATIONALE
Provide an exercise prescription that includes the mode, duration, frequency, and intensity of the activity.	Levels of tolerated activity are highly individualized, and interventions are aimed at tailoring the plan in any of the four areas of the exercise prescription. A regular program of exercise will reduce the risk of activity intolerance.
Refer to a supervised and/or monitored exercise program if more specific guidelines are needed due to existing pathophysiology.	Supervision or monitoring is warranted when there is an inability to perform self-monitored exercise or when the severity of cardiac or respiratory problems warrants more specific assessment of physiological parameters.
Teach self-monitoring skills for activity or exercise progression.	The heart rate or perceived exertion at peak effort can be used to monitor the intensity of activity or exercise. Increases in perceived exertion or heart rate for a given activity are early signs of activity intolerance. Perceived exertion can be rated on a scale of one to 10. Table 4, p. 7, provides the Borg Scale for rating perceived exertion.
Teach guidelines for including a five-minute warm-up prior to the prescribed exercise and concluding with a five-minute cooldown.	A warm-up gradually increases the cardiorespiratory response to activity and provides gradual stretching of the muscle fibers. The cooldown allows for a gradual return to baseline. In addition, cooldown provides for the removal of lactic acid from the working muscle, which reduces the potential for muscle soreness post exercise.

Inpatient

Monitor heart rate and systolic blood pressure response before, during, and after ambulation; range of motion exercise; or performance of an activity.	In the presence of cardiopulmonary disorders, peak response should be limited to 20 beats per minute and a 20 mm Hg over resting level or an increase of 125%. Any other change in heart rate or blood pressure indicates actual activity intolerance.
Monitor heart and lung sounds with activity.	Presence of an abnormal response indicates actual activity intolerance and warrants a decrease in the intensity or cessation of activity.

INTERVENTIONS	RATIONALE
Monitor oxygen saturation with activity.	An arterial oxygen saturation drop of more than 10% with activity indicates actual activity intolerance and warrants the use of supplemental oxygen with activity if a cardiopulmonary disorder is present.
Ambulate for increasing distances and/or increasing frequencies.	Increase tolerance of activity to prepare for the three MET level required for most activities of daily living.
Encourage chair rest rather than bed rest unless contraindicated due to pathophysiology.	Chair rest reduces the risk of postural hypotension and thromboembolism. Furthermore, chair rest can improve respiratory function.
Encourage participation in care.	Gradually increase tolerance of the activities needed for self care. These activities are at an intensity of one to three METs.
Perform passive, active assisted, or active range of motion exercises one to four times per day.	Range of motion activity reduces the risk of immobility hazards.
Teach ways to balance activity and rest during hospitalization and after discharge.	Adequate rest is required to provide the strength to maintain or increase activity tolerance.
Community Health/ Home Care	
Assess level of intensity of social, recreational, or occupational activity.	The activity level is quantified in terms of METs. Table 1, p. 34, provides this information for common activities and exercises. Determine if the activity level has changed since the appearance of risk factors for activity intolerance.
Maintain conditioning through participation in an ongoing exercise/activity program.	Maintenance is achieved when exercise entails an isotonic activity three times per week, for 30-minute duration at an intensity of 60% to 80% of the maximum heart rate response. Lower intensity may be recommended if the duration or frequency of the activity are increased. Maintaining conditioning reduces the risk of activity intolerance developing.

INTERVENTIONS	**R**ATIONALE
Teach self-monitoring skills for exercise and/or activity.	Self monitoring for increases in level of perceived exertion or heart rate for a specific activity are the initial signs of actual activity intolerance. Also, self-care knowledge increases control, satisfaction, and adherence to the exercise program.
Teach ways to modify the activity/exercise during environmental changes.	Wind resistance, extremes in temperature, or increased humidity increase the effort of a specific activity. Under these conditions, reduce the intensity of the activity. Maintain the same target heart rate or level of perceived exertion.

REFERENCES/BIBLIOGRAPHY

American College of Sports Medicine. (1986). **Guidelines for exercise testing & prescription.** Philadelphia: Lea & Febiger.

American Heart Association Special Report. (1990). Exercise standards: A statement for health professionals from the American Heart Association. **Circulation, 82,** 2286–2332.

Baas, L.S. (1991). Assessment and prescription of activity for the person with cardiovascular disease. In L.S. Baas. (Ed.). **Essentials of Cardiovascular Nursing,** 171–187. Rockville, MD: Aspen.

Borg, G., & Ottoson, D. (1986). **The perception of exertion in physical work.** Houndsmills, U.K.: MacMillan.

Kim, M.J., McFarland, G.K., & McLane, A.M. (1989). **Pocket guide to nursing diagnosis** (3rd ed.). St. Louis: Mosby.

North American Nursing Diagnosis Association. (1990). **Taxonomy I** (Rev. 1990). St. Louis: NANDA.

Olson, E.V. (1990). The hazards of immobility. **American Journal of Nursing, 90,** 43–46.

Pender, N.J. (1987). **Health promotion in nursing** (2nd ed.). Norwalk, CT: Appleton & Lange.

Wenger, N.K., & Hellerstein, H.K. (1984). **Rehabilitation of the coronary patient** (2nd ed.). New York: Wiley.

Winslow, E.H. (1985). Cardiovascular consequences of bedrest. **Heart and Lung, 14,** 236–246.

Adjustment, Impaired

A state in which an individual is unable to modify life style/behavior in a manner consistent with a change in health status (NANDA, 1990, p. 62).

M. Kathleen Eilers, R.N., M.S.N.

DEFINING CHARACTERISTICS

Exhibition of extended period of shock, disbelief, or anger regarding health status change
Lack of future-oriented thinking
Lack of movement toward independence
Non-existent or unsuccessful ability to be involved in problem-solving or goal-setting
Verbalization of non-acceptance of health status change

CONTRIBUTING FACTORS

Pathophysiological

None

Psychosociobehavioral

Altered locus of control
Assault to self-esteem
Disability requiring change in life style
Impaired cognition
Inadequate support systems
Incomplete grieving
Sensory overload

EXPECTED OUTCOMES

Client will modify lifestyle to coincide with change in health status.
   Awareness of changes in health status and its effect on lifestyle is verbalized.
   Active role is taken in identifying goals and the means to achieve these goals.
   Strategies are used that will assist in coping with limitations and losses.

47

INTERVENTIONS	RATIONALE
Universal	
Evaluate and monitor understanding of change in health status and the limitations it imposes.	Knowledge of health status and limitations is essential to appropriate adjustments.
Evaluate progress made in achieving goals. Encourage description of perceived change in health and feelings about change, especially limitations.	Verbalization of feelings leads to understanding and adjustment.
Support efforts at problem-solving and goal formulation.	Progress is dependent on reality-based problem-solving and realistic goals.
Focus on ways to exhibit more independence.	Independence leads to increased self-esteem.
Assist in identifying support systems available to offer assistance. Identify persistent interferences to goal achievement. Praise achievements.	Positive feedback reinforces new behaviors.
Assist in focusing on strengths, abilities and past achievements to increase self-confidence.	New behaviors are most easily learned if based on previously learned skills.
Assist in initiating activities that provide satisfaction. Encourage acceptance of the assistance of others when necessary.	Focusing on pleasurable activities can help provide a sense of control and diversion to deal with the current situation.
Inpatient	
With permission, include family or other potential support systems in discussion of limitations and lifestyle changes required.	Support by significant others fosters adjustment.

INTERVENTIONS	**R**ATIONALE
Encourage practice of new behaviors in a supportive environment.	New behaviors are most easily learned in a neutral/supportive environment.
Provide opportunities for increased independence.	As independence increases, so does self-esteem, coping skills and adjustments.
Community Health/ Home Care Monitor level of change in lifestyle.	
Evaluate role of support systems in achieving goals.	
Evaluate and monitor environmental factors that inhibit successful adaptation.	
Refer to psychiatric/mental health clinical nurse specialist or other appropriate therapist if adjustment continues to be impaired.	Problems in adjustment may require the specialized skills and training of a psychotherapist.

REFERENCES/BIBLIOGRAPHY

Kanter, F.H., & Goldstein, A. (Eds.). (1975). **Helping people change.** Elmsford, NY: Pergamon.

Kolb, L.C., Keith, H., & Brodie, H. (1982). **Modern clinical psychiatry** (10th ed.). Philadelphia: Saunders.

McFarland, G.K., & McFarlane, E.A. (1989). **Nursing diagnosis and intervention.** Philadelphia: Mosby.

Millon, T. (1969). **Modern psychopathology. A biosocial approach to maladaptive learning and functioning.** Philadelphia: Saunders.

North American Nursing Diagnosis Association. (1990). **Taxonomy I** (Rev. 1990). St. Louis: Author.

Robinson, L. (1977). **Psychiatric nursing as a human experience** (2nd ed.). Philadelphia: Saunders.

Stuart, G., & Sundeen, S. (1983). **Principles and practice of psychiatric nursing** (2nd ed.). St. Louis: Mosby.

Airway Clearance, Impaired

A state in which an individual is unable to clear secretions or obstructions from the respiratory tract to maintain airway patency (NANDA, 1990, p. 37).

Claudia M. West, R.N., M.S.

DEFINING CHARACTERISTICS

Adventitious breath sounds (crackles [rales], rhonchi, wheezing)
Changes in blood pressure
Chest tightness or wheezing
Cough, effective/ineffective, with or without sputum
Decreased or absent breath sounds
Decreased oxyhemoglobin saturation (obtained from arterial blood gases or oximetry)
Dyspnea
Hypoxemia with or without central cyanosis

Increased airway resistance (on mechanical ventilator)
Increased peak airway pressure (on mechanical ventilator)
Increased use of accessory muscles
Paradoxical abdominal motion
Restlessness or agitation
Retractions, intercostal or supraclavicular
Rhonchial fremitus
Tachycardia
Tachypnea, change in depth of respirations

CONTRIBUTING FACTORS

Pathophysiological

Cognitive or perceptual impairment
Decreased vital capacity related to:
 adult respiratory distress syndrome
 (fixed chest wall abnormalities or injury
 impaired respiratory muscle function

interstitial pulmonary fibrosis
large pleural effusions
obstructive pulmonary diseases
pain
pneumothorax
Endotracheal intubation
Impaired mucociliary blanket related to:
 anesthesia

50

dehydration
endotracheal suctioning
narcotics
Impaired respiratory muscle functions
    related to:
    diaphragm descended and flat
      (fixed diaphragm)
    hypomagnesemia and
      hypophosphatemia
    neuromuscular diseases

phrenic nerve injury
protein calorie malnutrition
respiratory muscle fatigue
surgical incisions
Production of copious secretions related to:
    bronchitic, chronic or acute
    cystic fibrosis
    inhalation injuries (e.g., smoke,
      thermal, or chemical)
    pneumonia

Psychosociobehavioral

Anxiety
Depression
Lack of motivation

EXPECTED OUTCOMES

Client will have patent airway.
    Diminished or absent rhonchial fremitus or wheezing are reported.
    More comfortable breathing (less dyspnea) is reported.
    Intensity of breath sounds increases.
    Adventitious breath sounds diminish or cease.
    Peak airway pressure and airway resistance decrease (on mechanical ventilator).
    Less restlessness or agitation is reported.
    PaO_2 and/or oxyhemoglobin saturation (oximetry) improve.
    Respiratory rate, pulse, and blood pressure return to baseline.
    Amount of secretions removed increases.
    Use of accessory muscles diminishes.
    Paradoxical abdominal motion diminishes.
    Retractions will diminish or cease.
    Proper coughing or huffing technique is demonstrated.
    Correct use of abdominal-diaphragmatic breathing is demonstrated.
    Correct use of positive expiratory pressure mask (if available) is demonstrated.
    Correct techniques for postural drainage, chest percussion, and chest vibration are
      demonstrated.
    Adaptations for performing chest physical therapy in the home are verbalized.
    Correct technique for tracheostomy care in the home is demonstrated.
    Correct technique of endotracheal suctioning and cleaning of equipment is demonstrated.

INTERVENTIONS

RATIONALE

Universal

Monitor the following:

1. Intensity of breath sounds and presence of adventitious breath sounds

   These are the most important indicators of airway patency.

2. Level of consciousness

   Restlessness, agitation, or diminished arousal may be related to hypoxemia or elevated carbon dioxide related to accumulated secretions.

3. Vital signs, including temperature

   Changes in vital signs may indicate increased respiratory and cardiac work related to increased airway resistance or hypoxemia (from accumulated secretions) or the presence of a respiratory infection.

4. Use of accessory muscles and paradoxical abdominal motion (inward motion of the abdomen with inspiration)

   Accumulation of secretions may increase the work of breathing, resulting in use of accessory muscles. Paradoxical abdominal motion is an important sign of respiratory muscle fatigue, usually as a result of severe or prolonged increase in work of breathing.

5. Elevations in peak airway pressure and airway resistance if on a mechanical ventilator

   Accumulated secretions will increase airway resistance and the pressure required by the ventilator to deliver each tidal volume.

6. Thoracic expansion and diaphragmatic excursion

   These test the ability to take a deep breath. The ability of the diaphragm to descend with a maximal inspiration will determine the ability to perform diaphragmatic breathing.

7. Arterial oxygen tension (PaO_2) or hemoglobin saturation (via oximetry)

   Hypoxemia or decreased hemoglobin saturation may be related to decreasing ventilation from accumulated secretions in the airways. Improvements in these values could be related to effective coughing or suctioning.

8. Ability to learn and use deep breathing and coughing strategies

   Cognitive impairment, fatigue, and dyspnea may prevent learning of or the ability to cooperate with these strategies.

9. The amount and quality of secretions

   These will indicate the effectiveness of treatment, presence of respiratory infection, and hydration of mucus blanket.

INTERVENTIONS	RATIONALE
10. Cough and gag reflex in neurologically impaired or comatose clients	These will indicate the risk of aspiration.
Determine causes of ineffective airway clearance.	The nurse will be able to direct nursing interventions more effectively.
Encourage deep breathing (with the diaphragm when possible), coughing,[1] and forced expiratory technique (huffing).	Deep breathing, especially using the diaphragm, allows for greater lung expansion and ventilation and provides for a more effective cough. Coughing in conjunction with deep breathing increases intrathoracic pressure and airflow velocity, which assist in mobilizing secretions toward the pharynx. Huffing is a series of one, two, or three short, forceful expirations performed after taking a deep breath and with the glottis open. Huffing can be a substitute for or an adjunct of chest percussion and drainage. Huffing may be more effective in clearing distal airways than coughing.
Encourage the use of deep breathing and coughing or huffing after the administration of bronchodilators.	Airways will be dilated allowing for greater lung volumes, better airflow, and more effective cough.
Perform postural drainage, percussion, and vibration (chest physical therapy) when secretions are present but cannot be cleared by coughing or suctioning.	Percussion and vibration loosen secretions from walls of airways, and gravity assists drainage. Chest physical therapy carries risks of bronchospasm and hypoxemia; a head down position is contraindicated in those with heart failure or increased intracranial pressure. Hence, the nurse must critically evaluate the need for this therapy.
Perform endotracheal suctioning when secretions are present and cough is ineffective.	Endotracheal suctioning removes secretions from larger airways, but it traumatizes the airways and may cause dangerous hypoxemia or arrhythmias. It should be done only when the real need for it exists.

[1] Coughing may cause airway collapse or bronchospasm resulting in worsening ventilation and dyspnea, and thus should be performed only when secretions are auscultated.

INTERVENTIONS	RATIONALE
Encourage intake of 2–3 L of fluids every 24 hours unless fluids are restricted.	Water is a major component of the mucus blanket and is necessary for ciliary motion. The water is provided by the vascular supply to the epithelium, which in turn is maintained by an adequate fluid volume. A dehydrated epithelium results in dried, viscous secretions that are difficult to mobilize.
Provide > 3 L of fluids every 24 hours if there is fever, increased respiratory rate, or an endotracheal tube present, and if not contraindicated.	Insensible water losses from the respiratory tract increase significantly under these conditions.
Provide humidification of oxygen at flow rates over 2 L/min or 30%, or in clients with bypassed upper airways or on mechanical ventilators.	Humidification prevents drying of the airways and secretions. If environmental humidity is adequate, additional humidity is not usually needed with low flow rates or low oxygen concentrations.
Avoid milk products.	These products may produce more sputum.
Splint incisions or painful areas during deep breathing and coughing.	Splinting minimizes the stretch of a locally painful area, allowing for deeper breathing and more forceful cough.
Change position in bed frequently.	This allows for drainage of secretions from dependent parts of the lungs and increases lung expansion.
Encourage ambulation as much as tolerated.	This encourages deeper tidal volumes and clearance of secretions.
Use the positive expiratory pressure (PEP) mask (if available) for 4–5 min., to a maximum of 4x/24 h.	The PEP mask applies positive pressure to the airways during expiration so that the airways remain open throughout expiration. This allows for greater lung volumes and a more effective cough.
Perform tracheostomy and stoma care.	This ensures patency of the artificial airway and removes mucous encrustation around the stoma. This may need to be done frequently if secretions are copious or thick.

INTERVENTIONS	RATIONALE
Keep an obturator and extra tracheostomy tube at the bedside.	In case of accidental decannulation, the new tracheostomy tube is readily available for quick insertion.
Teach about the health risks of cigarette smoking and recommend various strategies and programs of smoking cessation.	Besides risks of emphysema, lung cancer, and coronary artery disease, cigarette smoking chronically irritates the airways, resulting in increased production of mucus and paralysis and loss of cilia.

Inpatient

INTERVENTIONS	RATIONALE
Teach the proper techniques of chest physical therapy if it is to be performed at home, including any adaptations needed.	The client and caregiver must be able to demonstrate this procedure accurately before discharge in order to maximize clearance of secretions in the home.
Refer to appropriate home health or community health agencies for follow-up after discharge.	Complex respiratory care or health status follow-up in the home is necessary to assure that equipment is properly cared for and accurately used, that respiratory therapy techniques such as chest physical therapy are done properly, and that the client is responding to therapy.

Community Health/ Home Care

INTERVENTIONS	RATIONALE
Assess ability to perform respiratory therapy techniques and use equipment correctly.	The level of follow-up and need for resources will be determined by the client's ability to manage care and equipment in the home.
Assess resources and supports in the home setting.	Knowledge of these will assist in providing additional resources if needed.
Help to identify factors that could interfere with ability to adhere to prescribed therapies.	Knowledge of these factors helps the nurse to devise an individualized plan that promotes optimal adherence or to minimize the negative effects of these factors.
Assist to identify resources and strategies that could help overcome barriers to adherence.	The client and the nurse are able to optimize adherence with the treatment plan, including what is realistic or unrealistic to perform.

INTERVENTIONS	**R**ATIONALE
Teach to perform endotracheal suctioning with the following changes in the procedure as it is performed in the acute care setting: 1. No gloves or a single clean glove 2. Deep breaths before and after suctioning in the spontaneously breathing individual with a permanent tracheostomy 3. Suction catheter may be disposable or non-disposable 4. Soak non-disposable catheter in soapy water after use, and at the end of the day wash all catheters in warm soapy water, boil in water for 10 minutes and store in plastic bags or foil after air drying 5. Wash suction tubing and jar daily in warm soapy water, rinse and air dry 6. Disinfect catheters, tubing, and jar at least twice a week by soaking 30 minutes in a solution of one part white vinegar and three parts tap water. A double quaternary ammonium compound may also be used and has the advantages of being reusable up to 10 to 14 days and, thus, costing less.	A clean technique is adequate at home because the risk of cross-contamination is not present. The respiratory tract already is colonized with organisms natural to the client and the home setting. A battery-operated portable suction machine should be available in case of an electrical power failure.
Instruct in tracheostomy care with the following changes in the procedure as it is performed in the inpatient setting: 1. Clean, not sterile, technique is used	Clean technique is adequate in the home if tracheostomy care is provided by the client (see previous rationale).

INTERVENTIONS	RATIONALE
2. Inner cannula is removed and allowed to soak for 2–3 min in one part hydrogen peroxide to one part tap water. The inner cannula is then scrubbed with a pipe cleaner or small brush and rinsed with running tap water. Excess water is shaken off and the inner cannula is reinserted.	
3. The stoma is cleaned once a day or as needed with hydrogen peroxide and cotton applicators. A dressing is not used since it allows accumulation of mucus around the stoma.	
Teach chest physical therapy techniques using pillows, ironing board, or something similar to achieve gravity drainage.	Proper and creative uses of articles available in the home allow management of self-care activities more independently and at less cost.

REFERENCES/BIBLIOGRAPHY

*Amborn, S.A. (1976). Clinical signs associated with the amount of tracheobronchial secretions. **Nursing Research, 25,** 121–126.

Christensen, E.F., Nedergaard, T., & Dahl, R. (1990). Long-term treatment of chronic bronchitis with positive expiratory pressure mask and chest physiotherapy. **Chest, 97,** 645–650.

Connors, A.F., Hammon, W.E., Martin, R.J., & Rogers, R.M. (1980). Chest physical therapy. The immediate effect on oxygenation in acutely ill patients. **Chest, 78,** 559–564.

Kaminska, T.M., & Pearson, S.B. (1988). A comparison of postural drainage and positive expiratory pressure in the domiciliary management of patients with chronic bronchial sepsis. **Physiotherapy, 74,** 251–254.

Kersten, L.D. (1989). **Comprehensive respiratory nursing.** Philadelphia: Saunders.

Kim, M.J., & Larson, J.L. (1987). Ineffective airway clearance and ineffective breathing patterns: Theoretical and research base for nursing diagnosis. **Nursing Clinics of North America. 22**(1), 125–134.

Lucas, J., Golish, J.A., Sleeper, G., & O'Ryan, J.A. (1988). **Home respiratory care.** Norwalk, CT: Appleton-Lange.

Moody, L.E., & Martindale, C.L. (1978). Effect of pulmonary hygiene measures on levels of arterial oxygen saturation in adults with chronic lung disease. **Heart and Lung, 7,** 315–319.

North American Nursing Diagnosis Association. (1990). **Taxonomy I** (Rev. 1990). St. Louis: Author.

Oldenburg, F.A., Dolovich, M.B., Montgomery, J.M., & Newhouse, M.T. (1979). Effects of postural drainage, exercise, and cough on mucus clearance in chronic bronchitis. **American Review of Respiratory Disease, 120,** 739–745.

* Riegel, B., & Forshee, T. (1985). A review and critique of the literature on preoxygenation for endotracheal suctioning. **Heart and Lung, 14,** 507–518.

Shapiro, B.A., Kacmarek, R.M., Cane, R.D., Peruzzi, W.T., & Hauptman, D. (1991). **Clinical application of respiratory care** (4th ed.). St. Louis: Mosby Year Book.

Sutton, P., et al. (1983). Assessment of the forced expiration technique, postural drainage, and directed coughing in chest physiotherapy. **European Journal of Respiratory Disease, 64,** 62–68.

Anxiety

A state in which an individual experiences generalized feelings of unease and apprehension triggered by a perceived threat; it may be experienced in acute, chronic, or panic levels.

Karen Goyette Vincent, R.N., M.S., C.S.

. . . .

DEFINING CHARACTERISTICS

Acute Anxiety

Anger
Attends to only a specific
     detail
Change in appetite
Change in sleeping
     pattern
Chest tightness
Clinging
Crying
Diarrhea/constipation
Difficulty in expressing
     self

Distractable
Dizziness
Dry mouth
Facial tension
Faintness
Fatigue
Generalized increase in
     acuity of illness
Glancing about
Hand wringing
Headaches
Hyperventilation

Indecisive
Irritable
Nausea/vomiting
Palpitations
Pupil dilation
Selective inattention
Tachycardia
Trembling
Verbalizes/demonstrates
     inability to
     concentrate
Withdrawal

Chronic Anxiety — A constant state of anxiety. Defining characteristics are less severe than in the acute phase and continue for an extended period of time.

Attends only to immediate
     tasks
Belching
Fatigue during the day
Frequent sighing

Heartburn
 Increased number of so-
          matic complaints
Insomnia
Irritability

Jumpiness
Loneliness
Muscle tension
Ruminating
Worrying

Panic (severe) Anxiety

All behaviors as in acute
   anxiety
Increased sensitivity to
   envronmental
   stimuli
Paresthesia

Poor reality testing
Purposeless activity
Restlessness
Terror
Unable to determine
   cause/effect

relationships
Verbalizes feeling detached
   from one's
   physical body/
   environment

CONTRIBUTING FACTORS

Pathophysiological

Cardiac disease
Chronic obstructive pul-
   monary disease
Diagnosis of terminal
   illness

Early stage Alzheimer's
   disease
Excessive alcohol, caffeine
   intake
Hyperthyroidism

Impending surgery
Post head injury
Recent myocardial infarction
Threat to change in health
   status

Psychosociobehavioral

Addition to family
Change in job
Change in responsibility at
   work/school/
   home
Change in usual source
   of support

Conflict regarding basic
   values/beliefs
Death in family
Depression
Lack of knowledge
Life-threatening illness of
   family member
Marital difficulties

Multiple life stress events
Relocation
Son/daughter leaving home
Threat to change in socio-
   economic status
Threat to self concept
Uncertainty of control over
   illness

EXPECTED OUTCOMES

Client will demonstrate, both verbally and behaviorally, a decrease in anxiety.
   Subjective experience of anxiety is verbalized.
   Six to eight hours of sleep is obtained per night.
   Past successful coping methods are identified.
   Problem solving regarding conflictual life areas begins.
   Interactions with others are in a focused manner.
   A decisive course of action is chosen from a list of alternatives.
   A reduction in physical symptoms of anxiety (dilated pupils, chest tightness, etc.) is exhibited.
   Attention to more than one detail or task is achieved.
Client will utilize new methods of coping with stress and controlling anxiety.
   Sources of anxiety are identified.
   Long-term coping strategies (i.e. problem solving, relaxation techniques, exercise, etc.)
      are verbalized.
   Increasing anxiety symptoms can be identified.

Use of relaxation strategies with a decrease in blood pressure, pulse, and muscle tension
   is rehearsed.
An understanding of chronic or acute disease process, including prognosis and treatment
   options is verbalized.
Methods to enlarge or utilize existing social support system are identified.
Caffeine intake is decreased to two cups per day.

INTERVENTIONS	RATIONALE
Universal	
Monitor the ongoing anxiety level.	Ability to attend to directions, understand new information, perform tasks, etc. diminishes when anxiety increases. The efficacy of interventions depends on continually assessing anxiety level.
Evaluate and document response to antianxiety medication.	The goal of antianxiety medication is not to eliminate anxiety, but to decrease the symptoms to a manageable level so that there can be focus on its source and more successful coping.
Speak slowly and calmly in a low voice using short, simple sentences.	It is difficult to focus on conversations when anxiety is high. Speaking in short sentences will simplify the process. The tone of voice will convey calmness and a sense of security.
Be direct in focusing on specific topics.	Anxiety diminishes the ability to concentrate and attend to detail. An example of a verbal response may be, "We were just talking about what you wanted for dinner. Why don't we focus on that."
Assure that client is not "going crazy" or having a medical problem.	Many of the symptoms of anxiety mimic medical and psychiatric disorders. It is important to provide reassurance about the etiology.
Discuss personal sources of anxiety.	Identifying sources of anxiety aids in the analysis of the connection between events and the anxiety experience.
Help to identify symptoms of anxiety.	Recognizing the physical and emotional symptoms can lead to early intervention and can clarify what events trigger the feeling state.
Discuss past methods for coping with anxiety.	It is important to know what strategies have been used for dealing with stress/anxiety in the past. These techniques may no longer be useful

INTERVENTIONS	RATIONALE
	or may have been overwhelmed by the stressors involved. In the case of chronic anxiety, the coping skills themselves may be faulty.
Discuss past methods of problem-solving.	Problem-solving is a long-term coping strategy. Identifying a lack of knowledge regarding problem-solving techniques can direct interventions.
Teach relaxation techniques such as progressive relaxation, meditation, deep breathing, or guided imagery.	These methods of relaxation have been researched and are used frequently in helping people deal with any level of anxiety.
Teach a constructive model for problem-solving.	A step-by-step method for problem identification, alternative identification, analysis of alternatives, and selection is necessary, thus gaining control over process of solving problems.
Teach about the positive aspects of anxiety.	The goal of treatment is not elimination of anxiety from life but rather, keeping the level of anxiety manageable and using anxiety as a motivating force for learning and growth.
Inpatient *PANIC (SEVERE) ANXIETY* Monitor whether the behavior is being contained.	The basic goal of treatment is safety for the client and others.
Evaluate whether the cycle of anxiety is slowing or stopping.	Assessing the efficacy of interventions, both in behavior and medication, provides direction for continuing treatment.
Assure that the goal is to provide safety and control.	When in a panic state, hallucinations and poor reality testing may be present. Providing verbal boundaries and limits offer external security.
Stay at a close, safe distance.	Staying within view offers support and allows monitoring for physical safety. It also provides a feeling of space.
Place in a quiet area.	Anxiety can cause increased sensitivity to external stimuli. Decreasing environmental noise and interruptions will decrease agitation and enable focusing on specific details.

INTERVENTIONS	RATIONALE
Provide ample room to pace or move about to release energy.	Large muscle group movements help release excess energy and decrease cardiovascular symptoms.
MODERATE ANXIETY Evaluate understanding of the disease process, including treatment options.	Ongoing evaluation of understanding provides information for future educational needs.
Involve family and significant others in education about disease or diagnosis and needs upon discharge.	Uncertainty and lack of knowledge can be a major cause of anxiety. Education about the disease process and what may be expected when returning home give the family concrete information and an increased feeling of control over the situation.
Inform family about support groups within the community (e.g., Alliance for the Mentally Ill, Alzheimer's and Related Disorders, Support Groups, etc.).	Support groups in the community can provide a source of ongoing education and advocacy after discharge.
Include in educational groups with others having similar illnesses.	These groups can provide both factual information and dispel the myth of being alone with an illness. This intervention can be helpful in relieving anxiety.
Conduct family support group on the unit.	These groups will introduce the concept of mutual support and empowerment through collective action.
Teach about the disease process, including prognosis and treatment options.	Knowledge of the disease process can help to highlight misconceptions, myths about the illness, and in turn, decrease anxiety. Education empowers both client and family.
Community Health/ Home Care *PANIC (SEVERE) ANXIETY* Monitor the frequency of panic attacks between visits.	Determining the number of attacks evaluates the severity of the illness, impact on the family, and the efficacy of interventions.

INTERVENTIONS	RATIONALE
Evaluate understanding of stress reduction techniques (e.g., Are stress reduction techniques being used when the panic attack starts? Is there an awareness of the techniques used?)	The use of stress reduction techniques can prevent, slow, or stop an anxiety attack.
Evaluate and document the ongoing impact these panic attacks have on client and significant others' lifestyles.	The support of significant others is critical to recovery. Vital roles that the client plays within the family unit may be compromised by the panic attacks.
Assess the feelings described prior to a panic attack and help identify stressors or precipitants to the panic attack.	Identifying specific stressors may highlight beliefs or fears that are not based in reality. The intervention can help dispel those myths and give a greater sense of control over the client's life.
Involve the significant others in discussion about the panic attacks.	Education can decrease anxiety and elicit greater support.
Teach client to keep a journal with information on each panic attack with the events and emotions occurring before the attack, time of day, place, symptoms of the attack, etc.	This exercise may glean information about triggers for the attacks based on nonreality-based fears. It also can give a sense of control over the attacks when in similar situations.

REFERENCES/BIBLIOGRAPHY

*Boyd, C., & Munhall, P. (1989). A qualitative investigation of reassurance. **Holistic Nursing Practice, 4**(1), 61–69.

Chishom, M. (1988). Anxiety. In C. Beck, R. Rawlins, & S. Williams. (Eds.). **Mental health-psychiatric nursing: A holistic life-cycle approach.** St. Louis: Mosby.

Ganguli, R. (1983). Medical assessment. In M. Hersen, A. Kazdin, & A. Bellack. (Eds.). **The clinical psychology handbook.** New York: Pergamon.

Haber, J., Hoskins, P., Leach, A., & Sideleau, B. (1987). **Comprehensive psychiatric nursing.** New York: McGraw-Hill.

*Halm, M. (1990). Effects of support groups on anxiety of family members during critical illness. **Heart and Lung, 19**(1), 62–71.

*Renfroe, K. (1988). Effect of progressive relaxation on dyspnea and state anxiety in patients with chronic obstructive pulmonary disease. **Heart and Lung, 17**(4), 408–413.

*Webster, K., & Christman, N. (1988). Perceived uncertainty and coping post myocardial infarction. **Western Journal of Nursing Research, 10**(4), 384–400.

Aspiration: Risk

A state in which an individual is at risk for entry of gastrointestinal secretions, oropharyngeal secretions, or solids or fluids into tracheobronchial passages (NANDA, 1990, p. 43).

Georgene C. Siemsen, R.N., M.S., C.S.

RISK FACTORS

Internal

Age greater than 65 years
Cardiopulmonary arrest
Damage to the 5th, 7th, 9th, 10th, and 12th cranial nerves
Decreased esophageal motility
Depressed level of consciousness (sleep, coma)
Dysphagia
Facial or neck trauma or surgery

Gastric distention
Gastroesophageal reflux
Hiatal hernia
Incompetent lower esophageal sphincter
Nasogastric tube
Neuromuscular disease
Preexisting pulmonary disease
Pregnancy, labor, emergency cesarean section

Receiving central nervous system depressants, alcohol
Tardive dyskinesia
Tube feedings
Upper airway intubation
Ventilator dependency
Vomiting
Wired jaws

External

Cold tube-feeding formula
High nutrient density tube-feeding formula
Hypo- and hyper-osmolar tube-feeding solution
Situations resulting in an inability to elevate the upper body

EXPECTED OUTCOMES

Client will evaluate level of risk for aspiration.

> Predisposing risk factors for aspiration are listed.
>
> Existing aspiration risk is identified.

Aspiration will be prevented.

> Activity, function, and comfort are optimized within the limitations of aspiration risk to maintain quality of life.
>
> Adequate, safe nutrition is experienced.
>
> Optimum airway clearance is experienced.

INTERVENTIONS

RATIONALE

Universal

Assess for symptoms of swallowing difficulties, including:

1. Difficulty initiating a swallow, or, exaggerated swallow
2. Pocketing food into the cheeks
3. Drooling
4. Cough or throat clearing, especially after a swallow
5. An ineffective cough; weak or absent
6. Fluid passing from the nose after swallowing

Abnormal symptoms vary depending on location of brain or nerve injury.

Examples of the effect of damage to the cranial nerves:

a. Trigeminal nerve (5th cranial): Controls the muscles of mastication. Damage results in loss of sensation and inability to move the mandible.

b. Facial nerve (7th cranial): Provides the sense of taste, controls facial muscles. Damage results in increased salivation and pouching of food in cheeks.

c. Glossopharyngeal nerve (9th cranial): Transmits sensation to the tongue, pharynx, and soft palate. Damage results in decreased taste, decreased salivation or destroyed gag reflex.

d. Vagus nerve (10th cranial): Controls sensation of the pharynx and palate as well as the muscles in that area. Damage results in difficulty swallowing, nasal regurgitation, and reduced or loss of gag reflex.

e. Hypoglossal nerve (12th cranial): Controls the extrinsic and intrinsic muscles of the tongue. Damage results in difficulty positioning food for mastication, resulting in pouching of food. Ongoing evaluation for signs of impaired swallowing determines effectiveness of interventions and need for further evaluation by the speech/language pathologist.

INTERVENTIONS	RATIONALE
Evaluate gag and cough reflexes frequently; assist with feeding to provide the opportunity to observe tolerance.	Depressed gag and cough reflexes increase aspiration risk of oral secretions, thin liquids, or food. A persistent cough noted during meals may indicate aspiration.
Monitor and document vital signs and symptoms of respiratory failure.	Typically, respiratory distress is noted when aspiraton is experienced. Neuromuscular disease may cause an ineffective cough, decreased gag reflex, or impaired swallow that poses an aspiration risk. The common presentation of respiratory distress may not occur in the client with neuromuscular disease. Early warning signals of respiratory distress include increased pulse (greater than 120 beats/min) or pulse less than 70 beats/min, respiratory rate greater than 30 breaths/min with or without abnormal respiratory pattern. Aspiration may occur without obvious coughing or respiratory distress.
Auscultate breath sounds.	Rales, rhonchi, and decreased vesicular sounds are suggestive of aspiration.
Evaluate and monitor mental status.	Aspiration causes a decrease in oxygen available for cognitive and total brain functioning. Also, altered cognition affects response to meals and ability to swallow, increasing the aspiration risk.
Monitor oral cavity for accumulation of food or secretions.	Decrease oral sensation or impaired swallow may result in pocketing food in the mouth or pooling secretions in the oral cavity.
Determine fit and condition of dentures. Initiate dental referral as needed.	Dentures that need repair or do not fit properly result in the inability to prepare the bolus for the swallow and may impair the swallow itself. Weight loss over time affects denture fit.
Request a referral for a speech/language pathologist evaluation.	The speech/language pathologist has the tools and expertise for dysphagia assessment. Screening is important in determining the need for further workup, such as video fluoroscopy and treatment.

INTERVENTIONS	RATIONALE
Feed foods in the form of a bolus to facilitate swallowing.	Diminished oral sensation or weak mastication ability results in the inability to prepare food for swallow.
Provide meals in an upright position—in chair or elevate head of bed.	Elevating the head facilitates the movement of food to the stomach, lowering risk of reflux and aspiration.
When positioning in bed between meals, support comfortably with pillows while having the mouth dependent.	Side-lying with the mouth dependent prevents pooling of oral secretions that can be aspirated.
Provide suction equipment for oral or tracheal suctioning—suction as needed to maintain a patent airway.	Maintaining a clear airway decreases the risk of aspiration.
Perform chest physiotherapy.	Postural drainage, percussion, and vibration assist to mobilize secretions, thereby preventing aspiration from unassisted attempts to clear the airway or pooling of secretions.
Clear the mouth and pharynx of vomitus after emesis.	Altered level of consciousness or neurological deficits result in an inability to clear the oral cavity of material that can be aspirated.
Teach and supervise deep-breathing exercises and effective cough technique.	A strong controlled cough and deep-breathing exercises support effective airway clearance, decreasing risk of aspiration.
Teach and supervise safe feeding techniques, including: 1. Follow recommended dietary texture restrictions such as thickened liquids 2. Encourage a double swallow to clear the pharyngeal tract 3. Position in a sitting position during meals and at least fifteen minutes after eating 4. Remove any residual food from the mouth	Active participation in the prevention of aspiration decreases anxiety by providing control, and supports compliance with the recommended regime. Supervision of meals allows ample time for determining effectiveness of the plan of care.

INTERVENTIONS	**R**ATIONALE
5. Allow adequate time for effective swallowing	
Inpatient For the client receiving enteral feedings: Evaluate motility of the bowel, and withold feedings if symptoms of decreased gastric motility are present. 1. Auscultate bowel tones 2. Percuss the abdomen for air 3. Note nausea and vomiting	Decreased gastric motility increases risk of aspiration. Accumulated material in the stomach increases the risk of reflux or emesis.
Monitor for tube placement at regular intervals, including prior to each use. Techniques for checking tube placement include: 1. Aspirate for gastric contents. A 10-ml syringe may be helpful to accomplish this with small bore tubes, although they tend to collapse with syringe aspiration. Note: This test may be unreliable because the literature reports incidences in which formula was withdrawn from tubes of clients being fed inadvertently into the lungs. Also, tubes can pass the glottis without causing a cough or respiratory distress in severely ill clients. 2. Instill 10 ml of air into the tube and listen over the stomach for verification of placement. Note: The accuracy of this test is questioned in the literature due to lack of consistency in identifying tube placement using this technique.	A displaced nasogastric tube may move up and out of the stomach, allowing tube-feeding formula or gastric contents to enter the airway.

INTERVENTIONS	**R**ATIONALE
3. Monitor aspirate for glucose. Note: The presence of blood in the aspirated secretions may result in a false positive test for glucose. 4. After dislocating events such as coughing, vomiting or suctioning occur, and correct placement cannot be determined definitively by other methods, radiographic examination is indicated.	
Assess for ability to position with HOB at 30° to 45° or upright in a chair and position accordingly. Techniques for ensuring safe positioning include: 1. Stop feedings 30 minutes to one hour prior to head-down positioning procedures or suctioning. 2. If the head-up position is contraindicated, the client should be positioned on the right side as much as possible.	Head-up positioning aids in progression of feedings by gravity, thus minimizing the amount of fluid in the stomach at one time. Right side-lying facilitates passage of stomach contents into the pylorus and allows emesis to drain from the mouth rather than be aspirated.
Monitor for signs of aspiration, including sudden onset of respiratory distress, coughing, dyspnea, and wheezing.	Aspiration of gastric contents causes marked irritation in the airways. Note: Aspiration of small amounts of gastric contents may not be detected, especially in clients with decreased mental status or decreased ability of glottis closure.
Monitor vital signs, note and describe sputum, auscultate breath sounds, and evaluate for hypoxemia.	Clients with impaired mental status or decreased ability of glottis closure may not present typically after aspiration. A combination of the above clinical signs are suggestive of aspiration.

INTERVENTIONS	**R**ATIONALE
Evaluate for appropriate size of nasogastric tube. If large amounts of medications are to be given, a 12 or 14 French polyurethane or silicone feeding tube can be used.	Client comfort must be balanced with safety needs when considering tube size. Note: Small-bore weighted tubes are not free from risk of displacement. Gastrostomy tubes may be more comfortable for the client for long-term enteral nutrition, but aspiration remains a risk.
Monitor for gastric retention of tube feeding: 1. Gastric contents should be measured prior to intermittent bolus infusion. If more than 100–150 ml of fluid is present, the feeding should be held for approximately one hour and the residual volume rechecked. Elevated residual volumes on two successive checks necessitate discontinuation of the feedings. 2. With continuous tube-feedings: A residual that is 10% to 20% greater than the flow rate per hour is significant. Measure abdominal girth from one anterior iliac crest to the other. An increase of 8–10 cm above baseline is significant, indicating a need to temporarily stop the feedings.	Gastric retention of tube feeding results in reflux or emesis, increasing aspiration risk.
Evaluate for continued need for nasogastric feedings.	The presence of the nasogastric feeding tube may inhibit a normal swallow. Feeding tubes may interfere with closure of the lower esophageal sphincter resulting in reflux and high aspiration risk. Nasogastric feedings should be used only in the presence of intact gag and cough reflexes. A speech/language pathology referral is indicated if the condition improves with the possibility of beginning oral feedings.

INTERVENTIONS	RATIONALE
Add blue food coloring to formula.	Detection of blue color in pulmonary secretions indicates aspiration.
Do not restrain in a manner that would prevent protection of the airway should vomiting occur.	Mitts are preferable to wrist restraints for clients that attempt to pull out tubes. They allow greater mobility of the extremities. Try distracting with a second "dummy" tube taped to an arm or the chest.
Tape tube securely in place. Check markings to insure the tube did not slip.	Dislocation of the tube may occur after suctioning, coughing, or vomiting. It is imperative that tube position be checked frequently for proper placement.
Flush feeding tube with 20–50 cc of water after each feeding or administration of medication. Flush every four hours when feedings are given continuously.	Flushing insures patency of the tube as well as prevents interaction between medications and formula.
For the client with an endotracheal tube or tracheostomy: 1. Suction to insure a patent airway 2. Maintain good oral hygiene, ensuring oral cavity is free of secretions	The presence of an endotracheal tube interferes with the normal swallow, causing aspiration risk. The presence of a cuffed tube does not eliminate risk of aspiration.

Community Health/ Home Care

Teach proper positioning to decrease aspiration risk.	Proper positioning decreases risk of emesis, reflux, or pooling of secretions in the oral cavity.
Teach signs of impaired swallowing indicating a need for further evaluation.	Changes in cognition or physical status may result in a need to change the established plan of care for preventing aspiration.
Teach recommended feeding techniques and meal preparation.	Texture of food, temperature of food, timing of the swallow, and swallowing techniques help compensate for deficits resulting in dysphagia and aspiration risk.

INTERVENTIONS	**R**ATIONALE
Teach signs and symptoms of aspiration, including a cough, wheezing, hoarseness, gurgling speech, or dyspnea.	Individuals differ regarding the severity of aspiration and response to it. The signs of aspiration vary depending on these individual differences, as well as the amount and nature of the material aspirated. It is important to monitor for signs of aspiration to determine effectiveness of the plan of care for preventing aspiration and to determine need for further evaluation.
Teach suctioning techniques.	Keeping the airway free of secretions decreases risk of aspiration. Impaired swallowing results in an inability to handle oral secretions. Accumulation of material in the oral cavity and upper airway can be aspirated.
Teach emergency procedures in the event of aspiration.	Resources for emergency transportation and care need to be established to provide timely follow-up in the event of respiratory distress from aspiration. Severe aspiration can result in asphyxiation.

REFERENCES/BIBLIOGRAPHY

Alltop, S.A. (1988). Teaching for discharge: Gastrostomy tubes. **RN, 11,** 42–46.

*Ciocon, J.O., Silverstone, F.A., Graver, L.M., & Foley, C.J. (1988). Tube feedings in elderly patients: Indications, benefits, and complications. **Archives of Internal Medicine, 148,** 429–433.

Cogen, R., & Weinryb, J. (1989). Tube feeding: Providing the most nutrition with the least discomfort. **Postgraduate Medicine, 85**(5), 355–360.

Dodds, W.J. (1989). The physiology of swallowing. **Dysphagia, 3,** 171–178.

Donahue, P.A. (1990). When it's hard to swallow: Feeding techniques for dysphagia management. **Journal of Gerontological Nursing, 16**(4), 8–9.

*Elpern, E.H., Jacobs, E.R., & Bone, R.C. (1987). Incidence of aspiration in tracheally intubated adults. **Heart and Lung, 16**(5), 527–531.

George, M.R. (1988). Neuromuscular respiratory failure: What the nurse knows may make the difference. **Journal of Neuroscience Nursing, 20**(2), 110–117.

Hoffman, L.A. (1987). Ineffective airway clearance related to neuromuscular dysfunction. **Nursing Clinics of North America, 22**(1), 151–166.

Irwin, M.M., & Openbrier, D.R. (1985). Feeding ventilated patients–safely. **American Journal of Nursing, 85**(5), 544–546.

Kim, M.J., & Larson, J.L. (1987). Ineffective airway clearance and ineffective breathing patterns: Theoretical and research base for nursing diagnosis. **Nursing Clinics of North America, 22**(1), 125–134.

Logemann, J.A. (1990). Factors affecting ability to resume oral nutrition in the oropharyngeal dysphagic individual. **Dysphagia, 4,** 202–208.

McKay, S., & Mahan, C. (1988). How can aspiration of vomitus in obstetrics best be prevented? **Birth, 15**(4), 222–229.

McGee, L. (1987). Feeding gastrostomy: Part 1. Indications and complications. **Journal of Enterostomal Therapy, 14,** 73–8.

McGee, L. (1987). Feeding gastrostomy: Part 2. Nursing care. **Journal of Enterostomal Therapy, 14,** 201–211.

* Metheny, N.A., Eisenberg, P., & Spies, M. (1986). Aspiration pneumonia in patients fed through nasoenteral tubes. **Heart and Lung, 15**(3), 256–261.

North American Nursing Diagnosis Association. (1990). **Taxonomy I** (Rev. 1990). St. Louis: Author.

Pritchard, V. (1988). Tube feeding-related pneumonias. **Journal of Gerontological Nursing, 14**(7), 32–36.

Terry, P. B., & Fuller, S.D. (1989). Pulmonary consequences of aspiration. **Dysphagia, 3,** 179–183.

Bathing/Hygiene Deficit

A state in which an individual experiences an impaired ability to perform or complete bathing/hygiene activities for oneself (NANDA, 1990, p. 83).

Rosemary J. McKeighen, R.N., Ph.D., F.A.A.N
Carol Dickel, R.N.
Suellyn Ellerbe, R.N., M.N.
Peg. A. Mehmert, R.N., C., M.S.N.
Dianne C. Kolb, R.N., B.A.

DEFINING CHARACTERISTICS

Inability to obtain/access water source
Inability to perceive need for personal
  hygienic measures

Inability to regulate water temperature
  or flow
Inability to wash body or body parts

CONTRIBUTING FACTORS

Pathophysiological

Activity intolerance
Decreased strength and endurance
Discomfort
Mobility impairment

Musculoskeletal impairment
Neuromuscular impairment
Pain

Psychosociobehavioral

Agitation
Anxiety, severe

Depression
Perceptual or cognitive impairment

EXPECTED OUTCOMES

Client will achieve optimum functional level in bathing/hygiene activities in a safe and effective
  manner with skin clean and integrity intact.
    Maximum level of independence in performing total bathing/hygiene activities is
      demonstrated.

75

Maximum level of independence in performing partial bathing/hygiene activities is demonstrated.

Acceptance of limitations in performing bathing/hygiene activities is stated.

Correct use of adaptive device(s) is demonstrated—specify device(s).

Knowledge of altered lifestyle/functional ability is communicated.

INTERVENTIONS	**R**ATIONALE
Universal	
Assess functional ability for independence in bathing/hygiene activities.	Acute or chronic health problems increase the opportunity for decreased functional ability in performing activities of daily living.
Assess significant other's perception of client's limitations in self-care ability.	Knowledge of and accuracy in perception of functional level enhances acceptance of status and participation as care provider.
Establish maximum potential for independence in performing bathing/hygiene activities.	The alleviation of current health problem may restore level of functional ability.
Monitor and document progress in attaining maximum level of functional ability in bathing/hygiene.	Documentation provides a measurement level for evaluation of achievement of expected outcome(s) and legal records of results of nursing intervention.
Involve client/significant others in setting goals and plan to achieve maximum level of independent functioning and expected outcome(s).	Mutual planning between nurse and client enhances motivation for achievement of outcomes.
Establish a schedule for bathing/hygiene activities with client that is congruent with their personal needs and preferences.	Collaboration respects the ethical principle of autonomy, increases client's self-control, thus decreasing feelings of powerlessness.
Promote expression of feelings regarding limitations in self-care ability.	Expression of true feelings allows opportunity for nonjudgmental listening/dialogue, and the opportunity to receive input may enhance self-image and self-esteem.

INTERVENTIONS	RATIONALE
Provide assistive/adaptive device(s) and monitor appropriateness of use.	Devices may be used to enhance independence in mobility to achieve self-care, provide safety, and/or enhance manual dexterity in performance of bathing/hygiene.
Provide positive verbal reinforcement for advancement in performance of bathing/hygiene activities.	Self-esteem, self-confidence, and motivation towards achievement of maximum level of independence are reinforced.
Schedule bathing/hygiene activities following periods of rest.	Excessive physical and mental fatigue related to activity intolerance are inhibited.
Provide partial or total assistance with bathing/hygiene activities in a private environment.	Personal needs for comfort and cleanliness are met, as well as need for maintaining skin cleanliness and integrity, and cleanliness of oral cavity. The right to individual privacy is respected.
Instruct on: • Use of adaptive device(s) • Use of energy conservation techniques • Use of analgesic for comfort during bathing/hygiene activity • Necessity of maintaining body hygiene • Methods to modify environment	Correct use of devices promotes functional independence. Use of techniques reserves strength and endurance throughout period of activity. Analgesia decreases activity-induced pain/discomfort, which enhances functional ability. Hygiene preserves integrity of skin and enhances social acceptance. Minor environmental changes may promote maximum independence and safety.

Inpatient

Medicate with analgesic 15–30 min before initiating bathing/hygiene activities when indicated for pain associated with activity.	Analgesia decreases activity induced pain/discomfort and enhances functional ability.

INTERVENTIONS	**R**ATIONALE
Community Health/ Home Care	
Assess environment for safety and/or risk factors and necessity for adaptive/assistive devices.	Reduction/elimination of environmental hazards diminishes risk of injury.
Instruct on methods for reducing environmental hazards that are within the client's socio-economic means.	Education promotes safety using available material and economic resources.
Instruct on signs and symptoms of deteriorating functional ability and when to seek medical intervention.	Knowledge prevents exacerbation of preexisting chronic disease process and increased dependence.

REFERENCES/BIBLIOGRAPHY

See bibliography for "Feeding Deficit," Care Planning Guide, pp. 231–235.

Body Image Disturbance

A state in which an individual perceives an alteration in the mental picture of his or her physical self.

Jan A. Sheldon, R.N., M.S., C.R.R.N.
Mary A. Gollinger, R.N., M.S., C.R.R.N.

DEFINING CHARACTERISTICS

Change in social involvement
Change in spatial relationship of body
  to environment
Change in structure or function of
  a body part
Expression of feelings of powerlessness,
  helplessness or hopelessness

Expression of negative feelings about
  body
Fear of rejection
Ignores body part
Over exposes a body part
Trauma to a nonfunctioning body part
Verbalization of change in life-style

CONTRIBUTING FACTORS

Pathophysiological

Amputation of body part
Cerebral event altering perception of
  the body
Change in body structure due to surgery
Colostomy

Congenital deformity
Morbid obesity
Trauma to a body part, altering its
  structure or function
Urinary diversion

Psychosociobehavioral

Body scheme/perceptual disorders
Change in life-style
Demonstration of feelings of helplessness
Demonstration of feelings of hopelessness
Demonstration of feelings of powerlessness
Demonstration of feelings of worthlessness

Disruption of life routines due to actual/
  perceived impairment of
  body part
Dysfunctional grieving
Expressions of intense guilt
Impaired adjustment

79

Ineffective coping
Loss of job
Loss of significant other
Severe psychological event,
         e.g., suicide attempt

Social isolation
Stress disorder
Violent traumatic event, e.g., rape or
         murder of a significant other

EXPECTED OUTCOMES

Client will acknowledge changes in body and express feelings of self-worth reflecting a positive
         body image.
    Interest in caring for altered body part is demonstrated.
    A plan of care to meet physical needs of altered body part is developed.

INTERVENTIONS   RATIONALE

Interventions	Rationale
Universal	
Ascertain cause(s) of the body image disturbance.	Focusing the interventions on the nature and presentation of the body image disturbance enhances the opportunity to respond to teaching and coping mechanisms directly focused on the presentation of the altered body image.
Monitor for changes in perception of self (i.e., increased or decreased negative or positive verbalizations or actions related to the body image disturbance).	Subtle changes in thoughts, feelings, or actions toward the body part indicate the direction in which adaptation is moving.
Refer to appropriate discipline as needed (psychologist or psychiatrist, social worker, dietitian, pastoral care, MD).	The cause of the body image disturbance may require more intervention than nursing alone can provide. The interdisciplinary team approach provides professionals from varied backgrounds the opportunity to intervene based on areas of expertise. All disciplines focus on the same goal, but from different perspectives.
Establish an interdisciplinary approach to intervening based on the cause of the body image disturbance.	Communication among the interdisciplinary team is crucial to having a systematic approach to res-olve the body image disturbance. The interdisciplinary team approach works best when all team members are committed to sharing information that enhances care.

INTERVENTIONS	RATIONALE
Encourage verbalization of feelings about the loss of structure or function of the body part.	Establishing the meaning of the loss leads to focusing energy toward coping.
Involve significant others in treatment and care.	One's perception of oneself affects relationships and interactions with others; treatment and care offered to the client need to be offered to the significant others.
Teach to improve function and awareness of altered body part.	Overall feelings of self-worth are enhanced by improving function and awareness of body parts.
Inpatient Assess specific causes and presence of contributing factors of body image disturbance.	In order to develop an adequate treatment plan, the cause of the body image disturbance must be clearly defined. Focusing the treatment plan on the cause of the body image disturbance enhances the opportunity for teaching the necessary physical care and coping skills.
Monitor verbal and nonverbal indications of the meaning of the loss of structure or function.	Subjective and objective observations are necessary to assess the changing body image.
Set up client's room with teaching aids and personal care items to encourage use of affected body part.	An environment that directs attention to an altered body part aids in attending to the part.
Encourage use and conversation about altered body part in daily contacts.	Open discussion and acceptance enhance the acceptance of oneself again.
Protect altered body part from injury.	Disassociation of the body part predisposes it to injury.
Refer to other inpatient support services (psychology, pastoral care, social worker, dietitian) to establish an organized treatment plan to decrease disruption of body image.	A team approach provides consistency and assures a greater potential for a positive outcome.

INTERVENTIONS	RATIONALE
Emphasize remaining capabilities and strengths.	Acknowledging remaining capabilities promotes a positive self-image and facilitates seeing oneself as a whole being.
Reinforce any attempts to attend to body part.	Acknowledging attempts to care for the altered body part indicates beginning attempts to deal with the loss.
Reinforce any verbalization of feelings regarding actual or perceived loss.	Acknowledging thoughts and feelings enables the client to move through the grieving process.
Teach self management of affected body part (i.e., stump care, dressing changes).	Involvement in the self care of the altered body part enables adaptation to actual or perceived changes in structure or function and empowers self management of that care.
Teach significant others appropriate physical care techniques as a backup to client-managed care.	Significant others begin to view the client's capabilities in self care and support the client through adaptation.
Teach safety techniques to protect the altered body part (i.e., wheelchair safety, transfers, skin care, changes in response to environmental stimuli like heat and cold).	The impaired body part is predisposed to injury and additional complications resulting from further insult.

Community Health/ Home Care

Assess current coping strategies and adjustment process.	It is essential to continue to support the client by accurately assessing adaptation skills used in the past and present. Building on past and present coping successes enables movement toward adaptation.
Assess self care and management of the altered body part.	The reinforcement of learned skills is dependent upon the knowledge base. A return demonstration is helpful to assess techniques (i.e., dressing changes, stump care, dietary management, or stoma care).
Adapt inpatient treatment plan for home care.	Management in the home environment is based on the availability of supplies (i.e., a supplier or financial means to obtain supplies).

INTERVENTIONS	RATIONALE
Identify and refer to peer support groups (i.e., amputation groups, cancer groups, multiple sclerosis groups, ostomy groups, Overeaters Anonymous).	Support groups facilitate adaptation by decreasing the sense of aloneness.
Arrange home environment so that the client will be safe (i.e., rearrange furniture so home is accessible; rearrange cupboards so client can reach things; place night lights so client can see; eliminate throw rugs).	Injury prevention reduces the chance of complications or further deformity or disability.
Encourage involvement in social activities that reinforce perception of self as a whole.	Successful reintegration is contingent upon a sense of self as a whole and as a valued member of the community.
Reinforce teaching done in inpatient setting. 1. Dressing changes 2. Stump care 3. Ostomy Care 4. Techniques to augment self-esteem and to perceive self as whole 5. Meal planning and preparation	Building on previously learned behaviors and care enhances the self-esteem and creates an environment conducive to further learning.

REFERENCES/BIBLIOGRAPHY

Bern-Sira, Z. (1986). Disability stress and readjustment: The function of the professional's latest goals and effective behavior in rehabilitation. **Social Science Medicine, 23**(1), 43.

Craven, R., & Sharp, B. (1972). The effects of illness in family functions. **Nursing Forum, 11**(2), 186.

Dell Orto, A. (1984). Coping with the enormity of illness and disability. **Rehabilitation Literature, 43**, 7, Jan./Feb.

Dittmar, S. (1989). **Rehabilitation nursing process and application** (1st ed.). St. Louis: Mosby.

Goldiamond, B. (1981). Resocialization. In N. Martin, N.B. Holt, & D. Hicks. (Eds.). **Comprehensive rehabilitation nursing.** New York: McGraw–Hill.

North American Nursing Diagnosis Association. (1990). **Taxonomy I** (Rev. 1990). St. Louis: NANDA.

Body Temperature, Altered: Risk

A state in which an individual is at risk for failure to maintain core body temperature within normal range. Normal adult temperatures range from 36.7°C to 37.1°C (± .2°C) (97.3°F–98.8°F).

Sharon Summers, R.N., Ph.D.

RISK FACTORS

Advanced age
Burn injuries
Consumption of excess alcohol
Compromised immune system
Dehydration
Extreme activity or inactivity
Extremely overweight or underweight
Gain in heat by altered evaporation; high humidity and high temperature
Gain in heat by conduction; from skin in direct contact with warmer surfaces
Gain in heat by convection; from warm air currents moving across skin
Gain in heat by radiation; infrared radiation of heat from hot surroundings to the client

Impending surgery, head injuries, disease, or illness affecting the temperature regulation center
Loss of heat by conduction; from direct contact of the skin to cold surfaces
Loss of heat by convection; when wind currents move across the skin
Loss of heat by radiation; infrared radiation of heat from the warm, inappropriately clothed client to cold surroundings
Medications affecting temperature regulation
Susceptibility to heatstroke
Susceptibility to malignant hyperthermia

EXPECTED OUTCOMES

Client will maintain normal body temperature ranging from an early morning low of 36.7°C to 37.1°C (± .2°C) (97.3°–98.8°F) at peak diurnal metabolic periods.
Normal metabolism is maintained.
Normal cardiac rhythm is maintained.
Thermal comfort is maintained.

INTERVENTIONS	**R**ATIONALE
Universal Assess body temperature.	Body temperatures above or below normal values increase risk for altered body temperature. Core temperature measurement with tympanic thermistor thermometers, or by oral or rectal temperatures using electronic thermometers, is preferred rather than axillary temperature measurement.
Assess for infection.	Risk for altered body temperature may result from altered immune status. Determining underlying cause can expedite resolution.
Assess environmental conditions.	Extremes in either hot or cold weather increase the risk for heat gain or loss by conduction, convection, radiation, or evaporation.
Assess age level.	The elderly are at increased risk for altered body temperature related to aging process of thermoregulation center.
Assess level of physical activity.	Extreme physical activity in hot weather increases risk for altered body temperature related to inability to dissipate body heat to the environment. Extreme physical inactivity in cold weather increases risk for altered body temperature related to conductive heat loss from the body to the cold environment.
Assess clothing adequacy.	Inappropriate clothing in either hot or cold weather increases risk for altered body temperature. Wearing apparel needs to be appropriate for climatic conditions to prevent over/under exposure.
Assess alcohol, fluid, or medication intake.	Consumption of alcohol in cold weather will cause vasoconstriction followed by vasodilatation and increase risk for altered body temperature. Dehydration increases risk for increasing body temperature related to decreased fluid available for sweat production and insensible water loss. Medications, such as vasodilators, combined with exposure to cold increase risk for altered body temperature.

INTERVENTIONS	RATIONALE
Assess nutritional status.	Inadequate nutrition and loss of insulating fat contribute to decreased body temperature. Obesity, with its resultant increase in body fat, inhibits heat dissipation.
Assess medication regimen.	Vasodilators, barbiturates, or phenothiazines increase risk for altered body temperature from increased heat loss or gain by conduction from dilated vessels to the hot or cold environment.
Assess activity level.	Overactivity in hot weather decreases the temperature gradient from the client to the environment and increases risk for altered body temperature. Inactivity in cold weather increases risk for altered body temperature by conduction of heat from the client to the cold environment.
Measure body weight.	Extremes in body weight (both high and low) contribute to risk for altered body temperature: The underweight client has less body fat to insulate from the cold and less muscle mass for effective shivering; the overweight client has more body fat, which inhibits heat dissipation.
Inpatient	None
Community Health/ Home Care Assess housing and home maintenance.	Housing that provides inadequate protection from environmental extremes of hot and cold increases risk for altered body temperature. The homeless are subjected to extremes in temperature and are at risk for altered body temperature.
Assess financial needs.	Inadequate funds may contribute to factors leading to risk for altered body temperature.
Assess safety needs.	Fear for personal safety and security may prevent opening windows to improve ventilation in hot weather.

INTERVENTIONS	**R**ATIONALE
Evaluate mental status.	Senility/dementia distorts decision-making processes regarding clothing or housing needs appropriate for environmental temperatures.
Refer to social agencies as needed.	Referral to social agencies for weatherization, food, clothing, and appliances may be needed to prevent alterations in body temperature.

REFERENCES/BIBLIOGRAPHY

Carpenito, L.J. (1989). **Nursing diagnosis application to clinical practice.** Philadelphia: Lippincott.

Ganong, W.F. (1989). **Review of medical physiology.** Norwalk, CT: Appleton & Lange.

McFarland, G.K., & McFarlane, E.A. (1989). **Nursing diagnosis & intervention.** St. Louis: Mosby.

North American Nursing Diagnosis Association. (1990). **Taxonomy I** (Rev. 1990). St. Louis: NANDA.

Bowel Incontinence

A state in which an individual experiences a change in normal bowel habits characterized by involuntary passage of stool (NANDA, 1990, p. 23).

Kathleen Fitzgerald, R.N., M.S., C.E.T.N.

DEFINING CHARACTERISTICS

Involuntary passage of stool.

CONTRIBUTING FACTORS

Pathophysiological

Disorders of the anus and rectum:
>   Inflammation of the rectum due to inflammatory bowel disease, radiation proctitis, or severe chronic diarrhea related to AIDS
>   Ischemia
>   Rectal prolapse
>   Fistulae
>   Infection, e.g., herpes
>   Anorectal trauma, e.g., injury, previous surgery, childbirth, or sphincterotomy

Neurological disorders:
>   Central nervous system disorders including dementia, mental retardation, stroke, brain tumors, spinal cord injuries or tumors, multiple sclerosis, tabes dorsalis, sedative drug effect
>   Peripheral nerve disorders including diabetes mellitus, nerve injury from childbirth, pelvic fractures, prolonged straining at defecation, ideopathic incontinence
>   Altered rectal sensation due to fecal impaction

Psychosociobehavioral

Confusion
Physical barriers or disabilities that prevent access to acceptable toileting facilities
Psychological barriers that prevent access to acceptable toileting facilities
Sudden change in surroundings—especially for the elderly, confused, or demented

EXPECTED OUTCOMES

Client will follow treatment plan (bowel program, use of assistive devices, biofeedback, surgery) as recommended.
An understanding of the underlying cause or contributing factors for incontinence is verbalized.
Episodes of incontinence are decreased in number.
Perianal or more extensive skin breakdown is prevented.

INTERVENTIONS / RATIONALE

INTERVENTIONS	RATIONALE
Universal	
Elicit a description of the pattern of bowel incontinence and the presence of contributing factors.	A detailed history assists in determining the cause of bowel incontinence.
Inspect the perianal area and surrounding skin (buttocks, inner thighs) for presence of fistulae, skin breakdown, or infection.	Perianal fistula or infection may be a cause of incontinence (radiation proctitis, AIDS diarrhea, inflammatory bowel disease). Skin breakdown occurs frequently when there is incontinence to liquid stool.
Assess for possible fecal impaction by performing a digital rectal examination which would reveal hard, formed stool.	Advanced age; immobility; medications, e.g., as opiate pain relievers and iron supplements; and central nervous system disorders, particularly spinal cord injuries; may cause decreased bowel mobility, constipation, and fecal impaction. Liquid stool then leaks around the impaction.
Administer softening enemas, e.g., mineral oil; or extract the hard stool manually.	Mineral oil acts on the surface of the hard stool, softening it for easier removal. Soap-suds enemas may be used with caution as the soap may irritate the colonic mucosa causing colitis. In severe constipation, the entire colon may require evacuation. Physiological solutions, e.g., normal saline may be administered as enemas until all the stool in the colon is removed. Once this is accomplished, a bowel program can be established.

INTERVENTIONS	**R**ATIONALE
Develop a bowel program specific to the cause, functional capacity, and environment using a combination of medications, diet, and activity.	A bowel program for an active paraplegic will be different than one designed for an elderly resident of a nursing home. Basic diet recommendations include fiber and adequate fluid intake. Medications may include stool softeners, suppositories, or enemas. Determination of the usual time for defecation and planning consistent toileting at that time will aid in establishing a routine.
Discuss strategies and products to control symptoms.	Practical explanations and suggestions are beneficial to assist the adult in managing a chronic and embarrassing problem.
Provide emotional support, and preserve dignity, while assisting through the diagnostic and treatment phase.	Many elderly have some degree of bowel incontinence and may become socially isolated or withdrawn because of embarrassment. Because of difficulty discussing symptoms, treatment may be delayed and information regarding assistive products may not be obtained.
Provide information regarding the diagnostic testing procedures which may be required if the cause is not readily determined from the history and physical examination. Test may include lower gastrointestinal barium studies; sigmoidoscopy, colonoscopy; or anal, balloon manometry; and electromyography.	Providing both descriptive and sensory information—what will be seen, felt, and heard during the procedures—will help decrease anxiety and promote relaxation during the tests.
Provide information on the cause and proposed treatment plan.	In some cases, the treatment may include biofeedback or corrective surgery. Biofeedback has been successful when the client has some sensation of rectal distention, ability to contract the external anal sphincter voluntarily, and ability to follow detailed instructions.

INTERVENTIONS	RATIONALE
Provide a resource list of incontinence products, suppliers, and services available in the area.	Most hospital supply stores and pharmacies carry a wide variety of products including adult diapers, padded briefs, skin-care products, linen protectors, and underpads. HIP, Inc., an organization established to assist people with urinary incontinence, publishes a resource and product guide that contains information relevant for bowel incontinence (see References/Bibliography).
Inpatient Assess new onset incontinence or diarrhea for contributing factors, especially fecal impaction, antibiotic-induced diarrhea, Candida or Clostridium difficile infection, tube feeding intolerance, or other medication changes.	Severe diarrhea may be the cause of the incontinence. If the diarrhea is treated the incontinence may also improve.
Rearrange the hospital environment to provide ease in toileting.	Weakness or immobility combined with a new and strange environment may precipitate incontinence. Use of bedside commodes or nearby bedpans will assist in maintenance of control.
Apply fecal incontinence devices when liquid incontinence is frequent, large volume, and threatens skin integrity.	Large-volume liquid stool will quickly cause skin breakdown. Skin barriers and ointments may not be sufficient protection and fecal stream diversion is necessary. The fecal incontinence devices can be applied by carefully following the manufacturers' recommendations. The use of inflated Foley catheters as rectal tubes is controversial and may cause sphincter disruption.
Initiate a home health care referral for follow-up teaching and assistance in adaptation to home environment.	Products or devices may work in the hospital but do not fit in the home environment. The home care nurse can make further adjustments or recommendations.
Community Health/ Home Care	None

REFERENCES/BIBLIOGRAPHY

Alterescu, V. (1986). Theoretical foundations for an approach to fecal incontinence. **Journal of Enterostomal Therapy, 13,** 44–48.

Boulton, S.W., & Kazemi, M.J. (1984). Evaluating disposable briefs. **American Journal of Nursing, 84,** 1413–1439.

Burgio, L.D., Jones, L.T., & Engel, B.T. (1988). Studying incontinence in an urban nursing home. **Journal of Gerontological Nursing, 14,** 40–45.

Henry, M.M. (1987). Pathogenesis and management of fecal incontinence in the adult. **Gastroenterology Clinics of North America, 16,** 35–45.

Lincoln, R., & Roberts, R. (1989). Continence issues in acute care. **Nursing Clinics of North America, 24,** 741–755.

Krasner, D. (1990). Alterations in skin integrity related to continence management/incontinence: Some problems and solutions. **Ostomy/Wound Management, 28,** 62–63.

MacLeod, J.H. (1987). Management of anal incontinence by biofeedback. **Gastroenterology, 93,** 291–294.

North American Nursing Diagnosis Association. (1990). **Taxonomy I** (Rev. 1990). St. Louis: NANDA.

Peterson, M. (1988). Effective fecal collectors. **Journal of Enterostomal Therapy, 15,** 259.

Schiller, L.R. (1989). Fecal incontinence. In Sleisinger, M.H., & Fordtran, J.S. (Eds.). **Gastrointestinal disease.** Philadelphia: Saunders.

In addition to the above references, the following client educational materials are also available: HIP (HELP FOR INCONTINENT PEOPLE), P.O. Box 544, Union, SC 29379, (803) 585–8789.

Breastfeeding, Effective

A state in which a mother-infant dyad
exhibits adequate proficiency and
satisfaction with breastfeeding process
(NANDA, 1990, p. 82).

Vicki E. McClurg, R.N., M.N.
Ginna R. Wall, R.N., M.N.
Dona J. Lethbridge, R.N., Ph.D.
Mary Henrikson, R.N., C., M.N., A.R.N.P.

DEFINING CHARACTERISTICS

Adequate infant elimination patterns for age
Appropriate infant weight patterns for age
Eagerness of infant to nurse
Effective mother/infant communication patterns (infant cues, maternal interpretation and
    response)
Infant is content after feeding
Maternal verbalization of satisfaction with the breastfeeding process
Mother able to position infant at breast to promote a successful latch-on response
Regular and sustained suckling/swallowing at the breast
Signs and/or symptoms of oxytocin release (let down or milk ejection reflex, e.g., during feed-
    ing: uterine cramping, increased lochia flow, dripping from contralateral breast,
    tingling sensation in breasts, sound of infant swallowing; after feeding: noticeable
    softening of breasts)

CONTRIBUTING FACTORS

Physiological

Breastfeeding within first hour after birth
Exclusive and frequent breastfeeding until milk supply established
Infant gestational age greater than 34 weeks
Normal infant oral structure
Normal maternal breast structure

Psychosociobehavioral

Basic breastfeeding knowledge

93

Maternal confidence
Maternal determination to breastfeed
Support sources (e.g., encouraging partner, history of positive breastfeeding experiences among relatives and friends, access to support groups such as a local chapter of the La Leche League)

EXPECTED OUTCOMES

Client will maintain effective breastfeeding.
    Normal growth patterns of the infant are maintained.
    Satisfaction with breastfeeding process is verbalized.

INTERVENTIONS / RATIONALE

Universal	
Assess knowledge base regarding basic breastfeeding.	Knowledge of the psychophysiology of lactation is associated with successful breastfeeding.
Assess knowledge of prevention/treatment of common, breastfeeding problems.	Common problems can lead to early termination of breastfeeding.
Monitor breastfeeding process.	It is important to monitor positioning, latch-on and suckling patterns to detect any change in status.
Evaluate adequacy of infant intake.	Indications of adequate infant intake (eight feedings per 24 hours, feedings lasting five to ten minutes with audible swallowing, satiation after feedings, at least six wet diapers and one bowel movement per 24 hours) reassures that the breastfeeding is effective. The primary reason given for discontinuing breastfeeding is actual or perceived inadequate milk supply.
Assess support person network.	Encouragement by support persons is correlated positively with successful breastfeeding.
Give praise.	Verbally describing positive mother-infant interactions increases maternal confidence.
Reinforce and add to knowledge base regarding breastfeeding.	Knowledge of the psychophysiology of lactation is associated with successful breastfeeding.

INTERVENTIONS	RATIONALE
Provide education to support persons as needed.	A knowledgeable support person will be better able to help the breastfeeding mother.
Inpatient	
Assess breast and nipple structure.	Graspability of the nipple-areolar complex must be assessed, as flat or inverted nipples are a common cause of latch-on difficulties.
Assist with the first attachment at the breast within the first hour after birth.	Infant is most alert during the first period of reactivity. Research indicates that breastfeeding within the first hour after birth increases breast-feeding duration.
Avoid supplemental bottle feedings.	Colostrum provides all the necessary nutrients and fluids for the normal newborn in the first few days after birth. In families with a positive history for allergies, introduction of foreign proteins (cow's milk or soy formula) in the first three months may sensitize the infant. Artificial nipples require different oral motor mechanisms and may lead to a difficult transition back to the breast.
Do not provide samples of formula at discharge.	Several studies demonstrate a relationship between providing samples of formula at discharge and early termination of breastfeeding.
Avoid nipple shields.	The amount of milk the infant is able to extract from the breast is substantially reduced when a nipple shield is used.
Encourage rooming-in with breastfeeding on demand around the clock.	Rooming-in provides opportunities for mother to learn infant's cues and respond appropriately. Research indicates that mothers rest as well or better when infant is in the same room.
Teach to observe for infant's subtle hunger cues and to nurse whenever signs are apparent.	The infant nurses most readily in the quiet, alert state. Rooting, sucking, and hand-to-mouth activity are the first signs of hunger and may proceed to crying or a return to deep sleep in the newborn period. Infants who are fed in response to these early cues tend to feed more easily and more often.

INTERVENTIONS	**R**ATIONALE
Review guidelines for frequency of feedings.	Frequent breastfeeding (every two to three hours or at least eight feedings per 24 hours) increases milk supply.
Review guidelines for duration of feeding.	Duration should be determined by the infant's response (until suckling and swallowing slow down), since there is wide variation among mother/infant pairs and from feeding to feeding.
Provide anticipatory guidance about common infant behaviors.	Knowledge about infant growth spurts, temperament, sleep/wake cycles, and introduction of other foods increases confidence.
Provide anticipatory guidance about maternal concerns.	Knowledge about adequacy of milk supply, leaking, breastfeeding in public, expression and storage of breastmilk, and reproductive changes during lactation increases comfort with breastfeeding.
Community Health/ Home Care Evaluate current breastfeeding status.	New questions and concerns often arise in the first week at home with the new infant.
Provide for early and repeated contacts after discharge from the hospital.	Early and repeated postpartum breastfeeding support is effective in increasing the duration of breastfeeding.
Provide information about additional breastfeeding resources.	Knowledge of available resources increases confidence and problem-solving ability.

REFERENCES/BIBLIOGRAPHY

* Auerbach, K.G. (1990). The effect of nipple shields on maternal milk volume. **Journal of Obstetric, Gynecologic, and Neonatal Nursing, 19,** 419–427.
* Bernard-Bonnin, A., Stachtchenko, S., Girard, G., & Rousseau, E. (1989). Hospital practices and breastfeeding duration: A meta-analysis of controlled clinical trials. **Birth, 16,** 64–66.
* Frank, D.A., Wirtz, S.J., Sorenson, J.R., & Heeren, T. (1987). Commercial discharge packs and breastfeeding counseling: Effects on infant-feeding practices in a randomized trial. **Pediatrics, 80,** 845–854.
* Keefe, M.R. (1988). The impact of infant rooming-in on maternal sleep at night. **Journal of Obstetric, Gynecologic, and Neonatal Nursing, 17,** 122–126.
North American Nursing Diagnosis Association. (1990). **Taxonomy I** (Rev. 1990). St. Louis: NANDA.

Breastfeeding, Impaired

A state in which a mother, infant, or child experiences dissatisfaction or difficulty with the breastfeeding process (NANDA, 1990, p. 81).

Vicki E. McClurg, R.N., M.N.
Ginna R. Wall, R.N., M.N.
Dona J. Lethbridge, R.N., Ph.D.
Mary Henrikson, R.N., C., M.N., A.R.N.P.

DEFINING CHARACTERISTICS

Maternal

Actual or perceived inadequate milk supply

Inability to achieve latch on

No observable signs of oxytocin release (let down or milk ejection reflex, e.g., during feeding: uterine cramping, increased lochia flow, dripping from contralateral breast, tingling sensation in breasts, sound of infant swallowing; after feeding: noticeable softening of breasts)

Persistence of sore nipples beyond the first week of breastfeeding or for the duration of a feed in the first week after birth

Reluctance to put infant to breast

Unsatisfactory breastfeeding process

Infant

Arching and crying at the breast; resisting latching on

Fussiness and crying within the first hour after breastfeeding; unresponsive to other comfort measures (not associated with establishment of milk supply or growth spurts)

Insufficient opportunity for suckling at the breast

Nonsustained suckling/swallowing at the breast

Observable signs of inadequate infant intake (e.g., inadequate weight gain, inadequate elimination patterns, dehydration)

Sleepiness at the breast

CONTRIBUTING FACTORS

Pathophysiological

Maternal

Breast anomaly (e.g., inverted nipple)
Drugs
Engorgement
Fatigue

History of breastfeeding failure due to
  pathophysiological causes
Previous breast surgery
Sore nipples

Infant

Anomaly (e.g., abnormal oral structure)
Delayed initiation of breastfeeding
Illness
Inability to modulate states
  (sleep-wake cycles)

Poor sucking reflex
Prematurity
Receiving supplemental feedings with
  artificial nipple

Psychosociobehavioral

Anxiety or ambivalence
Depression
History of breastfeeding failure due to
  psychosociobehavioral causes

Knowledge deficit
Nonsupportive partner/family/health
  care provider

EXPECTED OUTCOMES

Client will achieve effective breastfeeding.
  Techniques to manage breastfeeding problems are verbalized and demonstrated.
  Infant manifests signs of adequate intake at the breast.
Client will manifest positive self-esteem in relation to the infant feeding process.
  If unable to continue exclusive breastfeeding, client learns a safe alternative method of
    infant feeding.

INTERVENTIONS	RATIONALE
Universal	
Assess for presence/absence of related factors or conditions which would preclude breast-feeding.	If underlying cause of ineffective breastfeeding is determined to be incompatible with breastfeeding, then nursing interventions will be directed toward a safe alternative method of infant feeding.
Evaluate and record the mother's ability to position, give cues, and help the infant latch on.	Correct positioning is essential for effective breastfeeding.

INTERVENTIONS	RATIONALE
Evaluate and record the infant's ability to properly grasp and compress the areola with lips, tongue, and jaw.	The infant must properly grasp and compress the areola in order to extract milk from the breast.
Evaluate and record the infant's suckling and swallowing pattern at the breast.	Audible swallowing is the most accurate indicator of breastmilk intake.
Evaluate and record signs of oxytocin release.	Oxytocin release is necessary for adequate milk ejection.
Evaluate and record infant's state at the time of feeding.	Infant's ability to modulate between states is essential for effective breastfeeding.
Assess knowledge base regarding psychophysiology of lactation and specific treatment measures for underlying problems.	Teaching should be based on the mother's current knowledge base.
Assess psychosocial factors which may contribute to ineffective breastfeeding (e.g., anxiety, goals, and values/life-style which contribute to ambivalence about breastfeeding).	Personalities, attitudes, and emotional states have measurable effects on breastfeeding success.
Promote comfort and relaxation to reduce pain and anxiety.	Milk flow can be inhibited by discomfort and tension.
Use alerting techniques (provide variety in auditory, visual, and kinesthetic stimuli such as unwrapping, placing upright, or talking to the infant) or consoling techniques as needed to bring the infant to a quiet, alert state.	The infant nurses most readily in the quiet, alert state.
Provide instruction in correct positioning.	Correct positioning is essential for effective breastfeeding.

INTERVENTIONS	RATIONALE
Enhance the flow of milk: when infant's swallowing slows down, teach mother to massage breast or burp infant and switch to other breast.	Research shows these techniques to be effective in increasing milk volume.
Discourage supplemental bottle feedings and encourage exclusive, effective breastfeeding.	Supplemental bottle feedings interfere with supply and demand regulation and are associated with early abandonment of breastfeeding.
Reinforce and add to knowledge base regarding psychophysiology of lactation and specific treatment measures for underlying problems.	Knowledge increases compliance and independence.
Provide education to support persons as needed.	Knowledgeable support people are better able to help the breastfeeding mother.
Strengthen new mother's self-esteem by acknowledging her frustration and disappointment, and supporting her decision to continue or choose an alternate plan.	Positive maternal self-esteem is necessary for optimal family adjustment and bonding.
Make appropriate referrals.	When intensive breastfeeding assistance is needed, benefit can be derived from an appropriate specialist, such as a lactation specialist, nutritionist, or physical therapist.
Help accept and learn an alternate method of infant feeding if unsuccessful in achieving effective breastfeeding.	Top priorities for nursing care are infant well-being and positive maternal self-esteem.
Inpatient	None
Community Health/ Home Care	None

REFERENCES/BIBLIOGRAPHY

North American Nursing Diagnosis Association. (1990). **Taxonomy I** (Rev. 1990). St. Louis: NANDA.

*Stutte, P.C., Bowles, B.C., & Morman, G.Y. (1988). The effects of breast massage on volume and fat content of human milk. **Genesis, 10,** 22–24.

Breathing Pattern, Impaired

A state in which an individual's inhalation and/or exhalation pattern does not enable adequate pulmonary inflation or emptying (NANDA, 1990, p. 38).

Claudia M. West, R.N., M.S.

DEFINING CHARACTERISTICS

Apnea
Asynchronous chest and abdominal motions
Biot's breathing (irregular periods of breathing at various depths and rates interrupted by periods of apnea)
Bradypnea
Cheyne-Stokes respirations (regular periods of accelerating and decelerating respirations interrupted by periods of apnea)
Decreased diaphragmatic excursion
Decreased thoracic expansion
Decreased vital capacity
Dyspnea
Hemoglobin desaturation (on arterial blood gas or oximetry)
Hypoxemia
Increased anterior-posterior chest diameter
Increased arterial carbon dioxide
Increased or decreased respiratory depth
Loud snoring
Paradoxical abdominal motion
Prolonged expiratory phase
Pursed lip breathing
Sleep apnea
Tachypnea
Use of accessory muscles

CONTRIBUTING FACTORS

Pathophysiological

Alveolar hypoventilation
Chest trauma (e.g., contusion, flail chest)
Heart disease
Impairment of the respiratory center in the medulla (related to narcotics, stroke, brain tumor, etc.)
Inappropriate mechanical ventilator settings
Morbid obesity
Neuromuscular disease (e.g., myasthenia gravis, Guillain-Barré syndrome)
Obstructive lung disease (i.e., emphysema, bronchitis, asthma, cystic fibrosis)

Pain
Protein-calorie malnutrition
Respiratory muscle fatigue
Restrictive lung disease (e.g., pneumonia,
      pulmonary fibrosis)

Sleep apnea syndrome
Vascular lung disease (e.g., pulmonary
      hypertension)

Psychosociobehavioral

Anxiety
Depression

EXPECTED OUTCOMES

Breathing pattern will improve.
      Dyspnea diminishes or disappears.
      Respiratory rate, depth, and rhythm return to normal or usual baseline.
      Accessory muscle use diminishes or disappears.
      Expiratory phase is normal or returns to baseline.
      Paradoxical or asynchronous breathing diminishes or disappears.
      Thoracic expansion increases.
      Diaphragmatic excursion increases.
      Intensity of breath sounds increases.
      Adventitious breath sounds returns to normal or baseline.
      Decreased muscle tension and anxiety is reported.
      Arterial blood gases are within normal range or usual baseline, including oxygen saturation
            on oximetry.
      Vital capacity or volume achieved with incentive spirometer is increased.
      Periods of sleep apnea and hemoglobin desaturation diminish or disappear.
      An increase in exercise tolerance and activities of daily living is reported.
      Strategies for reducing dyspnea are demonstrated.
Client will have improved nutritional status.
      Weight gain is achieved.
      Increased protein and calorie intake occur.
      Serum albumin is within normal range.
      Respiratory muscle strength and endurance increase.
      The 6- or 12-minute walking distance increases.
Weight loss will be achieved and maintained in the obese sleep apnea client.
      The relationship between weight and sleep apnea is verbalized.
      Barriers to weight loss are identified.
      The weight loss programs available in the community and those best suited to personality
            and life style are described.
      Methods of coping with the change in eating and food patterns are identified.
      Progressive weight loss is accomplished over periods of time specified by the weight loss
            program.
      Weight loss is maintained for at least one year.

Client demonstrates correct use of prescribed respiratory equipment.
>   The rationale and hazards of equipment are verbalized.
>   Proper method of disassembling, cleaning, and reassembling equipment is demonstrated.
>   Therapeutic effects are achieved (e.g., normal or baseline blood gases or oxygen saturation via oximetry, diminished or absent sleep apnea episodes, etc.).
>   Hazardous events or side effects are minimized.

INTERVENTIONS

RATIONALE

Universal

Monitor the following:

1. Respiratory rate, depth and rhythm while awake and during sleep

2. Use of accessory muscles

3. Length of expiratory phase of breathing, pursed lips breathing

4. Paradoxical abdominal motion and asynchronous chest and abdominal motions

5. Chest and abdominal wall motion during sleep

6. Presence of dyspnea at rest and with a variety of usual activities using a 0–10 rating scale (0 = no dyspnea, 10 = worst dyspnea)

7. Thoracic expansion and diaphragmatic excursion

Changes from usual breathing pattern will indicate improvement or worsening of the nursing diagnosis. Sleep apnea syndrome is characterized by apneic periods of over 20 seconds.

This will indicate changes in the work of breathing.

Changes will indicate improvement or worsening of airway resistance.

These are important indicators of respiratory muscle fatigue.

In sleep apnea syndrome there may or may not be chest and abdominal movement during apneic periods. If due to obstructive causes, there will be no airflow at the nose and mouth, though there may be chest movement.

Dyspnea is an important indicator of respiratory muscle work and may be associated with changes in arterial blood gases. Numerical rating of dyspnea will provide a sensitive and reliable index of the effects of exercise and the primary problem on these factors.

These will indicate the ability to breathe deeply and to move the diaphragm effectively. These are skills needed when using abdominal-diaphragmatic breathing.

INTERVENTIONS	**R**ATIONALE
8. Intensity of breath sounds and presence of adventitious sounds	These will indicate the quality of airflow throughout the lungs and the presence of airway obstruction.
9. Arterial blood gases or oxygen saturation (via oximetry)	These are the most important indicators of the effectiveness of the breathing pattern with rest or exercise. Nighttime oximetry is important for monitoring periods of sleep apnea and hemoglobin desaturation.
10. Vital capacity via bedside spirometer or incentive spirometer	This measurement is an important indicator of respiratory muscle function and progression of the etiology of impaired breathing pattern. An incentive spirometer is easy to use in the home or clinic setting and is useful for monitoring trends in vital capacity rather than absolute values. Serial measurements on a daily or more frequent basis are used to assess the extent and progression of respiratory muscle impairment in a variety of neuromuscular diseases (e.g., myasthenia gravis, muscular dystrophy, Guillain-Barré syndrome).
11. Use of dyspnea-reducing strategies found helpful by the client	Knowledge of these allows the nurse to reinforce their use as well as provide the nurse with a repertoire of strategies to assist other clients with dyspnea. Nursing research has found that clients use very unique strategies to manage their dyspnea that may be unfamiliar to others with the same problem.
12. Quality and amount of usual food intake, body weight, recent history of weight loss, and serum albumin	These are important indicators of nutritional status, which has an important effect on respiratory muscle mass, strength, and endurance. In addition, protein calorie malnutrition is associated with diminished respiratory drive, impaired immunity, and respiratory infection.
13. Complications of continuous positive airway pressure (CPAP) therapy in clients treated for sleep apnea, such as nasal dryness or congestion, epistaxis, and skin breakdown from improper mask fit	These problems often interfere with client acceptance of CPAP and can be treated or minimized.

Interventions	Rationale
14. Amount of exercise tolerated before dyspnea, fatigue, or significant changes in heart rate and blood pressure interfere with performance	This will provide a starting point for the implementation of a progressive exercise plan at home or in the hospital.
15. History of weight loss efforts and motivation to participate in a weight-loss program	Weight loss has been found to reduce or eliminate sleep apnea in morbidly obese persons. The nurse must assess past efforts to lose weight and current motivation before beginning to teach about the relationship between obesity and sleep apnea syndrome.
Introduce a variety of relaxation strategies and encourage their practice.	Practices such as progressive relaxation, guided imagery, meditation, or prayer may help reduce muscle tension and anxiety during acute dyspnea or as needed. Oxygen demand and respiratory muscle work, therefore, will be reduced.
Use pillows and/or elevate the head of the bed during sleeping hours.	Orthopnea is a significant problem that interferes with sleep. Keeping the head elevated allows gravity to pull the diaphragm and abdominal contents downward, providing for greater thoracic expansion.
Medicate the severely dyspneic client with narcotics or anxiolytics as prescribed and assess response.	Narcotics such as hydrocodone and morphine sulfate have been shown to relieve dyspnea by decreasing perception of respiratory muscle work, reducing ventilatory drive, and lowering anxiety. Anxiety associated with dyspnea can be treated with diazepam or other similar medications. The lowest doses possible to achieve relief should be used in order to prevent respiratory depression.
Obtain a dietitian consult to assess nutritional requirements and quality of usual intake.	Knowledge of nutritional requirements will increase the nurse's awareness of over- or undernutrition and what will be needed to meet nutritional needs.

INTERVENTIONS	RATIONALE
Encourage in the undernourished small, frequent meals high in calories and protein, such as milk shakes, peanut butter, and custard.	Small meals or snacks require less energy and oxygen demand, thus minimizing dyspnea and respiratory muscle work. Calorie- and protein-dense foods are necessary to ensure that energy and tissue maintenance requirements are met. Milk products should be avoided if they produce mucus. Gas-producing foods should be avoided since they may cause bloating and restrict breathing.
Provide hard candy before meals.	Anorexia is a common problem in dyspneic persons. A piece of hard candy will stimulate salivation, the taste buds, and peristalsis. Food will taste better and appetite will be stimulated.
Obtain physician order for a glass of wine before dinner.	Wine stimulates the appetite and will help reduce muscle tension.
Time bronchodilator medications 15 to 20 minutes before meals.	This will lower airway resistance and maximize ventilation so that there may be less dyspnea during eating.
Provide a restful and pleasant atmosphere at mealtimes, such as reducing noise, using soft music, and encouraging significant others to share the meal.	These strategies will help reduce muscle tension, anxiety and dyspnea. Mealtimes are often social in the American culture, and company while eating may enhance appetite and enjoyment of the meal.
Provide oxygen during the nighttime hours for those who have a history of desaturating during sleep such as those with sleep apnea, obesity hypoventilation, congestive heart failure, and chronic obstructive pulmonary disease.	Although daytime oxygenation is adequate for many individuals with these disorders, sleep normally causes a decrease in ventilation that may be sufficient to cause significant hemoglobin desaturation.
Teach the use of pursed-lips breathing and slow abdominal-diaphragmatic breathing during acute episodes of dyspnea.	Pursed-lips breathing during expiration slightly increases pressure in the airways, allowing them to remain open longer and resulting in more complete emptying of the lungs and improved oxygenation. If the client is able to move the

INTERVENTIONS	RATIONALE
	diaphragm, a slow deep pattern of abdominal-diaphragmatic breathing improves inspiratory volume and ventilation. This breathing pattern is also relaxing for many people and reduces anxiety.
Teach energy conservation techniques such as moving slower and grouping activities with periods of rest in between.	These strategies will reduce oxygen demand and dyspnea.
Caution the client with sleep apnea to avoid working with dangerous machinery and driving.	Hypersomnolence during the daytime is a significant problem with these individuals, because multiple periods of apnea cause frequent interruptions of their sleep. In addition, obesity hypoventilation syndrome, which is a similar disorder, causes elevated carbon dioxide levels and sleepiness. Accidents and serious injury are hazards of daytime sleepiness.
Educate the obese client with sleep apnea about the need for weight loss.	Sleep apnea results in progressive pulmonary artery hypertension, heart failure, and generalized hypoxia. It is vital that the client understand the relationship between obesity and sleep apnea, because significant weight loss will effectively treat this disorder.
Teach the client with sleep apnea about the use of continuous positive airway pressure (CPAP) mask therapy, par-ticularly how to monitor the amount of positive pressure and complications.	CPAP therapy can be applied via mask over nose or mouth. The principle behind its use is that the continuous positive pressure maintains the airways in an open position, including the soft tissues of the pharynx, which otherwise collapse during sleep and obstruct the upper airway. CPAP therapy replaces tracheostomy as the most immediate treatment of obstructive-type sleep apnea. It is important that the mask fit firmly, preventing air leak and loss of positive pressure. The amount of positive pressure is prescribed by the physician and should be checked on the pressure gauge before sleep. Common problems are nasal dryness and congestion, tissue trauma from a poorly fitting mask, and loss of positive pressure. The loss of positive pressure will result

INTERVENTIONS	RATIONALE
	in the signs of upper airway obstruction such as loud snoring, restless sleep, apnea, and daytime sleepiness.
Refer the obese sleep apnea client to a comprehensive weight loss program.	Weight loss is critical to the successful treatment of sleep apnea. A weight loss program that provides behavior modification approaches and group support will more likely increase adherence to the program and help the client maintain the weight loss.
Refer the dyspneic client to educational and/or support groups such as the local chapter of the Better Breather's Club.	Such groups assist the client in learning about the disease and developing strategies for managing symptoms. The support and companionship of the group help meet needs for affiliation and self-esteem.
Discuss with the physician referral to a local pulmonary rehabilitation program.	In addition to education and support, as mentioned previously, a pulmonary rehabilitation program provides an individualized exercise program that can improve respiratory efficiency, aerobic capacity, and functional ability in a safe environment. Another important outcome is that perception of dyspnea lessens and/or the client learns to be less frightened of dyspnea as ability to optimize function, despite it, is gained.

Inpatient

During acute episodes of dyspnea:

1. Place in a position of comfort, which is usually upright and leaning forward

2. Provide oxygen at the prescribed amount

Upright and leaning forward on bent elbows maximizes thoracic expansion and aids ventilation. Clients may experience relief from dyspnea in a variety of positions, however, and all these should be encouraged.

Significant hypoxemia may be inducing the dyspnea or worsened by the dyspnea. However, PaO_2 may be normal, since dyspnea does not always correlate with hypoxemia. Providing oxygen still may be beneficial, though, because it can relieve anxiety and tension.

INTERVENTIONS	RATIONALE
3. Remain with the client and encourage pursed lips and abdominal-diaphragmatic breathing	Dyspnea causes anxiety that may progress to panic. The nurse's presence and calmness provide reassurance that the client is not alone and helps to relieve anxiety. The breathing strategies are employed to maximize ventilation and to promote relaxation.
Provide a back rub after the acute dyspneic episode or at bedtime.	A back rub promotes further relaxation, encourages sleep, and helps build a trusting nurse-client relationship.
Teach a family member or friend to assist the client through episodes of dyspnea.	Involvement of family or friends will provide the support and consistency in managing dyspnea after discharge.
Instruct in the correct use and hazards of oxygen therapy.	Accurate use will optimize therapeutic effects of oxygen and prevent hazards such as hypoventilation, carbon dioxide accumulation, and fire.
Teach the correct use of negative or positive pressure ventilation and allow a period of several days before discharge to practice using the equipment.	Occasionally periods of respiratory muscle rest may be prescribed for use in the home, using one of several options for ventilating the client intermittently or through the night. The cuirass, which generates negative pressure over the chest, or a portable positive-pressure ventilator are commonly used in such situations. In order to maximize learning and adjustment, the client should become familiar with the equipment and its care in a safe environment with reinforcement and correction provided.
Provide referral to social services and appropriate community agencies, such as public health nursing, home health care, and respiratory care.	These services are important to assess resources and provide follow-up in the home setting, particularly for those needing specialized respiratory equipment or complex care.

INTERVENTIONS	**R**ATIONALE
Community Health/ Home Care	
Assess performance of the six- or 12-minute distance as follows: Walk at client's usual pace with accompanying 0_2 (if prescribed). Walk on level surface. Walk as long as possible before dyspnea forces client to stop. Note that time.	Walking with client provides information about exercise tolerance before dyspnea or fatigue interference and can be used to assess response to therapy. The degree of dyspnea can be assessed during and at termination of the walk with a numerical rating scale. Improvement in exercise tolerance is measured by an increase in the distance achieved before dyspnea becomes debilitating or by a decreased level of dyspnea for a certain distance.
Assess correct use and cleaning of respiratory therapy equipment such as nebulizers, oxygen delivery system, ventilators, cuirass, and CPAP system.	Correct use enhances therapeutic benefit and reduces the hazards of the equipment. Proper cleaning (see care planning guide for Airway Clearance, Impaired) prevents transmission of microorganisms and respiratory infections.

REFERENCES/BIBLIOGRAPHY

Donahoe, M., & Rogers, R.M. (1990). Nutritional assessment and support in chronic obstructive pulmonary disease. **Clinics in Chest Medicine, 11**(3), 487–504.

Finkelstein, S.M., Kujawa, S.J., Budd, J.R., & Warwick, W.J. (1987). An evaluation of incentive spirometers for following pulmonary function by self-measurement in the home. **IEEE Transactions on Biomedical Engineering, 34**(3), 212–216.

Foote, M., Sexton, D.L., & Pawlik, L. (1986). Dyspnea: A distressing sensation in lung cancer. **Oncology Nursing Forum, 13**(5), 25–31.

Hopp, L.J., & Williams, M. (1987). Ineffective breathing pattern related to decreased lung expansion. **Nursing Clinics of North America, 22**(1), 193–205.

Kersten, L.D. (1989). **Comprehensive respiratory nursing.** Philadelphia: Saunders.

Kim, M.J., & Larson, J.L. (1987). Ineffective airway clearance and ineffective breathing patterns: Theoretical and research base for nursing diagnosis. **Nursing Clinics of North America, 22**(1), 125–134.

* Kohlman-Carrieri, V., & Janson-Bjerklie, S. (1986). Strategies patients use to manage the sensation of dyspnea. **Western Journal of Nursing Research, 8**(3), 284–305.

Lareau, S., & Larson, J.L. (1987). Ineffective breathing pattern related to airflow limitation. **Nursing Clinics of North America, 22**(1), 179–191.

Larson, J.L., & Kim, M.J. (1987). Ineffective breathing pattern related to respiratory muscle fatigue. **Nursing Clinics of North America, 22**(1), 207–223.

Martin, L. (1989). Obstructive sleep apnea: Preventing complications. **Dimensions of Critical Care Nursing, 8**(2), 83–91.

* Montgomery-Hunter, S., & Strinden-Hall, S. (1989). The effect of an educational support program on dyspnea and the emotional status of COPD clients. **Rehabilitation Nursing, 14**(4), 200–202.

North American Nursing Diagnosis Association. (1990). **Taxonomy I** (Rev. 1990). St. Louis: NANDA.

Nino-Murcia, G., McCann-Crowe, C., Bliwise, D.L., Guilleminault, C., & Dement, W.C. (1989). Compliance and side effects in sleep apnea patients treated with nasal continuous positive airway pressure. **The Western Journal of Medicine, 150**(2), 165–169.

Openbrier, D.R., & Covey, M. (1987). Ineffective breathing pattern related to malnutrition. **Nursing Clinics of North America, 22**(1), 225–247.

Shapiro, B.A., Kacmarek, R.M., Cane, R.D., Peruzzi, W.T., & Hauptman, D. (1991). **Clinical application of respiratory care** (4th ed.). St. Louis: Mosby.

Suratt, P.M., McTier, R.F., Findley, L.J., Pohl, S.L., & Wilhoit, S.C. (1987). Changes in breathing and the pharynx after weight loss in obstructive sleep apnea. **Chest, 92**(4), 631–637.

Tiep, B.L., Burns, M., Kao, D., Madison, R., & Herrera, J. (1986). Pursed lips breathing training using ear oximetry. **Chest, 90**(2), 218–221.

Zerwekh, J.V. (1987, November). Comforting the dying dyspneic patient. **Nursing '87**, 66–69.

Cardiac Output, Altered

A state in which the blood pumped by an individual's heart is sufficiently reduced that it is inadequate to meet the needs of the body's tissues (NANDA, 1990, p. 35).

Colleen Creamer-Bauer, R.N., M.S., C.C.R.N.

DEFINING CHARACTERISTICS

Abnormal arterial blood gases
Abnormal chest film
Abnormal electrolytes
Abnormal heart sounds S3, S4
Abnormal hemoglobin and hematocrit
Adventitious breath sounds
Angina
Arrhythmias; electrocardiographic changes
Cough
Cyanosis; pallor of skin and mucous
    membranes
Decreased activity tolerance
Decreased peripheral pulses
Dizziness
Dyspnea
Edema
Ejection fraction < 40%
Elevated cardiac enzymes
Fatigue
Jugular vein distention
Oliguria: anuria
Orthopnea
Paroxysmal nocturnal dyspnea
Rales
Shortness of breath
Syncope
Variations in blood pressure readings (low
    blood pressure, orthostatic
    hypotension)
Variation in hemodynamic readings
Weakness
Weight gain

OTHER POSSIBLE CHARACTERISTICS

Abdominal distention
Anorexia
Ascites
Change in mental status
Confusion
Decreased attention span
Diaphoresis
Fear
Feeling of anxiety
Frothy sputum
Insomnia
Left parasternal lift
Memory loss
Palpitations
Pulsus alternans
Restlessness
Stress
Subcostal pain
Vertigo

CONTRIBUTING FACTORS

Pathophysiological

MECHANICAL

Alteration in preload
> Increased—e.g., congestive heart failure, fluid overload
> Decreased—e.g., hypovolemic shock, cardiac tamponade

Alteration in afterload
> Increased in left ventricle—e.g., systemic hypertension, aortic valve disease
> Increased in right ventricle—e.g., chronic obstructive pulmonary disease, pulmonary embolism
> Decreased in both ventricles—e.g., anaphylaxis, neurogenic shock

Alteration in contractility
> Increased—e.g., hyperdynamic states
> Decreased—e.g., myocardial infarction, hypoxia, acidosis, electrolyte imbalance

ELECTRICAL

Alteration in heart rate
> Increased—e.g., sympathetic nervous system stimulation, hypoxia, hypotension
> Decreased—e.g., parasympathetic nervous system stimulation, increased intracranial pressure

Alteration in heart rhythm—e.g., atherosclerosis, medications
Alteration in conduction—e.g., dysrhythmias

STRUCTURAL

Alteration in function of cardiac structures—e.g., papillary muscle rupture, ventricular septal defect

Psychosociobehavioral

Physical, emotional, environmental stress
Poor compliance with medical treatment

EXPECTED OUTCOMES

Client will demonstrate stabilization or improvement in systemic arterial blood pressure, heart rate and rhythm, quality of peripheral pulses, breath sounds, and mental status.
> There is an absence of extra heart beats.
> Blood pressure and pulse are stable with position.
> Normal respirations of 16–20/min. are present.
> Urine output is ≥ 30cc/H.
> Palpable peripheral pulses are felt.
> Sensorium is clear.
> Neck veins are flat.
> Lungs are clear to auscultation.
> A stable dry weight is maintained.

No shortness of breath is experienced.
An adequate appetite is maintained.
Chest pain is absent.
Increasing tolerance for physical activity is demonstrated.
A specified diet, medications, activity, and limitations can be described.
New signs and symptoms and when to call the doctor are verbalized.
A decrease in anxiety and fear is experienced.

INTERVENTIONS	**R**ATIONALE
Universal	
Assess mental status.	If the cerebral perfusion decreases, there will be a change in affect and orientation. When perfusion falls below a critical level, disorientation occurs.
Assess skin integrity (color, texture, turgor, temperature).	The skin normally receives 4% to 9% of the cardiac output. In times of stress, blood flow is shunted away from non-vital organs. The skin temperature reflects cutaneous perfusion. Presence of peripheral or central cyanosis may reflect the degree of altered cardiac output. Cardiac edema is soft, pitting, maybe symmetric in dependent parts of the body. It may progress to pre-sacral and genital areas. If ascites is present, measurement of daily abdominal girth is necessary.
Assess heart sounds.	Auscultation of the heart provides a means for clinically evaluating the mechanical and hemodynamic changes of the heart. Murmurs may reflect structural damage to the heart. The third heart sound may be the first and only clinical sign of left ventricular failure. The fourth heart sound is one of the first signs of mechanical dysfunction.
Assess jugular vein distention.	Observation of the internal and external venous pulsations are used to assess circulatory blood volume, right heart function, and central venous pressure.
Assess peripheral pulses.	Examination of the arterial pulses gives information about the cardiovascular system, such as arterial wall structure, magnitude of cardiac output, state of the aortic valve, and evidence

INTERVENTIONS	RATIONALE
	of heart failure. All major pulses need to be assessed for amplitude, contour, equality, rate and rhythm.
Monitor vital signs (temperature, heart rate, blood pressure).	It is necessary to establish a baseline for comparison. Temperature may reflect a cue to an identified stress, (e.g., fever). Tachycardia indicates compensation for the failure of the left ventricle to perfuse the rest of the body with an adequate cardiac output. Hypotension indicates an increase in afterload—the amount of pressure against the aorta due to peripheral resistance.
Confirm respiratory rate.	A rapid respiratory rate (tachypnea) may be an early sign of heart failure. Cheyne-Stokes respirations are frequently seen in severe heart failure. The mechanism of Cheyne-Stokes respirations seems to be a prolongation of circulation from the lungs to the respiratory centers of the brain.
Auscultate lung sounds.	When the heart fails, pressure inside the chambers increases. This increase in pressure is transmitted to the pulmonary circulation and may cause a leak of fluid from the pulmonary vessels into the surrounding lung fields. Fluid in the alveolar spaces inhibits gas exchange and increases the work of breathing. Alveolar fluid produces audible pulmonary rales.
Evalute the presence of chest pain/pressure.	Chest pain may reflect the presence of myocardial ischemia. It represents an imbalance of the myocardial oxygen supply and demand.
Evaluate weight daily (same time, clothing, and scale).	One kilogram of body weight reflects approximately one liter of fluid. Calculating a stable, dry weight is a goal for self-care.
Evaluate usual weight, appetite and eating patterns, food preferences.	Anorexia, nutrient loss, a hypermetabolic state, and impaired delivery of cellular nutrients are four factors that may lead to cardiac cachexia. Clients are often too tired to eat and reach a premature sensation of fullness due to delayed gastric emptying and fluid overload.

INTERVENTIONS	**R**ATIONALE
Monitor medication administration.	Prescribed drugs need to be monitored for side effects (e.g., nitroglycerin, furosemide, digoxin, morphine, hydralazine.) Nitroglycerin works by ausing vasodilatation, which (1) decreases venous return and workload on the heart by causing coronary vasodilation and (2) increases myocardial oxygen supply. Diuretics reduce circulating blood volume. Digoxin improves the contractility of the heart by increasing the force and velocity of contractions. Digoxin brings more calcium into the cell, maximizing the contractile process. Digitalis also exerts a vagal effect, controlling the heart rate. Morphine works to relieve anxiety and causes transient arterial and venous dilatation. Hydralazine works as a smooth muscle relaxant and causes vasodilatation of the arterial vascular bed. This action can increase cardiac output by lowering blood pressure and systemic vascular resistance (afterload).
Monitor serum potassium and magnesium levels.	Normal potassium levels are essential to salt balance, normal osmotic pressure, and impulse conduction. Magnesium is a cofactor for the enzyme that plays a major role in the regulation of intracellular potassium concentration in the myocardium.
Measure intake and output.	Charting the fluid balance daily helps to determine the progress of cardiac and renal function. Fluid balance estimates the effectiveness of varied interventions. Renal perfusion is assessed by measuring urinary output.
Provide a therapeutic environment.	Identify internal and environmental stressors. Some stressors which could compromise the ability to cope include sensory overload; sleep deprivation; alteration in comfort, anxiety, and fear. Clients who cannot cope with the crisis of illness may have a physiologic stress response that may increase myocardial oxygen demand and threaten the heart.

INTERVENTIONS	RATIONALE
Identify coping and sleeping patterns and support or enhance imagery and calm environment p.r.n. (music, relaxation, exercise, important rituals).	Emphasis on positive behaviors enhances cooperation and promotes hope for recovery.
Position in high Fowler's in bed or sitting in a chair.	This position decreases the work of breathing and enhances gas exchange. Blood pools in the extremities, decreases preload, and decreases the workload of the heart.
Allow for periods of physical and emotional rest.	Rest decreases the body's demands for oxygen and can provide for a redistribution of blood flow to non-vital organs (e.g., kidneys). Bedrest alone can often produce a diuresis, therefore reducing congestion.
Encourage rest periods following each activity.	The higher the metabolic level of activity, the higher the increase in oxygen demand. The additive effects of two or more metabolic demands at one time will probably decrease the ability to perform.
Progress activity levels as indicated.	The ability of the heart to respond to the increased demands of the activities of life is called the cardiac reserve. The normal response to increased activity is to increase the cardiac output by increasing the heart rate and stroke volume. Clients with altered cardiac output may have a deficit in this ability. Fatigue, dyspnea, tachycardia, and exertional hypotension may be experienced.
Administer oxygen therapy.	The administration of supplemental oxygen is an intervention to restore arterial oxygen saturation to normal levels. Measure results with an SvO_2 monitor or an arterial blood gas measurement.
Provide for a dietary consult, evaluation of anthropometric assessment, and evaluation of laboratory data.	A calorie count is necessary to assist the nurse in evaluating a basal calorie requirement. Anthropometric measurements give a more accurate measure of nutrition. Evaluation of serum albumin and lymphocyte counts assess protein depletion.

INTERVENTIONS	RATIONALE
Turn frequently and provide back rubs.	Complete bedrest has its associated hazards of immobility. Frequent repositioning provides comfort and attention. Giving back rubs and massaging pressure points provide a means of inspection for edema and encourage the use of therapeutic touch. This may foster a decrease in anxiety and an increase in trust.
Teach to take pulse.	Pulse monitoring can be used as a guide to activity. It increases self-care and provides empowerment.
Advise to monitor daily weight.	A careful watch of weight pattern will identify changes and allow early intervention for retention of fluid.
Guide to adhere to dietary restrictions (fluid and sodium).	An increase in body sodium leads to retention of water and extracellular fluid volume. Sodium restrictions are common. This may require total elimination of salt in food preparation and elimination of many foods high in salt.
Instruct to report abnormal response to medications.	Prompt reporting may avoid problems with noncompliance.
Review when to call the doctor.	Role playing is essential in order to understand what to do in the case of emergency. Rehearsal may provide a decrease in anxiety and confidence in the discharge plan. Teaching what symptoms to monitor enhances self-care.
Explain progressive activity schedule and signs of over-exertion.	Reviewing activities of daily living gives a sense of control and may prevent fatigue. The risks of stress and exercise can also be reviewed.

Inpatient

Monitor the EKG for baseline data, presence of arrhythmias, and response to interventions.	Atrial kick contributes 15% to 35% of ventricular filling to stroke volume. Atrial contribution may exceed 35% in cases of cardiac deterioration. Arrhythmias can compromise cardiac output and reduce myocardial tissue perfusion.

INTERVENTIONS	RATIONALE
Provide standardized care and observation of pulmonary artery catheter and insertion site.	Assessment of cardiac function, circulating blood volume, and physiological response to treatment can be obtained.
Measure CVP, PAP, PCWP, and cardiac output and report any significant changes.	The central venous pressure, pulmonary artery diastolic, and pulmonary capillary wedge pressures, are the clinical indications of preload assessment. Systemic vascular resistance, systolic blood pressure, and diastolic blood pressure are the clinical indicators of afterload measurement. Cardiac output, cardiac index, and ejection fraction are clinical indicators of contractility.
Evaluate laboratory data as necessary. (e.g., BUN, electrolytes, ABGs.)	BUN is a measurement of renal function; electrolytes are essential in optimal cardiac conduction and function. ABGs are a measure of arterial oxygenation.
Monitor SvO_2 continuously.	Decreased oxygen saturation of mixed venous blood (SvO_2) is coming to be accepted as one of the earliest indicators of a decreased cardiac output. An SvO_2 of less than 60% is a reliable cue for imbalances in tissue oxygen supply and demand.
Provide aseptic dressing change of pulmonary artery line as ordered.	Prevention of infection from invasive monitoring needs to be maintained.
Measure and regulate IV therapy as ordered.	The goal is to maintain optimal fluid volume.
Community Health/ Home Care	None

REFERENCES/BIBLIOGRAPHY

Bumann, R., & Spetlz, M. (1989). Decreased cardiac output: A nursing diagnosis. **Dimensions of Critical Care Nursing, 8**(1), 6–15.

Burke, L., Gabriel, L., Barber, L., & Zemke, S. (1986). Nursing diagnosis, indicators and interventions in an outpatient cardiac rehabilitation program. **Heart and Lung, 15**(70), 70–76.

Carpenito, L.J. (1989). **Nursing diagnosis—Application to clinical practice.** Philadelphia: Lippincott.

* Dalton, J. (1985). A descriptive study: Defining characteristics of the nursing diagnosis cardiac output. **Image: The Journal of Nursing Scholarship, 17,** 118–117.

* Dougherty, C.M. (1985). The nursing diagnosis decreased cardiac output. **Nursing Clinics of North America, 20,** 787–799.

* Dougherty, C.M. (1986). Decreased cardiac output: Validation of nursing diagnosis. **Dimensions of Critical Care Nursing, 5,** 182–188.

Doyle, B. (1988). Nursing challenge: The patient with end stage heart failure. In Kern, L. **Cardiac critical care nursing.** Rockville, MD: Aspen, 311–332.

Field, L. (1986). Terminology issues in nursing diagnosis; focus on cardiovascular nursing. **Cardiovascular Nurse, 6,** 31–36.

Futrell, A. (1990). Decreased cardiac output: Case for a collaborative diagnosis. **Dimensions of Critical Care Nursing, 9**(4), 202–209.

Gulanick, M., et al. (1990). **Nursing care plans, nursing diagnosis and intervention.** Philadelphia: Mosby.

* Hubalik, K., & Kim, M.J. (1984). Nursing diagnoses associated with heart failure in critical care nursing. In Kim, M.J., McFarland, G.K., & McLane, A.M. (Eds.). **Classification of nursing diagnoses: Proceedings of the fifth national conference.** St. Louis: Mosby, 139–149.

* Keller, C. (1990). Cardiovascular nursing research review, 1969-1988. **Progress in Cardiovascular Nursing, 5**(1), 26–33.

Kim, M.J. (1984). Physiologic nursing diagnosis: Its role and place in nursing taxonomy. In Kim, M.J., McFarland, G.K., & McLane, A.M. (Eds.). **Classification of nursing diagnoses: Proceedings of the fifth national conference.** St. Louis: Mosby, 60–62.

Kim, M.J., et al. (1984). Clinical validation of cardiovascular nursing diagnoses. In Kim, M.J., McFarland, G.K., & McLane, A.M. (Eds.). **Classification of nursing diagnosis: Proceedings of the fifth national conference.** St. Louis: Mosby, 128–137.

Lederer, J., Marculescu, G., Mocnik, B., & Seaby, N. (1988). **Care planning pocket guide: A nursing diagnosis approach.** Menlo Park, CA: Addison-Wesley, 32–33.

McLane, A. (1987). Measurement and validation of diagnostic concepts: A decade of progress. **Heart and Lung, 16**(6), 77–83.

North American Nursing Diagnosis Association. (1990). **Taxonomy I** (Rev. 1990). St. Louis: NANDA.

Roberts, S., (1987). **Nursing diagnosis and the critically ill patient**. Norwalk, CT: Appleton-Century-Crofts.

Roberts, S., (1988). Cardiogenic shock: decreased coronary artery tissue perfusion. **Dimensions of Critical Care Nursing, 7**(4), 196–208.

Rossi, L., Haines, V. (1979). Nursing diagnoses related to acute myocardial infarction. **Cardiovascular Nurse, 3,** 11–15.

Thelan, L., Davie, J., Urden, L. (1990). **Text book of critical care nursing—Diagnosis and management**. St. Louis: Mosby.

* Wessel, S., & Kim, M.J. (1984). Nursing functions related to the nursing diagnosis, decreased cardiac output. In Kim, M.J., McFarland, G.K., & McLane, A. (Eds.). **Classification of nursing diagnoses.** St. Louis: Mosby, 192–198.

Utz, S.W., & Grass, S. (1987). Mitral valve prolapse: Self-care needs, nursing diagnoses, and interventions. **Heart and Lung, 16**(1), 77–83.

Communication, Impaired Verbal

A state in which an individual experiences a decreased or absent ability to use or understand language in human interaction (NANDA, 1990, p. 50).

Joan Harkulich, R.N., M.S.N.

DEFINING CHARACTERISTICS

Blank expression on face
Difficulty forming words or sentences
Difficulty verbalizing messages
Disorientation
Dyspnea

Slurring, stuttering speech
Turns ear toward sound
Unable to follow simple directions
Unable to speak dominant language
Withdrawal from interaction

CONTRIBUTING FACTORS

Pathophysiological

Congenital anomalies or birth defects
Decrease in circulation to the brain
Head and neck tumors
Hearing loss
Neurological disorders—e.g., Alzheimer's disease, Parkinson's disease, cerebral palsy

Physical barriers—e.g., intubation, tracheostomy, laryngectomy, wired jaw
Speech impediments

Psychosociobehavioral

Cultural differences
Inability to read or write or speak English
Inadequate or unrealistic self-concept
Lack of stimuli (social isolation)

Poor communication skills
Psychological barriers—e.g., hysteria, depression, stress
Sensory overload

EXPECTED OUTCOMES

Client will send/receive understandable messages through congruent verbal and nonverbal means.

Alternate methods of communication are learned.

Reading of facial expressions, body language, and gestures is learned.

Ability to respond by a yes/no answer is learned.

Increasing ability to express needs is demonstrated.

Understanding of need to change method of communication is demonstrated.

Communication of needs is achieved with minimal frustration.

INTERVENTIONS	RATIONALE
Universal Assess for specific type of verbal impairment: 1. Acute expressive aphasia—a sudden usually transitory inability to convey verbal messages to others, e.g., physical barrier (wired jaw, intubation) or psychotic problem 2. Chronic expressive aphasia—a long-term inability to send understandable messages, e.g., neurological disorders, congenital anomalies 3. Language barrier—inability to communicate because different languages are spoken 4. Sensory receptive aphasia—inability to receive information from the communicator, preventing the receiver from interpreting or responding appropriately, e.g., hearing loss, sensory overload, hysteria 5. Receptive neurological aphasia—inability to receive or understand communication from the sender; however, the hearing mechanism is intact, but the ability to inter-	Identification of the specific type of impairment will guide appropriate interventions.

INTERVENTIONS	RATIONALE
pret or receive a meaningful message is impaired, e.g., dementia due to Alzheimer's disease or drug/alcohol abuse, cerebral insufficiency, atherosclerosis 6. Global aphasia—massive impairments in all language modalities. e.g., massive brain damage	
Assess for signs of hearing impairment, e.g., turning head in direction of sound, turning better ear toward sound, or cupping the ear with hands.	These behaviors are indicators of a hearing loss.
Assess for evidence of inappropriate responses to messages, puzzled expressions on the face, decreased memory and attention span, confusion over words, ignoring communication, and inability to follow instructions.	These behaviors are indicators that the hearing mechanism is intact, but the ability to receive or interpret a meaningful message is impaired.

Assess the use of devices to facilitate communication, e.g.,
    Hearing aid
    Eyeglasses, contact lenses
    Voice aids
    Computer
    Typewriter
    Magic slate
    Pad/pencil
	This information will enable use of the proper equipment to facilitate communication.

Check ear canal for buildup of wax.	Cerumen impaction causes a conductive hearing loss—a frequently overlooked, reversible condition.
Treat as a mature communicating adult.	Acceptance, regardless of the level of communication, conveys respect.

INTERVENTIONS	RATIONALE
Practice active listening.	Listening with a purpose, listening to the emotions with attention, having open verbal reception, and using an appropriate response communicates that what is said is important.
Reassure that frustration and anger are acceptable and expected.	Lack of communication skills causes tremendous frustration.
Encourage opportunities for socialization.	Lack of socialization will bring on isolation, depression, and further communication barriers.
Use a natural voice, speak distinctly, and do not destroy the rhythm of speech.	These strategies are necessary to communicate important information, because messages conveyed with a smooth rhythm and natural voice are easier to understand.
Speak in a lower voice to communicate with older clients. Do not speak louder.	In the process of aging, high tones are not easily heard, but low tones continue to be heard. Loud sounds tend to distort the quality.
Use familiar words and sentences and refrain from using medical or nursing jargon.	Understanding what is being said is more easily accomplished when familiar words and expressions are used.
Phrase questions in order to receive a yes/no answer.	Soliciting a yes/no answer conserves energy and lessens confusion. It also provides an opportunity for a nonverbal response.
Elevate the head of the bed and face client in a well-lit area.	It is difficult to follow directions unless gestures and facial expressions can be seen.
Communicate while facing client's unaffected side.	Clients with unilateral neglect resulting from, e.g., a CVA, may not perceive interaction on the affected side.
Ask one simple question at a time.	Understanding one concept, dealing with it, and going on to another increases communication.
Give clear simple directions when necessary.	Basic directions are easier to grasp and comprehend.

INTERVENTIONS	RATIONALE
Allow "listening spaces" during the flow of questions and explanations.	Allowing space between sending messages encourages processing time.
Communicate only after assistive devices are in working order and in place.	Glasses are necessary to see; hearing aids must be worn and turned on to be effective; and other tools such as the Vocaid need to have fresh batteries in place and be in the "on" position.
Anticipate needs and try to meet them.	Anticipation will eliminate the need for communication to occur.
Encourage and praise all attempts at communication.	Openness to any communication effort will encourage further attempts.
Use touch to reinforce messages.	Touch (holding clients' hand, hand-over-hand contact, and squeezing hands) will communicate a feeling of well-being, increase self-esteem, and reinforce a trusting communicating relationship.
Use body movements, gestures, and facial expressions to convey messages.	Nonverbal cues augment the understanding of oral communication.
Minimize all environmental distractions.	Environmental distractions such as the sound of a radio, TV, other voices, the smell of food, or the presence of other people diminish effective communication.
Never speak for, interrupt, or treat clients who have speech difficulties—as if they were not present.	Any of these practices will decrease self-esteem and discourage communication.
Encourage to speak slowly and pace communication.	Employing energy conservation measures will aid clients with dyspnea in conveying messages.
Interpret hand gestures and eye contact.	When oriented and alert, efforts to communicate will be made in nonverbal ways.
Provide paper, pencil slate, or magic slate.	When oriented, messages can be written if tools are available.

Iɴᴛᴇʀᴠᴇɴᴛɪᴏɴs	Rᴀᴛɪᴏɴᴀʟᴇ
Supply missing word(s).	Interjecting words when needed provides notification that the conversation is being followed and understood.
Sing a message or ask the client to sing a message.	Expression of ideas may be successfully conveyed by singing, as this ability is accomplished in an alternate area of the brain from speaking.
Play word games.	Supplying a missing word, a rhyming word, or finishing an idiomatic expression can increase verbal skill and bolster self-esteem.
Write out cards with common phrases and words.	Basic information can be sent and received with a minimal amount of effort. This information is useful to a non-English speaking client as well as significant others.
Gain eye contact or touch to get attention before communicating.	When things such as hearing loss or sensory overload are the cause of the impaired communication, inattention may be due to lack of awareness.
Use sign language as appropriate.	Understanding some basic signs will aid in communication.
Use art and other expressive media.	Communication and expression of thoughts can be conveyed in alternative ways.
Use a communication board, cards, pictures of food, family, etc. when discussing various subjects.	A picture may be easier to see and comprehend, especially when pictures are black on white.
Use short, repetitive directives or questions.	Disoriented or highly anxious clients may experience more confusion if information is paraphrased or restructured when repeated.
Demonstrate desired behavior and encourage client to mimic it.	A demonstration/return demonstration provides opportunities to learn using a minimal amount of verbal communication.

INTERVENTIONS	**R**ATIONALE
Obtain referrals from other professionals (speech pathologist, physician, audiologist, or physical therapist).	These professionals may have input in regard to strategies to use.
Inpatient Observe for nonverbal indications of problems, e.g., watch eyes for evidence of an inner focus, shutting out stimuli, and presence of tears. Watch movement for signs of pain, rubbing an area, trembling hands, cold sweaty palms, facial expressions, flushed face, or biting lips.	Observation of nonverbal cues will help recognition of pain, frustration, or misunderstanding.
Listen for vocalizations such as moaning, groaning, shouting, or noise on exhalation.	The presence of things such as pain, discomfort, and anxiety may be communicated even though the message sent is incomplete.
Explain exactly what is being done in the process of giving care.	Unfamiliar and invasive procedures can be very frightening when not carefully explained.
Encourage frequent visits by family/friends.	Communication efforts can be enhanced by the assistance of significant others.
Approach when client is rested and not fatigued.	Interactions are more effective when energy levels are at their best.
Provide continuity in care giving assignments.	Consistent caregivers will encourage the development of a trust relationship, reduce frustration, and maximize communication ability.
Establish a set routine for care and furnish a schedule for the day.	Consistency in care provided and an outline of activities will eliminate the exhausting need to communicate daily basic needs.
Use an interpreter if available.	Interpretation can speed communication and lessen frustration.

INTERVENTIONS	**R**ATIONALE
Community Health/ Home Care	
Educate family members in regard to communication techniques such as breathing exercises, word games, sound exercises, and use of reinforcements and rewards.	Family members can benefit from knowledge of a variety of strategies to make communication more effective and meaningful.

REFERENCES/BIBLIOGRAPHY

Bedford, J. (1985). Bridging the communication gap. **Nursing Times. 81** (5): 22–23.

Bulechek, G.M., & McClosky, J.C. (1985). **Nursing interventions and treatment for nursing diagnosis.** Philadelphia: Saunders.

Calvani, D. (1985). How well do your clients cope with hearing loss? **Journal of Gerontological Nursing, 11** (7), 16–20.

* Christian, E., Dluhy, N., & O'Neill, R. (1989). Sounds of silence: Coping with hearing loss and loneliness. **Journal of Gerontological Nursing, 15** (11), 4–9.

Diaz-Duque, O.F. (1982). Overcoming the language barrier: Advice from an interpreter. **American Journal of Nursing, 82** (9), 1380–1382.

Gorrie, M. (1989). Reaching clients through cross cultural education. **Journal of Gerontological Nursing, 15** (10), 29–31.

Hall, G.R. (1988). Alterations in thought process. **Journal of Gerontological Nursing. 14** (3), 30–37.

Hanawalt, A., & Troutman, K. (1984). If your patient has a hearing aid. **American Journal of Nursing, 84** (7), 900–901.

Harison, M., Blumetti, P.J., & Cohen, L.S. (1985). Rehabilitation of the communicatively impaired. **Cleveland Clinic Quarterly, 52** (3), 345–349.

Harkulich, J., & Calamita, B. (1988). **A manual for caregivers of Alzheimer's disease clients in long-term care.** (2nd. ed.). Mayfield Heights, Ohio: Embassy Printing.

* Harkulich, J., Voith, A.M., & Dreikosen, S. (1987). **Communication I and communication II.** Unpublished research.

Hollinger, L.M. (1986). Communicating with the elderly. **Journal of Gerontological Nursing, 12** (3), 8–13.

Kumin, L., & Rysticken, N. (1985). Aids to bridge the communication barrier. **Geriatric Nursing, 6** (6), 348–351.

Language breakdown in persons with Alzheimer's disease. (1987). **Geriatric Care, 19** (3), 1–4.

Lusky, K. (1989). Communicating without words. **Contemporary Long-Term Care, 12** (8), 4041.

Mahoney, D.F. (1987). One simple solution to hearing impairment. **Geriatric Nursing, 8** (5), 242–245.

North American Nursing Diagnosis Association. (1990). **Taxonomy I** (Rev. 1990). St. Louis: NANDA.

Peplau, H.E. (1960). Talking with patients. **American Journal of Nursing, 60** (7), 964–966.

Reedy, D.F. (1986). The client with aphasia—The nurse's assessment of language abilities. **Topics in Clinical Nursing, 8** (1), 67–73.

* Scura, K.W. (1988). Audiological assessment program. **Journal of Gerontological Nursing, 14** (10), 19–25.

Spencer, D. (1985). When your patient can't talk. **R.N. 48** (6), 19–20.

Weber, J. (1988). **Nurse's handbook of health assessment.** Philadelphia: Lippincott.

White, J. (1988). Touching with intent: Therapeutic massage. **Holistic Nursing Practice, 2** (3), 63–67.

Conflict: Decisional (Specify)

A state in which an individual experiences uncertainty about course of action to be taken when choice among competing actions involves risk, loss, or challenge to personal life values (NANDA, 1990, p. 69).

Elizabeth Hiltunen, R.N., M.S., C.S.

DEFINING CHARACTERISTICS

Delayed decision making
Physical signs of distress or tension
(increased heart rate, increased muscle tension, restlessness, etc.)
Questioning personal values and beliefs while attempting a decision
Self-focusing (statements focus on risks to self or caring for self)

Vacillation between alternative choices
Verbalization of undesired consequences of alternative actions being considered
Verbalized feeling of distress while attempting a decision
Verbalized uncertainty about choices

CONTRIBUTING FACTORS

Pathophysiological

None

Psychosociobehavioral

Lack of experience or interference with decision making
Lack of relevant information
Multiple or divergent sources of information

Perceived threat to value system
Support system deficit
Unclear personal values/beliefs

131

EXPECTED OUTCOMES

Client will report satisfaction or peace with decisions.

Choices, alternatives, and consequences are discussed.

Plan for decision making is stated.

Choice is informed and freely made.

Decisions are congruent with personal values.

The action in the decision plan is implemented.

INTERVENTIONS	RATIONALE
Universal Evaluate perception of problem, expectations, goals, and factors contributing to difficult decision making (e.g., knowledge, decision-making experience, support system, stress level).	Baseline data help to provide information about the etiology of the problem and guide the focus of the interventions. Data provide basis for evaluation of progress toward outcomes.
Utilize a therapeutic approach in interactions: • Utilize presence	Availability, attention, communication of empathy and caring help to provide support and comfort.
• Utilize active listening	Attending, focusing on the meaning of the communication, and giving feedback which demonstrates understanding assist in clarifying values and reducing tension.
Assist with values clarification: • Review values, goals, expectations, perceived alternatives, and consequences • Utilize a clarifying response during discussions • Utilize values clarification exercises, (e.g., rank ordering personal values and outcomes, values-actions review)	Understanding and prioritizing personal values serves as a basis for making important life choices.

INTERVENTIONS	**R**ATIONALE
Implement decision therapy: • Assist to review goals and valued outcomes • Provide information regarding alternatives and outcomes (avoid too numerous or inadequate options) • Review risks and benefits of each alternative (utilize decision aids, such as balance sheet or decision tree) • Assist to identify acceptable course of action incorporating values • Provide environment to choose freely • Assist to practice implementation of choice (role play, identify resources, develop contingency plan) • Provide support when implementing decision	Effective decision making incorporates important personal values, is informed, and includes implementation of the action in the plan. Guidance through an organized problem-solving process will aid in developing decision-making skills.
Assist with stress reduction: • Review and identify successful stress-reduction techniques • Provide opportunity and support in using effective stress-reduction strategies • Teach/review preferred relaxation techniques (e.g., rhythmic breathing, relaxation training, guided imagery, exercise)	Conflict in decision making about major life events is associated with stress. Uncertainty, perceived threats, risks, and losses contribute to personal stress. Stress-reduction techniques help to cope with the feelings and physical signs of stress.
Assist with exploration for new and relevant information about alternatives, risks, benefits, and outcomes desired if contributing	Lack of information may contribute to the conflict. Providing adequate information will facilitate improved understanding and decision making.

INTERVENTIONS	RATIONALE
factor is lack of relevant information: • Provide relevant information materials (e.g., pamphlets, articles, books) • Refer to appropriate health care team professionals • Assist to re-examine new information and to incorporate into decision-making process	
Assist to improve/increase support system if contributing factor is support system deficit: • Clarify social and personal resources available • Facilitate opportunities to have contact with support people • Provide information about resources, support groups • Refer to desired resources	A support system deficit may contribute to the conflict. Social support aids in decreasing uncertainty through feedback, clarification of issues, increased information, and assistance with tasks of daily living.
Assist to utilize information that is accurate, realistic, and relevant to client goals if contributing factor is multiple or divergent sources of information: • Assist to focus on viable options and valued outcomes • Assist to evaluate discrepancies in information in relation to current knowledge • Help to limit those involved in the decision-making process to those identified as preferred	Multiple or divergent sources of information may contribute to the conflict. Assisting to maintain control over participation of others will aid in decreasing conflict by utilizing those preferred. Focusing on current, valid information related to high priority client goals will also aid in decreasing the contributing factors.

INTERVENTIONS	RATIONALE
Teach problem-solving process starting with low intensity decisions if contributing factor is lack of experience in decision making: • Focus on one decision at a time • Help to focus on daily life decisions • Allow extra time to make decisions and practice actions (e.g., role play)	Inexperience in decision making may contribute to the conflict. Guidance through less stressful problem solving will help to increase knowledge and skills for more intense or complex decision making.
Inpatient Provide therapy for decisional conflict for family or significant others in acute or urgent situations: • Evaluate roles of family or significant others in decision making (e.g., participation in client decision making as proxy decision makers) • Monitor intensity of decisional conflict • Evaluate length of time needed for decision making • Institute therapy for decisional conflict with family/significant others • Facilitate a shortened decision-making process if decision outcome is urgent • Advocate for extended decision-making time if complexity of conflict is increased (e.g., in joint decision making, or in life and death decisions)	Family or significant others may share in decision making, or be primary decision makers in acute or urgent situations, and may experience conflict. Participation in decision making may require more intensive family decision therapy. Intervention by the nurse as an advocate will facilitate and support decision making by the family or significant others.

INTERVENTIONS

RATIONALE

- Incorporate advance directives (e.g., living wills, medical durable power of attorney) in decision-making process when available. Provide follow-up care after decision making if post-decisional regret is present

Community Health/ Home Care

Provide therapy for decisional conflict for family or significant others in long-term and home care situations.

- Evaluate roles of family or significant others as care givers and in decision making
- Evaluate length of time conflict has been present and time anticipated for future resolution
- Monitor level of stress in decision makers
- Institute therapy for decisional conflict with family/significant others
- Provide social support, resources for daily tasks (respite, homemaker), and assistance with stress management
- Provide continued care after decision making if post-decisional regret is present
- Refer to counseling or psychiatrist if needed

Family or significant others may be care givers in home situations and may share in decision making or make choices about treatment and resource utilization if the client is unable. Decision making by care givers may extend for long periods of time and be intensified because of conflict in making a decision for another. Additional physical and psychosocial supports will help to decrease the burden on the care givers/decision makers.

REFERENCES/BIBLIOGRAPHY

Bujorian, G.A. (1988). Clinical trials: Patient issues in the decision-making process. **Oncology Nurses Forum, 15,** 779–783.

Carroll-Johnson, R.M. (Ed.). (1989). **Classification of nursing diagnoses: Proceedings of the eighth conference.** (pp. 447–48). Philadelphia: Lippincott.

Feigen, J. (1983). Divided loyalties. **Geriatric Nursing. 4** 298–300.

* Frank, D.I. (1990). Factors related to decisions about infertility treatment. **Journal of Obstetric, Gynecologic, and Neonatal Nursing, 19,** 162–167.

Gardner, D.L. (1985). Presence. In G.M. Bulecheck, & J.C. McCloskey, **Nursing interventions: Treatments for nursing diagnoses.** (pp. 316–324). Philadelphia: Saunders.

Geary, C.B. (1987). Nursing grand rounds: Viral cardiomyopathy. **The Journal of Cardiovascular Nursing, 2** (1), 48–52.

Helms, J. (1985). Active listening. In G.M. Bulecheck, & J.C. McCloskey, **Nursing interventions: Treatments for nursing diagnoses.** (pp. 328–337). Philadelphia: Saunders.

Hiltunen, E. (1987). Decisional conflict: A phenomenological description from the points of view of the nurse and the client. In A.M. McLane, **Classification of nursing diagnoses: Proceedings of the seventh conference.** (p. 269). St. Louis: Mosby.

Janis, I.L., & Mann, L. (1977). **Decision making: A psychological analysis of conflict, choice, and commitment**. New York: Free Press.

McNutt, B.A. (1989). Measuring patient preferences for health outcomes: A decision analytic approach. **Patient Education and Counseling, 13,** 271–279.

Minogue, J.P., & Reedy, N.J. (1988). Companioning parents in perinatal decision making. **Journal of Perinatal and Neonatal Nursing, 1** (3), 25–35.

Mishel, M.H. (1988). Uncertainty in illness. **Images: Journal of Nursing Scholarship, 20,** 225–232.

* Morris, J., & Royle, G.T. (1988). Offering patients a choice of surgery for early breast cancer: A reduction in anxiety and depression in patients and husbands. **Social Science and Medicine, 26,** 583–585.

Neal, M.C., Paquette, M., & Murch, M. (1990). **Nursing diagnosis care plans for DRGs.** (pp. 314–316). Venice, CA: General Medical Publishers.

O'Connor, A.M., & O'Brien-Pallas, L.L. (1989). Decisional conflict (specify). In G.K. McFarland, & E.A. McFarlane. (Eds.). **Nursing diagnosis and intervention.** (pp. 573–587). St. Louis: Mosby.

Pender, N.J. (1987). **Health promotion in nursing practice.** (2nd ed.). Norwalk, CT: Appleton & Lange.

Scandrett, S., & Uecker, S. (1985). Relaxation training. In G.M. Bulecheck, & J.C. McCloskey. **Nursing interventions: Treatments for nursing diagnoses.** (pp. 22–48). Philadelphia: Saunders.

Snyder, M. (1985). Progressive relaxation. In M. Snyder, **Independent nursing interventions.** (pp. 47–68). New York: Wiley.

Sodergren, K.M. (1983). Guided imagery. In M. Snyder, **Independent nursing interventions.** (pp. 103–124). New York: Wiley.

Tauer, K.M. (1983). Promoting effective decision making in sexually active adolescents. **Nursing Clinics of North America, 18** (2), 275–292.

Wilberding, J.Z. (1985). Values clarification. In G.M. Bulecheck, & J.C. McCloskey. **Nursing interventions: Treatments for nursing diagnoses.** (pp. 173–184). Philadelphia: Saunders.

* Zarit, S.H., Todd, P.A., & Zarit, J.M. (1986). Subjective burden of husbands and wives as caregivers: A longitudinal study. **Gerontologist, 26** (3), 260–266.

Zotti, M.E. (1987). Nursing intervention to assist patient's decision making with respect to family planning. **Public Health Nursing, 4** (3), 146–150.

Constipation

A state in which an individual experiences a change in normal bowel habits characterized by a decrease in frequency/passage of hard, dry, stools (NANDA, 1990, p. 19).

Kathleen Herman Scanlon, R.N., M.S.N.

DEFINING CHARACTERISTICS

Abdominal distention or bloating
Back pain
Cramping abdominal pain or discomfort
Decreased bowel sounds
Decreased frequency of defecation
Hard, formed, dry, or marble-sized stools

Headache
Interference with usual ADL's
Palpable fecal mass in rectum
Sensation of pressure in rectum
Straining during defecation
Use of laxatives, suppositories, or enemas

CONTRIBUTING FACTORS

Pathophysiological

Decreased ability to defecate due to abdominal pain as in recent surgery, or fatigue or dyspnea when attempting to defecate
Diagnostic procedures, i.e., lower or upper GI radioscopic examination
Diet changes related to hospitalization, illness, etc., which decrease intake of fruit, vegetables, fiber, or coffee
Electrolyte imbalance, i.e., hypercalcemia, hypokalemia
Inadequate fluid intake
Inadequate physical activity
Ingestion of medications which promote constipation
Mechanical problems, i.e., diverticulosis, ovarian hyperstimulation syndrome secondary to use of fertility drugs, polyps or tumors, pregnancy
Metabolic imbalance, i.e., hypothyroidism

Neuromuscular impairment
Painful perineal conditions

Psychosociobehavioral

Change in usual routine related to hospitalization, vacation, or living situation
Chronic use of stimulant laxatives, suppositories, or enemas
Dietary fiber intake < 20–25 gm of fiber daily due to insufficient finances; lack of fresh fruits,
    vegetables, and whole grains in diet; or poorly fitting dentures
Emotional disturbances which decrease or increase activity
Health beliefs
Ignoring the urge to defecate
Lack of privacy

Expected Outcomes

Client will evacuate soft, formed stool without undue straining at least every third day.
    The regular use of stimulant laxatives is avoided.
    2000–3000 cc of fluid is ingested daily.
    Aerobic exercises at a target heart rate for 20 min 3 times weekly, or physical activity
        including walking, as tolerated, is completed.

Interventions	Rationale
Universal	
Assess usual bowel pattern for frequency, size, shape, consistency, ease of passage, and color of stools.	Assessment determines the exact nature of the problem which provides information for intervention. Normal bowel patterns include defecation at least 3 times per week.
Assess oral intake of fiber via typical eating pattern or 24-hour recall, while utilizing nutritional tables to calculate fiber (see Table 1).	Assessment of usual patterns of eating provides information on the adequacy of dietary fiber, which leads to the determination of further intervention. Whole grains (bread and cereals), fruits, vegetables, psyllium-containing cereals, nuts, bran, and bran-containing cereals are sources of fiber.
Encourage not to avoid the urge to defecate.	The defecation reflex is weakened or lost if repeatedly ignored. The strongest urge occurs after meals, especially breakfast, because of increased peristalsis secondary to the gastrocolic and duodenocolic reflexes.

Table 1: Foods to Provide 25 Grams Dietary Fiber per Day

Fruits: about 2 g of fiber per serving: use 4 or more per day.

Apple, 1 small	Orange, 1 small
Banana, 1 small	Peach, 1 medium
Strawberries, ½ c	Pear, ½ small
Cherries, 10 large	Plums, 2 small

Grains and Cereals: about 2 g of fiber per serving: Use 4 or more per day.

Whole wheat bread, 1 slice	All Bran, 1 T
Rye bread, 1 slice	Cornflakes, ⅔ c
Cracked wheat bread, 1 slice	Oatmeal, dry, 3 T
Shredded Wheat, ½ biscuit	Wheat bran, 1 tsp
Grape-Nuts, 3 T	Puffed Wheat, 1 ½ c
Barley, ½ c	

Vegetables: about 2 g of fiber per serving: use 4 or more per day. These values are for cooked portions.

Broccoli, ½ stalk	Lettuce, raw, 2 c
Brussel sprouts, 4	Green beans, ½ c
Carrots, ⅓ c	Potato, 2-in. diameter
Celery, 1 c	Tomato, raw, 1 medium
Corn on the cob, 2 -in. piece	

Legumes: about 8 g of fiber per portion.

Garbanzo beans, ½ c	Baked beans, canned, ½ c
Kidney Beans, ½ c	

Miscellaneous: about 1 g of fiber per portion.

Peanut butter, 2 ½ tsp	Pickle, 1 large
Peanuts, 10	Strawberry jam, 5 T
Walnuts, ¼ c	

Taken from Whitney, E.N., Cataldo, C.B., & Rolfes, S.R. (1987). **Understanding normal and clinical nutrition** (2nd ed.). St. Paul, MN: West Publishing. An adaptation from recommendations for a high-fiber diet, **Nutrition and the MD**, July 1981, in turn adapted from Southgate, D.A.T., et al. A guide to calculating intakes of dietary fiber, **Journal of Human Nutrition**, (1976), **30**, 303-313. Reproduced with permission.

INTERVENTIONS

RATIONALE

INTERVENTIONS	RATIONALE
Encourage to facilitate defecation by sitting up, leaning forward, and flexing knees. Advise to use a small stool to promote knee flexion.	Effective utilization of abdominal muscles and gravity to promote defecation is enhanced by this position.

INTERVENTIONS	**R**ATIONALE
Provide privacy for defecation.	Defecation is considered a private activity, and lack of privacy enhances constipation.
Using tables in a nutrition manual, help plan daily menus which include 20–30 g/fiber. As necessary, increase fiber gradually.	Compliance is enhanced when foods selected have personal appeal. Too rapid an increase in dietary fiber causes nausea, bloating, and flatulence, and the experience of these negative results adversely influences compliance. Note: A high fiber diet is contraindicated in irritable bowel syndrome. (See above for fiber sources.)
Assist to evaluate bulk laxatives for:	
1. Type of agent contributing bulk	Agents differ in terms of personal taste, cost, convenience, and effectiveness.
2. Texture and form	Compliance is affected by taste, texture, and forms of products. Some products come in wafer form or have a gritty or smooth consistency.
3. Flavored or unflavored products	Unflavored products may be diluted in water, juice, milk, or other preferred liquid, while flavored products are generally diluted in water. Compliance is influenced by taste.
4. Fiber content per dose (especially if switching brands)	Fiber content per dose is not equal among brands and therefore affects response.
5. Calorie content per dose	Flavored products contain sugar or artificial sweetners and require consideration in diabetes or calorie-controlled diets.
6. Sodium content per dose	Effervescent bulk laxatives contain significant amounts of sodium and are contraindicated in edema, heart failure, and other fluid imbalance disorders.
Teach to recognize high-fiber foods by reading product labels.	Whole grain breads and cereals are a rich source of fiber but product appearances can be deceiving. Bread products that do not contain whole grain flour may contain caramel coloring to make them look healthier. Ingredients which indicate

INTERVENTIONS

RATIONALE

INTERVENTIONS	RATIONALE
	whole grains include 100% whole wheat flour, cracked wheat, rolled oats, wheat germ sprouted wheat, wheat berries, corn meal, unprocessed bran, bulgur wheat, barley, brown rice, and 100% rye flour. Psyllium-containing cereal has the same ingredient as the bulk laxative Metamucil.
Teach to add bran to the diet.	Bran is a very economical way to add fiber to the diet. It can be sprinkled onto cold or cooked cereal, as well as other dishes. Note: Bran is contraindicated in hypocalcemia and iron absorption deficits.
Teach to include fresh vegetables and fruits, especially with skins on, to the diet.	The source of fiber in vegetables is cellulose, hemicellulose, and lignin. Lignin is indigestible and adds bulk to the stool. Prune juice and prunes contain dihydroxyphenyl isatin, which is a laxative; but only prunes are high in fiber.
Institute teaching regarding the use of over-the-counter medications for constipation.	Informed decisions enable the appropriate meeting of needs.
Teach to avoid the use of stimulant laxatives, osmotic laxatives, and enemas.	Stimulant laxatives and enemas affect normal physiologic functioning of the colon, and long-term use results in dependence. Phenolphthalein and biscodyl are systemically absorbed and produce prolonged effect. Osmotic agents affect sodium retention and can cause fluid and electrolyte imbalances.
Teach pregnant and breast-feeding mother regarding the dangers of laxative use.	Stimulant laxatives, especially castor oil, precipitate labor. Cascara and danthron are transmitted through breast milk and can cause diarrhea in infants.
Teach how to take biscodyl laxatives if indicated.	Severe gastric distress is caused by destroying the enteric coating on biscodyl laxatives, and this is done by chewing, taking with milk, antacids, or a hydrogen blocker, i.e., cimetidine or ranitidine.
Teach to avoid magnesium- and phosphate-based products in renal failure.	Hypermagnesemia and hyperphosphatemia may occur with the use of laxatives, such as Milk of Magnesia or sodium phosphate.

INTERVENTIONS	**R**ATIONALE
Teach to avoid sodium-based laxatives in heart failure or edema.	The increase in sodium affects sodium retention and can worsen fluid and electrolyte imbalances.
Advise to use a bulk laxative if one is needed to prevent constipation, but teach that the effects are not immediate.	Bulk laxatives are the most physiologic and do not alter physiologic function of the colon or produce dependence, but effects may take as long as 72 hours to be seen. Fiber is not systemically absorbed; it absorbs fluids and promotes softer, bulkier stools. Note: Bulk laxatives are contraindicated in stricture or dysphagia.
Teach to drink an additional glass of fluid with bulk laxatives.	Bulk laxatives work by absorbing fluid and require an adequate intake of fluid; less than the recommended amount may result in obstruction.
Teach that psyllium can cause an allergic response in the one taking the laxative as well as the one preparing it.	Symptoms of shortness of breath or wheezing related to inhalation of the product are indications for discontinuation.
Teach that stool softeners such as docusate reduce straining.	Stool softeners facilitate the mixing of fat and water in stools, making them softer and easier to expel. This is especially helpful when straining is contraindicated as in cardiac disease.

Inpatient

Respect the need for maintenance of the normal routine for defecation when possible, e.g., client must have a cup of coffee or sit on the toilet after breakfast.	The defecation reflex is lost if repeatedly ignored.
Utilize digital stimulation of the rectum or rectal suppositories, i.e., glycerine or Dulcolax every other day for constipation in spinal cord injury. Digital stimulation is accomplished by inserting a lubricated gloved finger into the rectum and moving it in a circular or side-to-side manner. Teach to continue this technique upon discharge.	These techniques stimulate bowel evacuation within a short period of time, which promotes the scheduled elimination of stool and prevents evacuation at socially unacceptable times.

INTERVENTIONS	RATIONALE
Request dietitian consult regarding the modification of the hospital diet and diet teaching.	The dietitian is skilled in modifying the current hospital diet to promote bowel regularity. This is accomplished by incorporating fruits, vegetables, and whole grain products within the confines of the therapeutic diet and through the utilization of teaching and written materials.
Teach to include 30–60 cc of a low-cost fiber supplement daily.	Brown and Everett (1990) utilized a recipe consisting of two cups of Kellogg's All-Bran cereal, two cups of apple sauce, and one cup of prune juice; 30 cc of this recipe provide 2.2 g dietary fiber. The use of this recipe reduced laxative use among elders in an extended care facility. The initial dose of 30 cc was increased to 60 cc if needed.
Community Health/ Home Care Teach not to take a laxative in the presence of acute abdominal pain, nausea, vomiting, distention, or rectal bleeding	Appendicitis, bowel obstruction, or other health deviation which requires prompt medical attention may be made worse by the administration of a laxative.
Instruct about foods which have a natural laxative effect.	Prunes are high in fiber and contain dihydroxyphenyl isatin which has a laxative effect. Prune juice, however, is not high in fiber but still contains dihydroxyphenyl isatin.
Instruct to avoid mineral oil as a laxative, especially in the presence of impaired swallowing or decreased level of consciousness.	Mineral oil inhibits the absorption of fat-soluble vitamins (A,D,E, and K). If aspirated, mineral oil causes aspiration pneumonia.
Teach to seek medical attention if there has been a recent change in bowel habits which persists longer than two weeks.	Recent but persistent changes may indicate conditions requiring prompt medical attention, e.g., cancer of the colon.
Teach exercises to strengthen the abdominal and rectal muscles unless contraindicated by other health problems.	Tightening abdominal muscles, flexing each thigh to bring the knees up to the chest while in a recumbent position, performing bent knee sit-ups and straight leg lifts several times a day strengthen the muscles utilized in the process of defecation.

INTERVENTIONS	**R**ATIONALE
Advocate the use of regular aerobic exercise for 20 minutes three times a week. A monitored exercise program, i.e., hospital- or YMCA-based program, should be advised in the presence of heart or lung disease or lack of previous physical fitness.	Even slight increases in activity level stimulate gastrointestinal motility. A monitored program begins with an assessment of the level of fitness and is designed to meet individual needs.
In cases when medication which causes constipation is essential, i.e., major tranquilizers or analgesics, teach measures to promote good bowel habits.	Six to eight large glasses of liquid daily, increased activity, and additional fiber, as tolerated, enhance gastrointestinal motility and the evacuation of soft, formed stool.
Provide instruction on obtaining laxatives and advise to purchase the smallest quantity available or to ask the physician to order a small amount. Teach to check for generic equivalents for prescription items.	The appropriate, convenient, and pleasing use of laxatives is often dependent upon trial and error of several different products. When a small amount is purchased initially, needless cost and waste is avoided.

REFERENCES/BIBLIOGRAPHY

Basch, A. (1987). Changes in elimination. **Seminars in Oncology Nursing, 3** (4), 287–292.

Bradford, L., & Dunbar, J. (1987). Behavioral home management of cathartic withdrawal in a laxative-dependent elderly woman. **Archives of Psychiatric Nursing, 1** (5), 359–365.

Brown, M.K., & Everett, I. (1990). Gentler bowel fitness with fiber. **Geriatric Nursing, 11** (1), 26–27.

Brucker, M.C. (1988). Management of common minor discomforts in pregnancy: Part III: Managing gastrointestinal problems in pregnancy. **Journal of Nurse-Midwifery, 33** (2), 67–73.

Ellickson, E.B. (1988). Bowel management plan for the homebound elderly. **Journal of Gerontological Nursing, 14** (1), 16–19.

Groth, F. (1988). Effects of wheat bran in the diet of postsurgical orthopedic patients to prevent constipation. **Orthopedic Nursing, 7** (4), 41–46.

Kim, M.J., McFarland, G.K., & McLane, A.M. (1989). **Pocket guide to nursing diagnoses.** (3rd ed.). St. Louis: Mosby.

Kuhn, M.M. (1991). **Pharmacotherapeutics: A nursing process approach.** (2nd ed.). Philadelphia: Davis.

McMillan, S.C., & Williams, F.A. (1989). Validity and reliability of the constipation assessment scale. **Cancer Nursing, 12** (3), 183–188.

McShane, R.E., & McLane, A.M. (1988). Constipation: Impact of etiological factors. **Journal of Gerontologic Nursing, 14** (4), 31–34.

North American Nursing Diagnosis Association. (1990). **Taxonomy I** (Rev. 1990). St. Louis: NANDA.

Potter, P.A., & Perry, A.G. (1989). **Fundamentals of nursing: Concepts, process and practice.** (2nd ed.). St. Louis: Mosby.

Schlafer, M., & Marieb, E.N. (1990). **The nurse, pharmacology and drug therapy**. Menlo Park, CA: Addison-Wesley.

Taylor, C., Lillis, C., & LeMone, P. (1989). **Fundamentals of nursing: The art and science of nursing care**. Philadelphia: Lippincott.

Tremaine, W.J. (1990). Chronic constipation: Causes and management. **Hospital Practice, 25** (4a), 89–100.

Whitney, E.N., Cataldo, C.B., & Rolfes, S.R. (1987). **Understanding normal and clinical nutrition.** (2nd ed.). New York: West Publishing.

Yakabowich, M. (1990). Prescribe with care: The role of laxatives in the treatment of constipation. **Gerontological Nursing, 16** (7), 4–11.

Yen, P.K. (1988). Nature's laxative: Fiber. **Geriatric Nursing, 9** (6), 361–362.

Constipation: Colonic

A state in which an individual's pattern of elimination is characterized by hard, dry stool which results from a delay in passage of food residue (NANDA, 1990, p. 21).

Kathleen Herman Scanlon, R.N., M.S.N

DEFINING CHARACTERISTICS

Blood-tinged stools or blood noted on toilet tissue after wiping rectal area
Decreased frequency of defecation
Hard, formed, dry, or marble-sized stools
Impaction

Inability to pass stool
Oozing liquid stool around impaction
Palpable fecal mass in rectum
Rectal pain during defecation
Sensation of rectal fullness or pressure

CONTRIBUTING FACTORS

Pathophysiological

Electrolyte imbalance, i.e., hypokalemia or hypocalcemia

Hypothyroidism
Irritable bowel syndrome

Psychosociobehavioral

Change in usual routine
Depression
Inadequate fluid or fiber intake

Inadequate physical activity
Lack of privacy
Stress

EXPECTED OUTCOMES

Client will evacuate soft, formed stool without undue straining at least every third day.
   The regular use of stimulant laxatives is avoided.
   2000–3000 cc/fluid is ingested daily.

147

Aerobic exercises at a target heart rate for 20 min 3 times weekly, or physical activity including walking, as tolerated, is completed.

INTERVENTIONS	RATIONALE
Universal Assess rectum for presence of impaction.	The designation of therapeutic intervention is based on the determination of the cause of the constipation. Laxatives are contraindicated in impaction because they can take up to 72 hours to work and can cause bowel perforation.
Administer an oil retention enema prior to disimpaction.	The oil is absorbed by the hard stool, which softens and facilitates removal.
Using lubricated, gloved finger, break up and remove impaction. Monitor pulse during disimpaction.	Manual removal is more effective than suppository insertion, since the suppository is usually placed within the impaction rather than in contact with the rectal wall. Rectal manipulation stimulates a vagal response which slows the heart rate.
After disimpaction administer a tap water enema, but be certain all water is expelled and do not repeat.	Manual disimpaction removes only the stool in the lower rectum. A tap water enema stimulates peristalsis through distention of the colon which enhances feces expulsion. Tap water enemas can cause hyponatremia if repeated or if not expelled.
Refer for medical evaluation of the GI system if problem is chronic or represents a recent change in bowel habits.	Evaluation will rule out disease processes as a cause of colonic constipation and pinpoint the contributing factors. This information is essential to the determination of intervention. For example, increased fiber is contraindicated in irritable bowel syndrome and would, therefore, be eliminated as a teaching option.
Encourage not to avoid the urge to defecate and respect the usual routine for evacuation, e.g., must have a cup of coffee or sit on the toilet after breakfast.	The defecation reflex is weakened or lost if repeatedly ignored. Defecation after breakfast because of increased peristalsis secondary to the gastrocolic and duodenocolic reflexes, is common.
Encourage to facilitate defecation by sitting up, leaning forward, and flexing knees. Advise to use a small stool to promote knee flexion.	Effective utilization of abdominal muscles and gravity to promote defecation is enhanced by this position.

INTERVENTIONS	RATIONALE
Provide privacy for defecation.	Defecation is considered a private activity, and lack of privacy enhances constipation.
Using tables in a nutrition manual, help plan daily menus which include 20–30 g/fiber. As necessary, increase fiber gradually.	Compliance is enhanced when foods selected have personal appeal. Too rapid an increase in dietary fiber causes nausea, bloating, and flatulence, and the experience of these negative results adversely influences compliance. Note: A high-fiber diet is contraindicated in irritable bowel syndrome. Foods high in fiber include whole bran, whole wheat breads and cereals, psyllium-containing cereal, legumes, and nuts.
Assist to evaluate bulk laxatives for:	
1. Type of agent contributing bulk	Agents differ in terms of personal taste, cost, convenience, and effectiveness.
2. Texture and form	Compliance is affected by taste, texture, and forms of products. Some products come in wafer form or have a gritty or smooth consistency.
3. Flavored or unflavored products	Unflavored products may be diluted in water, juice, milk, or other preferred liquid, while flavored products are generally diluted in water. Compliance is influenced by taste.
4. Fiber content per dose (especially if switching brands)	Fiber content per dose is not equal among brands and therefore affects response.
5. Calorie content per dose	Flavored products contain sugar or artificial sweetners and require consideration in diabetes or calorie-controlled diets.
6. Sodium content per dose	Effervescent bulk laxatives contain significant amounts of sodium and are contraindicated in edema, heart failure, and other fluid imbalance disorders.

INTERVENTIONS	RATIONALE
Teach to recognize high-fiber foods by reading product labels.	Whole grain breads and cereals are a rich source of fiber, but product appearances can be deceiving. Bread products that do not contain whole grain flour may contain caramel coloring to make them look healthier. Ingredients which indicate whole grains include 100% whole wheat flour, cracked wheat, rolled oats, wheat germ sprouted wheat, wheat berries, corn meal, unprocessed bran, bulgur wheat, barley, brown rice, and 100% rye flour. Psyllium-containing cereal has the same ingredient as the bulk laxative Metamucil.
Teach to add bran to the diet.	Bran is a very economical way to add fiber to the diet. It can be sprinkled onto cold or cooked cereal, as well as other dishes. Note: Bran is contraindicated in hypocalcemia and iron absorption deficits.
Teach to include fresh vegetables and fruits, especially with skins on, to the diet.	The sources of fiber in vegetables are cellulose, hemicellulose, and lignin. Lignin is indigestible and adds bulk to the stool. Prune juice and prunes contain dihydroxyphenyl isatin which is a laxative; but only prunes are high in fiber.
Institute teaching regarding the use of over-the-counter medications for constipation.	Informed decisions enable the appropriate meeting of needs.
Teach to avoid the use of stimulant laxatives, osmotic laxatives, and enemas.	Stimulant laxatives and enemas affect normal physiologic functioning of the colon, and long-term use results in dependence. Phenolphthalein and biscodyl are systemically absorbed and produce prolonged effect. Osmotic agents affect sodium retention and can cause fluid and electrolyte imbalances.
Teach pregnant and breast-feeding mother regarding the dangers of laxative use.	Stimulant laxatives, especially castor oil, precipitate labor. Cascara and danthron are transmitted through breast milk and can cause diarrhea in infants.

INTERVENTIONS	RATIONALE
Teach how to take biscodyl laxatives if indicated.	Severe gastric distress is caused by destroying the enteric coating on biscodyl laxatives, and this is done by chewing, taking with milk, antacids, or a hydrogen blocker, i.e., cimetidine or ranitidine.
Teach to avoid magnesium- and phosphate-based products in renal failure.	Hypermagnesemia and hyperphosphatemia may occur with the use of laxatives such as Milk of Magnesia or sodium phosphate.
Teach to avoid sodium-based laxatives in heart failure or edema.	The increase in sodium affects sodium retention and can worsen fluid and electrolyte imbalance.
Advise to use a bulk laxative if one is needed to prevent constipation, but teach that the effects are not immediate.	Bulk laxatives are the most physiologic and do not alter physiologic function of the colon or produce dependence, but effects may take as long as 72 hours to be seen. Fiber is not systemically absorbed; it absorbs fluids and promotes softer, bulkier stools. Note: Bulk laxatives are contraindicated in stricture or dysphagia.
Teach to drink an additional glass of fluid with bulk laxatives.	Bulk laxatives work by absorbing fluid and require an adequate intake of fluid; less than the recommended amount may result in obstruction.
Teach that psyllium can cause an allergic response in the one taking the laxative as well as the one preparing it.	Symptoms of shortness of breath or wheezing related to inhalation of the product are indications for discontinuation.
Teach that stool softeners such as docusate reduce straining.	Stool softeners facilitate the mixing of fat and water in stools, making them softer and easier to expel. This is especially helpful when straining is contraindicated as in cardiac disease.
Teach to include 30–60 cc of a low-cost fiber supplement daily.	Brown and Everett (1990) utilized a recipe consisting of two cups Kellogg's All Bran cereal, two cups apple sauce, and one cup prune juice; 30 cc of this recipe provide 2.2 g of dietary fiber. The use of this recipe reduced laxative use among elders in an extended care facility. The initial dose of 30 cc was increased to 60 cc if needed.

INTERVENTIONS	**R**ATIONALE
Instruct about foods which have a natural laxative effect.	Prunes are high in fiber and contain dihydroxyphenyl isatin which has a laxative effect. Prune juice, however, is not high in fiber but still contains dihydroxyphenyl isatin.
Instruct to avoid mineral oil as a laxative, especially in the presence of impaired swallowing or decreased level of consciousness.	Mineral oil inhibits the absorption of fat-soluble vitamins (A,D,E, and K). If aspirated, mineral oil causes aspiration pneumonia.
Teach exercises to strengthen the abdominal and rectal muscles unless contraindicated by other health problems.	Tightening abdominal muscles, flexing each thigh to bring the knees up to the chest while in a recumbent position, performing bent knee sit-ups and straight leg lifts several times a day strengthen the muscles utilized in the process of defecation.
Advocate the use of regular aerobic exercise for 20 min 3 times a week. A monitored exercise program, i.e., hospital- or YMCA-based program should be advised in the presence of heart or lung disease or lack of previous physical fitness.	Even slight increases in activity level stimulate gastrointestinal motility. A monitored program begins with an assessment of the level of fitness and is designed to meet individual needs.
In cases when medication which causes constipation is essential, i.e., major tranquilizers or analgesics, teach measures to promote good bowel habits.	Six to eight large glasses of liquid daily, increased activity, and additional fiber, as tolerated, enhance gastrointestinal motility and the evacuation of soft, formed stool.
Provide instruction on obtaining laxatives and advise to purchase the smallest quantity available or to ask the physician to order a small amount. Teach client to check for generic equivalents for prescription items.	The appropriate, convenient, and pleasing use of laxatives is often dependent upon trial and error of several different products. When a small amount is purchased initially, needless cost and waste is avoided.

INTERVENTIONS

RATIONALE

Inpatient	None
Community Health/ Home Care	None

REFERENCES/BIBLIOGRAPHY

Brown, M.K., & Everett, I. (1990). Gentler bowel fitness with fiber. **Geriatric Nursing, 11,** 26–27.

Ellickson, E.B. (1988). Bowel management plan for the homebound elderly. **Journal of Gerontological Nursing, 14** (1), 16–19.

Groth, F. (1988). Effects of wheat bran in the diet of post surgical orthopedic patients to prevent constipation. **Orthopedic Nursing, 7** (4), 41–46.

Kim, M.J., McFarland, G.K., & McLane, E.M. (1989). **Pocket guide to nursing diagnoses.** (3rd ed.). St. Louis: Mosby.

Kuhn, M.M. (1991). **Pharmacotherapeutics: A nursing process approach.** (2nd ed.). Philadelphia: Davis.

North American Nursing Diagnosis Association. (1990). **Taxonomy I** (Rev. 1990). St. Louis: NANDA.

Potter, P.A., & Perry, A.G. (1989). **Fundamentals of nursing: Concepts, process and practice.** (2nd ed.). St. Louis: Mosby.

Schlafer, M., & Marieb, E.N. (1990). **The nurse, pharmacology and drug therapy**. Menlo Park, CA: Addison-Wesley.

Taylor, C., Lillis, C., & LeMone, P. (1989). **Fundamentals of nursing: The art and science of nursing care**. Philadelphia: Lippincott.

Tremaine, W.J. (1990). Chronic constipation: Causes and management. **Hospital Practice, 25** (4a), 89–100.

Whitney, E.N., Cataldo, C.B., & Rolfes, S.T. (1987). **Understanding normal and clinical nutrition.** (2nd ed.). New York: West Publishing.

Yakabowich, M. (1990). Prescribe with care: The role of laxatives in the treatment of constipation. **Gerontological Nursing, 16** (7), 4–11.

Yen, P.K. (1988). Nature's laxative: Fiber. **Geriatric Nursing, 9** (6), 361–362.

Constipation: Perceived

A state in which an individual makes a self-diagnosis of constipation and ensures a daily bowel movement through abuse of laxatives, enemas and suppositories (NANDA, 1990, p. 20).

Kathleen Herman Scanlon, R.N., M.S.N.

DEFINING CHARACTERISTICS

Health belief that bowel evacuation must occur daily or at a specific time each day
Inability to pass stool without laxatives, enemas, or suppositories
Preoccupation with daily bowel movements
Reported anxiety until anticipated defecation occurs
Reported interference with activities or daily living until anticipated defecation occurs
Sensation of pressure or fullness in rectum, abdominal discomfort, bloating, or headache until anticipated defecation occurs

CONTRIBUTING FACTORS

Pathophysiological

Changes in colon function related to chronic laxative/cathartic use

Psychosociobehavioral

Family or cultural belief system which stresses daily elimination
Knowledge deficit regarding normal bowel patterns and physiologic methods for promoting normal bowel function

EXPECTED OUTCOMES

Client will avoid use of laxatives, enemas, or suppositories and substitute non-pharmacologic measures to promote bowel function.

154

Client will evacuate soft, formed stool at least every third day.
2000–3000 cc/fluid is ingested daily.
Aerobic exercise at target heart rate for 20 min three times weekly, or a physical activity including walking, as tolerated, is completed..

INTERVENTIONS	RATIONALE
Universal Assess bowel pattern: 1. Color, consistency, frequency, size, shape, difficulty with stool passage 2. Method used to promote defecation, including type of agent (laxatives, enemas, or suppositories) 3. Frequency of use 4. Duration of use 5. Factors which influence decision to use agent 6. Effects of agent 7. Effects of not using agent 8. Attempts to discontinue agent or prolong period of time between uses of agent	Appropriate nursing intervention is dependent upon the provision of information regarding the specific pattern of laxative, enema, or suppository abuse.
Assess beliefs and knowledge about normal bowel function and the use of laxatives, enemas or suppositories to promote bowel function.	Both beliefs and knowledge influence behavior. When a knowledge deficit exists, teaching can be focused in the areas of deficit. When the individual, family, or cultural belief system subscribes to a certain set of beliefs about "normal" bowel function, then interventions can be designed to help the client or family unit modify the belief system in a way that is not offensive.
Refer for a medical evaluation of the gastrointestinal system.	Chronic abuse of laxatives may cause atrophy of colonic smooth muscle, neural damage, dilation and loss of motor activity which may require medical intervention and occasionally even surgery. Evaluation will also rule out disease processes as a contributing factor to abuse of laxatives, enemas, or suppositories. Once underlying medical problems have been ruled out or dealt with, nursing interventions aimed at the withdrawal from laxatives, enemas, or suppositories can proceed.

INTERVENTIONS	**R**ATIONALE
Allow to verbalize feelings/ anxiety about withdrawal from laxatives, enemas, or suppositories.	Breaking a pattern of dependency that is long-standing can be quite anxiety provoking. In the absence of a "daily" bowel movement, anxiety may prompt seeking relief in the form of a laxative, enema, or suppository. It is just as critical to deal with anxiety as it is to deal with constipation.
Avoid negative reinforcement if a laxative, enema, or suppository is taken during the withdrawal program.	Negative reinforcement promotes feelings of inadequacy. Reflecting on how difficult it is to change a long-term behavior, then focusing on changes in the plan for the next few days is more therapeutic. This approach encourages honesty in reporting responses to the withdrawal program, including laxative use, and increases willingness to stick with the program.
Provide positive feedback when there is avoidance of the use of laxatives, enemas, or suppositories for even one day.	The urge to return to old habits may be strong. Positive feedback encourages continuance with the withdrawal program. Each small step facilitates achievement of the larger goal.
Contact weekly or more often, if necessary, to evaluate the effectiveness of the plan, modify the plan and provide support.	Frequent contact is essential to assure continuation with the program, change a chronic behavior pattern, and modify the program to eliminate ineffective interventions.
Attempt laxative, enema, or suppository withdrawal by substituting other measures which promote bowel elimination. These include providing 2000–3000 cc fluid/day, increasing the intake of dietary fiber, and increasing the activity levels. (see Constipation care planning guide.)	Fluids increase the amount of liquid available to keep stools soft. Fiber increases stool bulk and activity stimulates peristalsis. These interventions promote bowel elimination.
Explain the purpose, procedure, and preparation for diagnostic tests, such as sigmoidoscopy or colonoscopy with biopsy, barium enema, and/or bowel transit studies.	Changes such as neuronal damage, atrophy of colonic smooth muscle, dilation, and loss of motor activity can be demonstrated with these tests. Sigmoidoscopy and colonoscopy allow direct visualization of the colon. Barium enema can reveal dilation. Bowel transit studies utilize

INTERVENTIONS	**RATIONALE**
	x-rays to determine how quickly radiopaque markers move through the GI system. Normally, some of the markers are excreted within two days and 80% of them are excreted within five days.
Teach that laxative abuse contributes to chronic constipation.	Chronic laxative abuse causes changes such as neuronal damage, atrophy of colonic smooth muscle, dilation, and loss of motor activity.
Using tables in a nutrition manual help client plan daily menus which include 20 to 30 grams of fiber. Increase fiber intake gradually.	Compliance is enhanced when the client participates in choosing palatable foods and planning meals with increased fiber content. Too rapid an increase in dietary fiber may cause nausea, bloating, and flatulence which may decrease compliance. Increasing fiber content gradually allows the GI system time to adapt to fiber intake and may promote compliance. A high-fiber diet is not recommended for irritable bowel syndrome. Foods high in fiber include whole grain, whole grain breads and cereals, psyllium-containing cereal, legumes, nuts, and bran.
Teach to recognize high-fiber foods by reading product labels.	Whole grain breads and cereals are a rich source of fiber but product appearances can be deceiving. Bread products that do not contain whole grain flour may contain caramel coloring to make them look healthier. Ingredients which indicate whole grains include 100% whole wheat flour, cracked wheat, rolled oats, wheat germ, sprouted wheat, wheat berries, corn meal, unprocessed bran, bulgur wheat, barley, brown rice, and 100% rye flour. Psyllium-containing cereal has the same ingredient as the bulk laxative Metamucil.
Teach to include bran in the diet.	Bran is a very economical way to add fiber to the diet. It can be sprinkled onto cold or cooked cereal, as well as other dishes. These foods can worsen hypocalcemia and may reduce iron absorption.

INTERVENTIONS	RATIONALE
Teach to include fresh vegetables and fruits, especially with the skins on, as a rich source of fiber.	The source of fiber in vegetables includes cellulose, hemicellulose, and lignin. Since lignin is indigestible, it contributes bulk to the stool. Although prunes are high in fiber, prune juice is not. Both prunes and prune juice, however, contain dihydroxyphenyl isatin which has a laxative effect.
Teach that bulk laxatives are the most physiologic and do not alter physiologic function of the colon or produce dependence but may take up to 72 hours to be effective. They are useful for preventing constipation.	Since the fiber is not systemically absorbed, it absorbs fluids and promotes softer bulkier stools. They are contraindicated if stricture or dysphagia exist.

Teach to evaluate bulk laxatives for:
 	
1. Type of agent contributing bulk
   a. Psyllium hydrophilic mucilloid (Metamucil)
   b. Methylcellulose (Cologel & Citrucel)
   c. Malt soup extract (Matsupex)
   d. Polycarbophil (Mitrolan chewable tablets)
	Agents vary in terms of palatability, cost, convenience, or effectiveness.

2. Texture and form of bulk laxative	Some products that are mixed in liquid taste gritty; whereas others are smooth textured. Other products come in wafer form. This may affect compliance.
3. Preference for flavored or unflavored product	Unflavored products may be diluted in any fluid. Flavored products are generally diluted in water. Compliance increases with increased palatability.
4. Fiber content per dose (especially if switching brands)	Fiber content per dose is not equal among brands and affects response.

INTERVENTIONS	**R**ATIONALE
5. Caloric content per dose	Flavored products may contain sugar or artificial sweeteners. In diabetes or a calorie-controlled diet, calorie content is a consideration.
6. Sodium content per dose	Sodium content may be restricted in edema, heart failure, or other disorders. Effervescent bulk laxatives contain significant amounts of sodium.
7. Required dilution and palatability	Bulk laxatives require an adequate fluid intake to work which necessitates taking them with 8 oz/ fluid. An additional glass of fluid is also recommended. The bulk laxatives can be diluted with any palatable liquid (water, juice, or milk). Taking them with less than the recommended amount of fluid may result in obstruction.
Warn client that psyllium causes an allergic response in a small percentage of individuals, which may include shortness of breath and wheezing. This reaction may also occur in a family member who prepares the product.	Inhalation of the product during preparation has produced this reaction in nurses. The product should be discontinued if allergic symptoms develop. If these symptoms develop in a family member, that individual should not prepare the product.
Teach strengthening exercises for abdominal and rectal muscles unless contraindicated by other health problems. Tightening the abdominal muscles, flexing each thigh to bring the knees up to the chest while in a recumbent position, bent knee sit-ups, and straight leg lifts should be done several times daily.	Abdominal and rectal muscle exercises strengthen the muscles which are utilized in the process of defecation.
Encourage regular physical aerobic exercise for 20 minutes three times a week. If physically out of shape or if there is a history of heart or lung disease, encourage a monitored exercise program (hospital based, YMCA based).	Monitored programs begin with assessment of the level of fitness. The program is designed to meet individual activity needs. These programs are safer than unmonitored programs. Even slight increases in activity level can stimulate gastrointestinal motility.

INTERVENTIONS	**R**ATIONALE
Help to identify and implement adaptive responses to the stress that laxative withdrawal creates (walking, hobbies, calling a friend, gardening, shopping, etc.).	Lack of adequate problem-solving skills or difficulty recognizing alternatives are barriers to alleviating stress. Recognition of previously effective strategies and the development of new strategies alleviate stress.
Teach to keep a log of food and fluid intake, bran intake, activity level, and laxative use.	The log provides ongoing data for evaluation of progress, facilitates modification of the nursing care plan, and provides for active participation in the decision-making process.
Inpatient	None
Community Health/ Home Care	None

REFERENCES/BIBLIOGRAPHY

Bradford, L., & Dunbar, J. (1987). Behavioral home management of cathartic withdrawal in a laxative-dependent elderly woman. **Archives of Psychiatric Nursing, 1** (5), 359–365.

Doenges, M.E., Townsend, M.C., & Moorehouse, M.F. (1989). **Psychiatric care plans: Guidelines for client care**. Philadelphia: Davis.

Ellickson, E.B. (1988). Bowel management plan for the homebound elderly. **Journal of Gerontological Nursing, 14** (1), 16–19.

Kim, M.J., McFarland, G.K., & McLane, E.M. (1989). **Pocket guide to nursing diagnoses.** (3rd ed.). St. Louis: Mosby.

Kuhn, M.M. (1991). **Pharmacotherapeutics: A nursing process approach.** (2nd ed.). Philadelphia: Davis.

McFarland, G.K., & McFarlane, E.A. (1989). **Nursing diagnosis and intervention**. St. Louis: Mosby.

North American Nursing Diagnosis Association. (1990). **Taxonomy I** (Rev. 1990). St. Louis: NANDA.

Potter, P.A., & Perry, A.G. (1989). **Fundamentals of nursing: Concepts, process and practice.** (2nd ed.). St. Louis: Mosby.

Shlafer, M., & Marieb, E.N. (1990). **The nurse, pharmacology and drug therapy**. Menlo Park, CA: Addison-Wesley.

Stuart, G.W., & Sundeen, S.J. (1983). **Principles & practice of psychiatric nursing**. St. Louis: Mosby.

Taylor, C., Lillis, C., & LeMone, P. (1989). **Fundamentals of nursing: The art and science of nursing care**. Philadelphia: Lippincott.

Tremaine, W.J. (1990). Chronic constipation: Causes and management. **Hospital Practice, 25** (4a), 89–100.

Whitney, E.N., Cataldo, C.B., & Rolfes, S.R. (1987). **Understanding normal and clinical nutrition.** (2nd ed.). New York: West Publishing.

Yakabowich, M. (1990). Prescribe with care: The role of laxatives in the treatment of constipation. **Gerontological nursing, 16** (7), 4–11.

Coping: Defensive

A state in which an individual repeatedly projects false positive self evaluation based on a self protective pattern which defends against underlying perceived threats to positive self regard (NANDA, 1990, p. 63).

Kay Koneazny, R.N., M.S.N.

DEFINING CHARACTERISTICS

Denial of obvious problems/weaknesses
Difficulty establishing/maintaining
    relationships
Difficulty in reality testing perceptions
Display of anger when authority/opinion
    is questioned
Grandiosity
Hostile laughter or ridicule of others
Hypersensitivity to slight criticism

Lack of follow-through or participation
    in treatment
Projection of blame/responsibility
Rationalization of failures
Rejection of advice
Superior attitude toward others
Use of manipulation
Withdrawal/rebellion when placed in
    a dependent role

CONTRIBUTING FACTORS

Pathophysiological

Acute/chronic disability

Acute/chronic illness

Psychosociobehavioral

Dysfunctional family system
Maturational crisis

Personal vulnerability
Situational crisis

EXPECTED OUTCOMES

Client will project realistic self-evaluation.
> Threats to self-esteem are verbally identified.
> Own strengths and weaknesses are realistically identified.
> Clarity of self-concept in decision making, accepting own limits is demonstrated. ·
> Acceptance of own role and role performance is verbalized.
> Acceptance of identified real self is verbalized.
> Functioning in a responsible manner is demonstrated.

Client will choose an interactional style which promotes health for self and others.
> Understanding of codependent behavior is verbalized.
> Own feelings are identified.
> Ability to clarify communication from others, versus assuming own perceptions are accurate, is demonstrated.
> Personal feedback regarding own behavior is accepted.
> Own behavior is accurately described as aggressive, assertive, or passive.
> Behavioral alternatives for use in threatening interpersonal situations are discussed.
> Individual and interpersonal outcomes of behavior are evaluated individually and in a group setting.

INTERVENTIONS / RATIONALE

INTERVENTIONS	RATIONALE
Universal	
Assess for behaviors which have caused interpersonal problems in the past.	Emergence of patterns may promote increased self-awareness and responsibility for own behavior.
Evaluate progress toward established outcomes.	Timely, ongoing evaluation of progress ensures an effective plan of care.
Establish a trusting relationship through listening and offering positive acceptance.	Trust is essential to enable therapeutic self-disclosure.
Involve the client and significant others in decisions regarding care and therapy.	Follow-through is more likely if this involvement is present.
Assist to identify individual strengths.	A recognition of one's strengths can increase the likelihood that one will draw successfully upon them.
Assist to identify feelings.	Feelings generate behavior.

INTERVENTIONS	RATIONALE
Assist to identify high-threat situations.	Identification of major stressors provides a focus for nursing intervention.
Assist to identify own behavioral responses to feelings during interactions.	Such analysis can increase self-awareness and a sense of personal responsibility.
Set limits on manipulative behavior.	Setting limits can eventually render these behaviors useless and open the client to alternative behaviors which may be more effective.
Help to identify appropriate behaviors and reinforce their use.	Appropriate behavior elicits a more positive response from others, which may decrease the need for defensive coping.
Formulate feedback using "I" statements; avoid evaluative statements.	Evaluative statements sound like criticism and can increase defensive coping behaviors. Sharing personal responses can provide a model for self-expression and self-responsibility.
Help to set realistic goals.	Client goals may be based on a grandiose self-evaluation and may predispose to failure.
Reframe failures as learning opportunities.	Reframing can decrease the threat to self-esteem and demonstrate that all life experiences can be useful.
Acknowledge yourself in an accepting manner.	Demonstrated self-acceptance provides useful role modeling.
Teach method for clarifying communication from others.	Often the client may have misperceived another's words to have negative meaning not intended, e.g., rejection.
Teach concept of codependency; identify codependent behaviors.	Integration of this concept can increase self-awareness of own behavior as being pathologically referenced to others.
Teach assertiveness concepts, communication.	Assertiveness skills are nondefensive coping tools.
Inpatient	None

INTERVENTIONS

RATIONALE

Community Health/ Home Care	
Assess quality of interpersonal dynamics with family and significant others.	Interpersonal dynamics will reveal attitudes and potential for client support.
Assist family and significant others to understand and to support client's healthy behavior.	In family systems, even healthy behavioral change can pose a threat and produce a non-supportive response.

REFERENCES/BIBLIOGRAPHY

Charron, H.S. (1990). Repetitive and ineffective neurotic defenses. In Varcarolis, M. (Ed.). **Foundations of psychiatric mental health nursing.** (pp. 339–384). Philadelphia: Saunders.

* Norris, J., & Kunes-Connell, M. (1988). A multimodal approach to validation and refinement of an existing nursing diagnosis. In **Archives of Psychiatric Nursing, 2** (2), 103–109.

North American Nursing Diagnosis Association. (1990). **Taxonomy I** (Rev. 1990). St. Louis: NANDA.

Pelletier, L.R. (1987). **Psychiatric nursing: Case studies, nursing diagnoses, and care plans.** Springhouse, PA: Springhouse Corp.

Task Force on Standards of Addictions Nursing Practice. (1988). **Standards of addictions nursing practice with selected diagnoses and criteria.** Kansas City, MO: American Nurses' Association.

Coping, Family: Compromised

A state in which a usually supportive and well-functioning family is having difficulty utilizing resources and positive adaptive strategies to simultaneously manage the care of an ill/dependent member and other developmental or situational stressors.

Marilyn A. McCubbin, R.N., Ph.D.

. . . .

DEFINING CHARACTERISTICS

Altered decision making
Anticipatory grief
Anxiety
Complaints and dissatisfaction with care
Confusion and uncertainty
Disruption of family routines
Disruption of sleep, eating schedules, and social contacts
Fatigue
Fear
Feelings of inadequacy
Feelings of regret about inability to attend to care
Guilt
Inability or reluctance to recognize signs and symptoms

Inadequate knowledge base about condition and care
Lack of coordination of appropriate community resources
Lack of knowledge of available formal support systems
Lack of use of support systems due to need for privacy and independence
Less than optimal care for dependent member
Overprotective and overmonitoring behaviors
Primary caregiver role overload
Restricted communication patterns among members
Somatic complaints

CONTRIBUTING FACTORS

Pathophysiological

Chronic illness in other family members
Deteriorating disease course

Frail health of primary caregiver
Terminal illness stage

165

Psychosociobehavioral

Geographical distance of extended family
Isolation of members from each other
Lack of availability or access to community
   resources
Limited financial resources

Limited insurance coverage or uninsured
   status
Long-term care situation
Multiple stressors and demands occurring
   simultaneously

EXPECTED OUTCOMES

Family will continue to provide care which is safe and appropriate.
   Knowledge about health problem is accurately verbalized.
   Prescribed treatment regimen and care is done in a safe manner.
   Symptoms and changes in condition are appropriately reported.
   Physical and emotional needs, i.e., nutrition, sleep, exercise, hygiene, social interaction
      are met.
   Fears and concerns about care and condition are freely discussed.
Family members will perform care without compromising own physical and emotional health.
   Stress associated with caregiving is identified.
   Feelings about the impact of caregiving on life situations are expressed.
   Community resources, i.e., home health aide, homemaker, visiting nurse are utilized.
   Effective coping behaviors are seen.
   Health needs, i.e., nutrition and rest, receive attention.
   Feelings of control and optimism increase.
The family unit will utilize resources and effective coping strategies to reduce stress and
      manage developmental and situational stressors.
   Stressors are identified.
   Realistic expectations of situation and roles are formed.
   Problem-solving abilities (accurate definition of the problem, identification of alternate
      solutions, and consensus) increase.
   Open communication is maintained.
   Flexibility in roles, rules, and decision making increases.
   Predictable family routines continue.
   Physical and emotional support is seen.
   A hopeful outlook is maintained.

INTERVENTIONS	RATIONALE
Universal (Note: All interventions in this care plan are listed as universal, since the place of intervention is variable and dependent upon each family situation—as the dependent member may or may not be hospitalized.) Assess if basic physical and emotional needs are being met.	Attention to all family members acknowledges their contribution and importance. Well-being is essential to dealing with stress.
Monitor continued ability to carry out treatment regimen and care.	Ongoing assessment promotes early detection of complications and provides feedback.
Monitor extent to which dependent member's needs are being met.	(Same as above)
Assist family to define present situation and assess for the need for additional community resources, i.e., home health aide, homemaker, respite care, extended family and friend support.	The gathering and utilizing of resources decreases the burden, provides assistance, and expands existing resources which will be useful in future need.
Help to assess the benefits and costs of existing support network.	Extended family and friend support may be given with an expectation of reciprocity. Obtaining a clear picture of the benefits and costs of existing supports assists the family to sort out needs and available resources and energy levels.
Assess receptivity to making changes in day-to-day functioning.	The initial reaction to crisis and stress may be to rely on previous patterns of behavior and interaction; these may need to be altered to manage current stressors.
Explore financial status and payment sources; consider referral to social services.	Financial resources are quickly exhausted in long-term care.

Interventions	Rationale
Develop a trust relationship.	Trust creates a climate of caring concern and provides a foundation for further intervention.
Discuss management of emotional outbursts, personality changes, mood swings.	Emotional upsets, and their tendency to involve everyone, are frequently more difficult to manage.
Encourage family conferences with health care providers.	Family conferences give current information and a realistic picture of the condition and caregiving requirements.
Encourage family members to express how caregiving has altered plans, goals, daily routines, and life situation; encourage the ventilation of feelings, emotions, and concerns.	The release of feelings represents the first step in identifying options for management. The validation of feelings, i.e., anger, fatigue, resentment, guilt allays additional stress by preventing the build up of feelings perceived as negative or not normal.
Help in the identification of current stressors and strains.	Identification of specific stressors is the first step toward solution. Family unity is promoted when members see that what happens to one impacts on all. Unresolved past strains, i.e., work difficulties, in-law or ex-spousal relationship problems, are often exacerbated in times of increased stress and crisis.
Encourage realistic expectations of role performances.	A better match between abilities and expectations of role performance promotes greater satisfaction with performance and recognition that "less than perfect" is acceptable.
Provide support and promote coordination for linkage to community resources.	Outside resources are essential to family unit functioning. Families benefit from and contribute to the community resource network. Sharing of information for family treatment plans with all agencies involved minimizes the duplication, disruption, and disorganization that can diminish trust and alienate the family.
Promote increased flexibility of roles, rules, and decision making. Address changes in one prioritized area at a time.	Coping requires the ability to try alternative ways of task management and responsibilities.

INTERVENTIONS	RATIONALE
Reinforce and provide feedback on continued utilization of problem-solving skills and prioritization, option identification, and decision making.	Long-term illness places exhausting and overwhelming demands on families due to the number and intensity of inherent stressors. Assistance with problem-solving skills is useful to sort out priorities for the immediate crisis and in future situations. Positive feedback reinforces behavior and increases self-esteem.
Encourage the maintenance of predictable routines whenever possible.	Routines provide stability and predictability in times of stress and crisis.
Encourage the inclusion of the dependent member in activities as health and conditions permit.	Involvement decreases isolation and increases feelings of self-worth and belonging.
Reinforce knowledge about disease processes, signs and symptoms, treatment modes, and reportable adverse effects.	Knowledge promotes autonomy, increases responsibility for self-care, and reduces anxiety about the unknown.
Teach coping strategies to manage tension and strain if previous techniques are no longer effective.	Alternative ways of coping provide strategies to reduce anxiety and increase feelings of control.

REFERENCES/BIBLIOGRAPHY

See bibliography for "Coping, Family: Disabled." (pp. 164–165).

Coping, Family: Disabled

A state in which a family demonstrates severe inability to utilize resources and positive adaptive strategies to simultaneously manage the care of an ill/dependent member and other developmental or situational stressors. The family situation, in turn, endangers the physical and emotional well-being of individual family members and the functioning of the family as a unit.

Marilyn A. McCubbin, R.N., Ph.D.

DEFINING CHARACTERISTICS

Blaming or scapegoating in family interactions
Communication patterns that tend to escalate rather than resolve conflict
Denial about existence or severity of health problem or developmental needs
Family members (especially caregiver) report or express:
  Aggressive intentions or actions
  Agitation
  Anger
  Depression
  Excessive guilt
  Extreme fatigue
  Feelings of despair, hopelessness, or inadequacy
  Hostility at present situation
  Ignoring or minimizing other members' needs
  Inability to engage in outside activities
  Inability to recognize symptoms, understand disease processes, and/or seek appropriate
    care for dependent member
  Manipulative or controlling behaviors

       Over monitoring of symptoms and treatment
       Prolonged over concern for ill member
       Role overload
       Severe disruption of life plans
       Withdrawal from social interaction
High level of conflict and strain in relationship between family members
Inflexibility and rigidity in role responsibilities, decision making, and power structure
Intolerance, rejection, abandonment, desertion of any member
Lack of clear rules, routines, and role expectations (chaotic, disorganized environment)
Neglectful care for either basic needs or illness treatment
Unrealistic or inaccurate picture of health problem or developmental needs

CONTRIBUTING FACTORS
Pathophysiological

Chronic mental or physical illness in other members
Clinical depression
Developmental disabilities
Learning disabilities

Psychosociobehavioral

Alcohol or other substance abuse patterns
Geographic/social isolation
Impaired social and problem-solving skills
Lack of availability or access to community resources
Limited formal and informal support systems
Major disruptions in routines due to caregiving demands
Previous history of physical, emotional, or sexual abuse
Severely strained financial resources
Simultaneous occurrence of multiple developmental/situational stressors

EXPECTED OUTCOMES

Family will provide care which is safe and appropriate without occurrence or reoccurrence of
      neglect or abuse.
       Knowledge about health problem is accurately verbalized.
       Prescribed treatment regimen and care is done in a safe manner.
       Symptoms and changes in condition are appropriately reported.
       Physical and emotional needs (i.e., nutrition, sleep, exercise, hygiene, social interaction)
         are met.
Family members will perform care without compromising own physical and emotional health.
       Stress associated with caregiving is identified.
       Feelings about the impact of caregiving on life situations are expressed.
       Community resources (i.e., home health aide, homemaker, visiting nurse) are utilized.
       Effective coping behaviors are seen.
       Physical needs (i.e., nutrition and rest) of all family members receive attention.

The family unit will utilize resources and effective coping strategies to reduce stress and manage developmental and situational stressors.

Stressors are identified.

Realistic expectations of situation and roles are formed.

Problem-solving abilities (accurate definition of the problem, identification of alternate solutions, and consensus) increase.

Flexibility in roles, rules, and decision making increases.

Predictable family routines which provide stability continue.

Physical and emotional support are seen.

Community resources to improve family interaction and coping abilities (i.e., social services, family crisis centers, crisis/abuse hotlines, mental health centers, abuse-specific treatment programs) are utilized.

(It should be noted that in families with long-term disabling coping patterns, these desirable outcomes will take time to achieve and most likely require multidisciplinary interventions.)

INTERVENTIONS	**R**ATIONALE
Universal (Note: All interventions in this care plan are listed as universal, since the place of intervention is variable and dependent upon each family situation—as the dependent member may or may not be hospitalized.) Monitor ability to continue to carry out treatment and illness regimen.	Ongoing assessment promotes early detection of complications and provides feedback.
Monitor extent to which physical and emotional needs are being met.	Ongoing assessment promotes early detection of complications and provides feedback. Also, attention to all family members acknowledges their contribution and importance, and is essential to family-centered care.
Assess for the need for additional community resources, i.e., home health aide, homemaker, respite care.	The gathering and utilizing of resources decreases the burden, provides assistance, and expands existing resources which will be useful in future need.
Assess receptivity to making changes in day-to-day functioning.	The initial reaction to crisis and stress may be to rely on previous pattens of behavior and inter-action; these may need to be altered to manage current stressors.

INTERVENTIONS	**R**ATIONALE
Assist to define present situation it terms of what capabilities and resources can be used to manage stressors and demands.	The definition of the situation provides the basis for guiding intervention and supporting or expanding existing resources.
Assist to assess existing resources and support systems for emotional support and task assistance.	Extended family and friend support may be given with an expectation of reciprocity. Obtaining a clear picture of the benefits and costs of existing supports helps to sort out needs and available resources and energy levels.
Develop a trusting relationship while remembering that in abuse situations it is necessary to carefully explain the legal requirements for reporting and the need to involve other agencies.	A trusting relationship provides a foundation for further intervention and creates a climate of caring concern for well-being.
Encourage family conferences with health care providers.	Family conferences give current information and a realistic picture of the condition and caregiving requirements.
Encourage family members to express how caregiving has altered plans, goals, daily routines, and life situation; encourage the ventilation of feelings, emotions, and concerns.	The release of feelings represents the first step in identifying options for management. The validation of feelings, i.e., anger, fatigue, resentment, guilt allays additional stress by preventing the buildup of feelings perceived as negative or not normal.
Help in the identification of current stressors and strains.	Identification of specific stressors is the first step toward solution. Family unity is promoted when members see that what happens to one impacts on all. Unresolved past strains, i.e., work difficulties, in-law or ex-spousal relationship problems are often exacerbated in times of increased stress and crisis.
Encourage realistic expectations of role performances.	A better match between abilities and expectations of role performance lessens the chances of abuse or exploitation and promotes greater role performance satisfaction.

INTERVENTIONS	**R**ATIONALE
Provide linkage to community resources and promote coordination among all resources involved.	Outside resources are essential to family unit functioning. Families benefit from and contribute to the community resource network. Sharing of information for family treatment plans with all agencies involved minimizes the duplication, disruption, and disorganization that can diminish trust and alienate the family.
Promote increased flexibility of roles, rules, and decision making. Address changes in one prioritized area at a time.	Coping requires the ability to try alternative ways of task management and responsibilities.
Refer to protective services in cases of abuse or neglect.	Protective services provide for meeting the legal requirements of the nurse and giving a specific source of help for intervention.
Reinforce and provide feedback on continued utilization of problem-solving skills and prioritization, option identification, decision making, and coping.	The development of problem-solving skills is useful to sort out priorities related to immediate crises and in future need. The number and intensity of stressors and demands placed on families can be overwhelming. Positive feedback reinforces behavior and increases self-esteem.
Develop some predictable routines whenever possible, but address a routine in one mutually decided area at a time, i.e., daily mealtime together, bedtime routine, etc.	Routines provide stability and predictability in times of stress and crisis.
Reinforce knowledge about disease processes, signs and symptoms, treatment modes, and reportable adverse effects.	Knowledge promotes autonomy, increases responsibility for self-care, and reduces anxiety about the unknown.
Teach coping strategies to manage tension and strain.	Alternative ways of coping provide strategies to reduce anxiety and increase feelings of control.
Teach how to utilize relative and friend support for task assistance and comfort.	Task completion and comfort are more easily provided when the load is distributed among family and friends who provide instrumental and emotional support.

REFERENCES/BIBLIOGRAPHY

Bomar, P. (1989). **Nurses and family health promotion: Concepts, assessment, and interventions**. Baltimore: Williams & Wilkins.

* Carey, P., Oberst, M., McCubbin, M., & Hughes, S. (in press). Correlates of caregiving demand and distress in family members caring for patients receiving chemotherapy. **Oncology Nursing Forum**.

Dolan, M. (1990). **Community and home health care plans**. Springhouse, PA: Springhouse Corp.

Friedman, M. (1986). **Family nursing: Theory and assessment.** (2nd ed.). Norwalk, CT: Appleton-Century-Crofts.

Gettrust, K., Ryan, S., & Engelman, D. (Eds.). (1985). **Applied nursing diagnosis: Guides for comprehensive care planning**. Albany, NY: Delmar.

Houldin, A., Saltstein, S., & Ganley, K. (1987). **Nursing diagnosis for wellness: Supporting strengths**. Philadelphia: Lippincott.

Keating, S., & Kelman, G. (1988). **Home health care nursing: Concepts and practice**. Philadelphia: Lippincott.

* McCubbin, M., & Huang, S. (1989). Family strengths in the care of handicapped children: Targets for intervention. **Family Relations, 38,** 436–443.

* McCubbin, M. (1989). Family stress and family strengths: A comparison of single- and two-parent families with handicapped children. **Research in Nursing and Health, 12,** 101–110.

McCubbin, M., & McCubbin, H. (1989). Theoretical orientations to family stress and coping. In C. Figley. (Ed.). **Treating stress in families.** (pp. 3–43). New York: Brunner Mazel.

* McCubbin, M. (1989). Family stress, resources and family types: Chronic illness in children. **Family Relations, 37,** 203–210.

Oberst, M., Hughes, S., Chang, A., & McCubbin, M. (in press). Self care burden, stress appraisal, and mood among persons receiving radiotherapy. **Cancer Nursing**.

Coping, Family: Potential for Growth

A state in which the family is effectively managing the utilization of resources and positive adaptive strategies to simultaneously manage the care of an ill/dependent member and other developmental or situational stressors; the physical and emotional well-being of family members and family system functioning is being maintained.

Marilyn A. McCubbin, R.N., Ph.D.

DEFINING CHARACTERISTICS

Ability to make decisions
Accurate knowledge about condition
and care
Adequate knowledge of available
community resources
Appropriate use of formal and informal
support systems
Asking questions about condition and care
Control over outcomes of life events and
situations
Flexibility in family task assignments so that
work usually gets done

Involvement of dependent member in
decisions affecting care
Maintenance of daily routines
Minimal fatigue
Open communication
Optimism
Realistic priorities in goals and daily
activities
Recognition and reporting of adverse symp-
toms or complications in care
Satisfaction with care
Sense of mastery of home care regimen

CONTRIBUTING FACTORS

Pathophysiological

Minimal health impairment of other members

Psychosociobehavioral

Ability to see new situations as challenges and opportunities for growth

Adequate financial resources and insurance coverage

Clear rules and expectations

Expressions of caring and concern

Openness to new information and resources

Successful management of previous life events and transitions

Work together as unit to problem solve and resolve difficulties

EXPECTED OUTCOMES

The family will continue to deliver care which is safe and appropriate.

Knowledge about health problem is accurately verbalized.

Prescribed treatment regimen and care are done in a safe manner.

Symptoms and changes in condition are appropriately reported.

Physical and emotional needs (i.e., nutrition, sleep, exercise, hygiene, social interaction) are met.

Fears and concerns about care and condition are freely discussed.

Family members will perform care without comprising physical and emotional health.

Stress associated with caregiving is identified.

Feelings about the impact of caregiving on life situations are expressed.

Community resources (i.e., home health aide, homemaker, visiting nurse) are utilized.

Effective coping behaviors are seen.

Health needs (i.e., nutrition and rest) receive attention.

Feelings of control and optimism are maintained.

The family unit will utilize resources and effective coping strategies to reduce stress and manage developmental and situational stressors.

Stressors are identified.

Realistic expectations of situation and roles are maintained.

Problem-solving abilities (accurate definition of the problem, identification of alternate solutions, and consensus) are preserved.

Open communication is maintained.

Flexibility in roles, rules, and decision making is supported.

Predictable family routines continue.

Physical and emotional support is seen.

A hopeful outlook is maintained.

INTERVENTIONS   RATIONALE

Universal

(Note: All interventions in this care plan are listed as universal, since the place of intervention is variable and dependent upon

Interventions	Rationale
each family situation—as the dependent member may or may not be hospitalized.)	
Monitor continued ability to carry out treatment regimen and care.	Ongoing assessment promotes early detection of complications and provides feedback.
Monitor extent to which dependent member's needs are being met.	(Same as above)
Assist family to define present situation and assess the need for additional community resources, i.e., home health aide, homemaker, respite care, extended family, and friend support.	The gathering and utilizing of resources decreases the burden, provides assistance, and expands existing resources which will be useful in future need.
Assist to assess the benefits and costs of existing support network.	Extended family and friend support may be given with an expectation of reciprocity. Obtaining a clear picture of the benefits and costs of existing supports assists the family to sort out needs and available resources and energy levels.
Assess receptivity to making changes in day to day functioning.	The initial reaction to crisis and stress may be to rely on previous patterns of behavior and inter-action; these may need to be altered to manage current stressors.
Explore financial status and pay-ment sources. Consider referral to social services.	Financial resources are quickly exhausted in long term care.
Develop a trust relationship.	Trust creates a climate of caring concern and provides a foundation for further intervention.
Discuss management of emo-tional outbursts, personality changes, mood swings, and memory loss.	Acknowledgement of the upsetting nature of behavior changes and practical suggestions for management eases family strain.

INTERVENTIONS	**R**ATIONALE
Encourage family conferences with health care providers.	Family conferences give current information and a realistic picture of the condition and caregiving requirements.
Encourage family members to express how caregiving has altered plans, goals, daily routines, and life situation; encourage the ventilation of feelings, emotions, and concerns.	The release of feelings represents the first step in identifying options for management. The validation of feelings, i.e., anger, fatigue, resentment, guilt allays additional stress by preventing the buildup of feelings perceived as negative or not normal.
Reemphasize importance of maintaining health promoting behaviors of all family members.	Showing concern acknowledges the contribution and importance of each member. Health promoting behaviors are essential to maintain adequate health and energy levels in this stressful situation.
Help in the identification of current stressors and strains.	Identification of specific stressors is the first step toward solution. Family unity is promoted when members see that what happens to one impacts on all. Unresolved past strains, i.e., work difficulties, in-law or ex-spousal relationship problems are often exacerbated in times of increased stress and crisis.
Encourage realistic expectations of role performances.	A better match between abilities and expectations of role performance promotes greater satisfaction with performance and recognition that "less than perfect" is acceptable.
Provide support and promote coordination for linkage to community resources.	Outside resources are essential to family unit functioning. Families benefit from and contribute to the community resource network. Sharing of information for family treatment plans with all agencies involved minimizes the duplication, disruption, and disorganization that can diminish trust and alienate the family.
Promote ongoing flexibility of roles, rules, and decision making. Address changes in one prioritized area at a time.	Coping requires the ability to try alternative ways of task management and responsibilities.

INTERVENTIONS	**R**ATIONALE
Reinforce and provide feedback on continued utilization of problem-solving skills and prioritization, option identification, and decision making.	Long-term illness places exhausting and overwhelming demands on families due to the number and intensity of inherent stressors. Assistance with problem-solving skills is useful to sort out priorities for the immediate crisis and in future situations. Positive feedback reinforces behavior and increases self-esteem.
Encourage the maintenance of predictable routines whenever possible.	Routines provide stability and predictability in times of stress and crisis.
Encourage the inclusion of the dependent member in activities as health and conditions permit.	Involvement decreases isolation and increases feelings of self-worth and belonging.
Reinforce knowledge about disease processes, signs and symptoms, treatment modes, and reportable adverse effects.	Knowledge promotes autonomy, increases responsibility for self-care, and reduces anxiety about the unknown.
Teach coping strategies to manage tension and strain if previous techniques are no longer effective.	Alternative ways of coping provide strategies to reduce anxiety and increase feelings of control.

REFERENCES/BIBLIOGRAPHY

See bibliography for "Coping, Family: Disabled." (pp. 164–165).

Coping, Impaired Individual

A state in which an individual demonstrates adaptive behaviors and problem solving abilities which are inadequate in meeting life's demands and roles (NANDA, 1990, p. 61).

Kay Koneazny, R.N., M.S.N.

DEFINING CHARACTERISTICS

Alteration in societal participation
Change in usual communication patterns
Destructive behavior toward self or others
Frequent accidents
Frequent illnesses
Inability to meet basic needs

Inability to meet role expectations
Inability to problem solve
Inappropriate use of defense mechanisms
Verbal manipulation
Verbalization of inability to cope or to ask for help

CONTRIBUTING FACTORS

Pathophysiological

Acute/chronic disability
Acute/chronic illness

Psychosociobehavioral

Dysfunctional family system
Inadequate support system
Lack of pertinent knowledge
Maturational crisis

Personal vulnerability
Situational crisis
Unresolved grief

EXPECTED OUTCOMES

Client will demonstrate effective coping behaviors.

Stressor is identified.

Need for a change in coping behaviors is verbalized.

Individual strengths are identified.

Usual coping behaviors are identified.

Coping resources, e.g., written materials, persons who possess the coping skills, are utilized.

Coping alternatives are discussed.

A chosen coping strategy is rehearsed.

The rehearsed coping strategy is utilized in an actual situation.

Feelings and coping effectiveness are discussed with an individual or group.

Client will effectively solve an identified problem.

The steps in the problem-solving process are identified.

The problem is defined.

Application of the steps of the problem-solving process to the problem is outlined.

The problem-solving plan is discussed with an individual or group for feedback and support.

The problem-solving plan is implemented.

Client will make a necessary decision.

Decision to be made is identified.

At least three decision options are identified with another individual or group.

The forces for and against each option are listed.

An option to implement is chosen.

Support/validation for decision made is sought.

INTERVENTIONS   RATIONALE

Universal	
Assess for individual problems/stressors.	Effective solutions/coping strategies cannot be identified if there is not correct identification of the problem or stressor.
Assess individual for usual coping behaviors.	Identification of personal coping behaviors can lead to strengthening of the effective behaviors and elimination of those which are not effective.
Assess perception of significant others as sources of emotional support.	These data are essential in order to effectively utilize significant others to support recovery/growth.
Evaluate response to limit setting.	Response will indicate effectiveness of limits chosen.

INTERVENTIONS	RATIONALE
Monitor for changes in coping behavior.	If there is no change, the reason for this must be evaluated and new interventions introduced.
Monitor how perceptions are validated prior to conclusions being drawn.	Inaccurate perceptions may lead to choice of inappropriate coping behaviors.
Provide an attitude of acceptance.	Acceptance promotes trust, which is needed as a basis for taking the risk to try new behaviors.
Assist to identify and utilize individual strengths.	An awareness of one's own strengths can increase the likelihood that one will draw upon them.
Provide outlet for expression of fears/anxieties using one-to-one time, journaling.	Fears and anxieties are obstacles to change. Expression can provide relief and may result in additional emotional support.
Set limits on inappropriate coping behaviors.	Consistent limit setting can decrease ineffective coping behaviors.
Assist to role play/rehearse coping behaviors.	Practice builds not only skill but also personal confidence.
Assist to identify coping/ decision options.	Often one's perception of personal options is limited. Another person or group can usually identify many others to provide wider choice.
Encourage to self-acknowledge coping successes.	Self-acknowledgement is part of the process of integration of new behavior into one's repertoire.
Assist to identify probable sabotage behavior.	Since personal sabotage is inevitable in behavior change, it is beneficial for the client to identify the sabotage behavior beforehand for increased self-awareness when the sabotage behavior is employed.
Provide materials on assertive-ness and discuss these.	When coping is impaired, there is often a knowledge deficit related to assertiveness.
Teach relaxation techniques.	Relaxation reduces stress and, once learned, constitutes an independent coping strategy.

INTERVENTIONS	**R**ATIONALE
Teach steps of the problem-solving process.	Problem solving is one effective coping strategy.
Inpatient Evaluate effectiveness of coping strategy role plays/rehearsals.	Correction here can increase potential effectiveness in the actual situation.
Encourage/provide physical outlets for stress release.	Physical exercise can discharge stress and produce mood elevating endorphins.
Point out effective/ineffective coping behaviors as they appear.	Over time, identification of behaviors can increase the accuracy of self-monitoring for coping effectiveness.
Community Health/ Home Care	None

REFERENCES/BIBLIOGRAPHY

Doenges, M.E., Townsend, M.C., & Moorhouse, M.F. (1989). **Psychiatric care plans: Guidelines for client care**. Philadelphia: Davis.

Gettrust, K.V., Ryan, S.C., & Engleman, D.S. (Eds.). (1985). **Applied nursing diagnosis: Guides for comprehensive care planning**. Albany, NY: Delmar.

North American Nursing Diagnosis Association. (1990). **Taxonomy I** (Rev. 1990). St. Louis: NANDA.

Denial, Impaired

A state in which an individual consciously or unconsciously attempts to disavow the knowledge or meaning of an event to reduce anxiety/fear to the detriment of health (NANDA, 1990, p. 64).

M. Kathleen Eilers, B.S.N., M.S.N.

DEFINING CHARACTERISTICS

Delay in seeking or refusal of health care attention
Denial of anxiety and fear when in a threatening situation
Expression of concerns and questions but no acknowledgement of anxiety or fear
Lack of perception of danger of symptoms
Minimization or lack of acknowledgement of presence of symptoms

CONTRIBUTING FACTORS

Pathophysiological

None

Psychosociobehavioral

Reception of information perceived as personally threatening

EXPECTED OUTCOMES

Client will have low or moderate anxiety.
    Denial as a short-term response to life-threatening illness is considered beneficial.
    Denial which allows for positive thinking and hopefulness is supported as an important psychological resource.
    Client remains defended with anxiety under control.
Client will be able to utilize facts of health status to achieve full health potential.
    Communication of the facts of illness takes place in a supportive context.

185

Information about health status is used in a way that allows for compliance with appropriate medical/nursing regimen.

INTERVENTIONS

RATIONALE

Interventions	Rationale
Universal	
Evaluate and monitor degree of denial and its effectiveness as a coping strategy.	At certain stages in the adaptation process, denial is a useful and healthy coping mechanism which permits hope to remain.
Never confront with the fact that denial is being used.	Confrontation leads to high levels of anxiety which are counter-therapeutic to the healing process.
Support appropriate behaviors. Provide opportunities to express any conscious fears or anxieties.	Verbalization allows for catharsis and development of a sense of mastery.
Provide with specific information or reassurance as requested or as appropriate.	Information and reassurance reduce anxiety.
Provide an environment that is supportive of movement between full and partial denial, as appropriate.	Some degree of denial is useful in adaptation.
Refer to psychiatric/mental health clinical nurse specialist if level of denial interferes with seeking or utilizing appropriate health care.	Specialized skills and/or training may be required to deal with significant psychopathology.
Inpatient	None
Community Health/ Home Care	None

REFERENCES/BIBLIOGRAPHY

Kanter, F.H., & Goldstein, A. (Eds.). (1975). **Helping people change**. Elmsford, NY: Pergamon.

Kolb, L.C., Keith, H., & Brodie, H. (1982). **Modern clinical psychiatry.** (10th ed.). Philadelphia: Saunders.

McFarland, G.K., & McFarlane, E.A. (1989). **Nursing diagnosis and intervention**. Philadelphia: Mosby.

Millon, T. (1969). **Modern psychopathology. A biosocial approach to maladaptive learning and functioning**. Philadelphia: Saunders.

North American Nursing Diagnosis Association. (1990). **Taxonomy I** (Rev. 1990). St. Louis: NANDA.

Robinson, L. (1977). **Psychiatric nursing as a human experience.** (2nd ed.). Philadelphia: Saunders.

Stuart, G., & Sundeen, S. (1983). **Principles and practice of psychiatric nursing.** (2nd ed.). St. Louis: Mosby.

Diarrhea

A state in which an individual experiences an increased stool liquidity and increased frequency of passage of stool.

Kathleen Fitzgerald, R.N., M.S., C.E.T.N.

DEFINING CHARACTERISTICS

Abdominal cramping
Increase in the fluid content of the stool characterized by liquid, semi-liquid, loose, pasty, or mushy stools
Increases in the number of bowel movements per day

CONTRIBUTING FACTORS

Pathophysiological

Altered motility as caused by increased transit time through the intestine, which may result in diarrhea but seldom results in significant malabsorption. Examples are:
  Anal sphincter dysfunction
  Cancer of gastrointestinal tract
  Diabetic neuropathy
  Fecal impaction
  Gastrointestinal hemorrhage from peptic ulcer or esophageal varices
  Ileal-cecal valve resection
  Ileus
  Irritable bowel syndrome (also called functional bowel disease)
  Medications, e.g., Quinidine, Digoxin, Reglan
  Surgery: post-gastrectomy, post-vagotomy, ileal resection
Osmotic diarrhea as caused by the presence in the gastrointestinal tract of poorly absorbable substances with high osmolality. Examples are:
  Disaccharidase deficiencies: sucrase or lactase deficiency
  Excess sorbitol or mannitol ingestion: chewing gum or artificial sweeteners
  High osmolality tube feeding products

Malabsorption syndromes: chronic radiation enteritis, chronic inflammatory bowel disease, short bowel syndrome, chronic pancreatic insufficiency

Medications: lactulose, magnesium sulfate, antacids containing magnesium

Post gastrectomy/vagotomy

Secretory diarrhea as caused by decreased fluid absorption in the intestine and increased intestinal secretion of fluid. Examples are:

AIDS enteropathy: diarrhea in AIDS clients without known infectious cause

Antibiotic-induced enterocolitis (Pseudomembranous colitis)

Bile acids not absorbed due to ileal resection

Cancer treatment: acute radiation enteritis, chemotherapeutic agents

Enterotoxins: viral, bacterial, parasitic, protozoal, fungal infections commonly include viral (flu), Campylobacter, Shigella, Salmonella, Enterotoxigenic E. coli, (traveler's diarrhea), Giardia, Clostridium difficile, Candida, Entamoeba histolytica, Cryptosporidium, and CMV (cytomegalovirus)

Laxative overuse or abuse

Other diseases that may exhibit secretory diarrhea as a symptom include: inflammatory bowel disease; intestinal lymphoma; hyperthyroidism; Zollinger-Ellison syndrome; carcinoid syndrome; medullary carcinoma of thyroid; collagen vascular diseases such as scleraderma or systemic lupus erythematosus

Psychosociobehavioral

Anxiety, stress

Irritable bowel syndrome is frequently exacerbated by stress

Laxative abuse

EXPECTED OUTCOMES

Acute diarrhea:

Diarrhea will resolve with a return to normal stool consistency and frequency.

Adequate hydration and nutrition is maintained during the acute phase of the illness.

The signs and symptoms requiring further medical attention are recognized.

Practices which will prevent the spread of infectious diarrhea are performed.

Chronic diarrhea:

Strategies will be developed for symptom control that will enhance the quality of life.

Understanding of the cause of the diarrhea is verbalized.

Complications such as perianal skin breakdown and infection are prevented.

Understanding of the medical treatment regime, i.e., medications and dietary alterations, is verbalized.

Signs and symptoms of exacerbation of chronic illness that would necessitate seeking medical attention are recognized.

INTERVENTIONS	RATIONALE
Universal	
Assess the description of the diarrhea in regards to the timing; gradual or sudden onset, frequency of stools, volume, jaundice, and aggravating or relieving symptoms such as certain foods or medications.	A detailed description of the diarrhea and its onset will provide valuable information in the diagnosis of the cause.
Monitor the vital signs and hydration status by measuring the temperature, orthostatic (lying, sitting, standing) blood pressure and pulse, daily weight, oral intake, and urine and stool volume. Symptoms of lightheadedness or dizziness need to be identified.	Large volume of stool lost will cause dehydration. A sudden weight loss over a few days is a sensitive indicator of dehydration. Postural hypotension occurs in dehydration and is seen as a drop in the blood pressure with a rise in pulse when moving from a lying to sitting or standing position. Fever may indicate an infectious etiology or may be a manifestation of severe dehydration.
Institute enteric isolation practices when etiology is unknown.	Infections diarrhea is transmitted by fecal-oral contamination.
Provide instructions about the cause and treatment of the diarrhea using printed client education or written instructions if they are available.	Clients benefit from written instructions that contain specific treatment information. There is a list in the bibliography of publications that can be obtained from a variety of organizations.
Assist in adapting the treatment and dietary plans into the daily routine by offering suggestions, such as taking the antidiarrheal medication before leaving the house to prevent sudden bathroom stops while out shopping.	Clients benefit by information provided with realistic examples of application to their lives.
Inpatient:	
ACUTE DIARRHEA: Assess for the cause of sudden onset of diarrhea in the hospitalized client by determining if risk	Some causes of hospital-acquired diarrhea can be prevented or treated by nursing interventions.

INTERVENTIONS	**R**ATIONALE
factors such as medication therapy, especially antibiotics or antacids, tube feedings, ileus, or fecal impaction exist.	
Assess for antibiotic-associated diarrhea by sending stool samples for fecal leukocytes, culture and sensitivity, and Clostridium difficile toxin. Consult the laboratory for proper collection of the sample.	Fecal leukocytes, presence of white cells in the stool, indicate inflammation and possible infection in the colon. Untreated hospital-acquired infections such as Clostridium difficile may result in pseudomembranous colitis, which has a high mortality rate in the acutely ill. Candida albicans, a possible cause of diarrhea, can be treated easily with medication.
Assess for possible fecal impaction by performing a digital rectal examination which reveals hard, formed stool.	Advanced age, immobilty, and medications such as opiate pain relievers and iron supplements may cause decreased bowel motility, constipation, and fecal impaction. Liquid stool then leaks around the impaction.
Administer softening enemas, e.g., mineral oil, or extract the hard stool manually.	Mineral oil acts on the surface of the hard stool, softening it for easier removal. Soap suds enemas may also be used with caution, as the soap may irritate the colonic mucosa causing colitis.
Administer stool softeners, bulk-forming medications, or modify the diet to include more fluid and fiber to prevent constipation and fecal impaction.	Preventing constipation will prevent fecal impaction.
Collaborate with the dietitian in tube feeding-induced diarrhea to adjust the type of the product, rate, or concentration of formula.	Diarrhea associated with tube feedings is usually related to hyperosmolar formula concentrations (>500 mosm/kg water), rapid infusions (>80 ml/min), bacterial contamination, low albumin levels (<2.0), and medications, e.g., magnesium-containing antacids, sorbitol-based drugs, and Reglan.

INTERVENTIONS	RATIONALE
Initiate, in cases of severe diarrhea, bowel rest (NPO or clear liquid diet), intravenous hydration, and comfort measures during the diagnositic testing phase to decrease bowel stimulation and restore hydration status.	Acute diarrhea usually responds to elimination of stimulation to the gastrointestinal tract for a short period of time. Adequate hydration by oral or intravenous route must be achieved during this time. In the cases where prolonged bowel rest is required or malnutrition is moderate to severe, total parenteral nutrition may be needed.
Administer anti-diarrheal agents once the etiology has been determined.	The antidiarrheal agents will provide comfort and minimize stool volume loss.
Administer the least amount of medication needed to stop the diarrhea.	Bulk-forming and pectin-based medications are not recommended with tube-fed clients because of tube clogging. Other types of medications decrease bowel motility and overusage may cause ileus or constipation.
Provide sitz baths, witch hazel compresses, ointments containing lidocaine anesthetic agents or hydrocortisone when mild perianal irritation or swollen, burning, or itching hemorrhoids occur.	Frequent diarrhea causes perianal irritation and swelling of hemorrhoids. Consistency in local care can alleviate irritation and prevent complications such as infection.
Protect the perianal skin by gentle cleansing with water, mild soap, or periwash products and the application of skin barrier ointments, creams, or spray-on protective barriers.	Perianal skin breakdown frequently occurs with diarrhea in both the continent and incontinent. Immunocompromised clients have delayed healing and are at risk for perianal infections, especially herpes and candida.
Collaborate with the dietitian in the advancement of the diet from clear liquids to a soft, lactose-free, caffeine-free, low-fiber diet.	Caffeine, fresh fruits and vegetables, and other high-fiber foods can be irritating and stimulating to the bowel, causing increased peristalsis and exacerbation of the diarrhea. In acute diarrheal disorders, the lactose sugar found in milk products is poorly absorbed and may cause gas, bloating, and diarrhea.

INTERVENTIONS	RATIONALE
Instruct on diet advancement, e.g., add one new food at a time, observing the effect if any on the stool frequency or liquidity. Provide a written list of the high-fiber and bowel-stimulating foods that should be added gradually back to the diet.	Providing specific guidelines will increase the ability to make informed decisions on diet.
Provide guidelines regarding the administration of the medications in relation to the diarrheal symptoms, e.g., appropriate timing for the antidiarrheal medications in daily routines.	Clients benefit by information provided with realistic examples of application to their daily routines.
Discuss the signs and symptoms of exacerbation or complications, specifically those requiring immediate medical attention.	Providing information on potential problems and resources available will assist in decision making regarding the illness and may prevent the development of complications of dehydration and malnutrition.
Initiate a home health care referral when further diet or medication instruction or monitoring of hydration, nutritional status, or tube feeding tolerance is required.	The elderly, handicapped, individual living alone without support from friends or family may require assistance in following the prescribed medical treatment plan or diet.

Inpatient:

CHRONIC DIARRHEA:
Assess for signs and symptoms of weight loss and nutritional deficiencies.

Chronic diarrhea with weight loss and nutritional deficiencies usually indicates a disruption of the gastrointestinal tract caused by a malignancy; malabsorptive disorder, e.g., pancreatic insufficiency, AIDS enteropathy or opportunistic infection, short bowel syndrome, scleraderma, chronic inflammatory disease; previous surgery; cancer therapies; eating disorders; or other diseases. Chronic diarrhea with minimal or no weight loss is usually psychosociobehavioral.

INTERVENTIONS	RATIONALE
Provide information regarding the diagnostic testing procedures in the diagnostic workup. Test may include the upper and lower gastrointestinal barium x-rays, upper and lower gastrointestinal endoscopic procedures with biopsies, abdominal CT scans or ultrasound, small bowel biopsy, pancreatic function tests, multiple stool collections, fecal fat collections, and hydrogen ion lactose or Dxylose breath test.	Providing both descriptive and sensory (what will be seen, felt, and heard) information will decrease anxiety.
Collaborate with the dietitian to maximize nutritional intake, e.g., high protein, high-calorie foods that will not exacerbate the diarrhea when malabsorption is present.	Chronic diarrhea frequently results in significant malabsorption with weight loss, debilitation, and multiple nutritional deficiencies. Combining medications to treat the underlying disorder and specialized formulas to supplement the diet are usually necessary to nutritionally replete and maintain the undernourished. Home total parenteral nutrition is utilized for severe malnutrition and/or malabsorption.
Provide information on the etiology and treatment of malabsorption disorder including diet and medication instructions.	Comprehension of the effect of the malabsorption disorder on the intestinal tract may assist in the understanding of the complex treatment and diet plan.
Discuss strategies to control symptoms and incorporate the treatment and diet plan into the daily routines.	Practical explanations and suggestions are beneficial to assist in managing a chronic, debilitating illness and still maintain quality of life.
Initiate a home health care referral when moderate to severe disability or malnutrition is present.	Reinforcement of the medical and dietary treatment plan once home is optimal especially if it is a complex regimen requiring reorganization of lifestyle and necessitates the support of others in the home. If home total parenteral nutrition is instituted, extensive teaching is required.

INTERVENTIONS	RATIONALE
Assist in identification of the relationship of the diarrhea to aggravating factors, e.g., stress, particular foods, and anxiety in those cases where there is minimal nutritional deficit.	Chronic irritable bowel syndrome (IBS)is a condition of altered colonic motility that is frequently exacerbated with medications, stress, anxiety, and foods.
Provide information on diet modification (high fiber, low lactose), life-style alterations (stress reduction strategies), and medicaitons to control the diarrhea.	High-fiber diets, bulk-forming agents, antispasmotic medications, and decrease in nervous stimulation (stress reduction) to the bowel assist in controlling hypermotility.
Provide the elderly with information on establishing a bowel program, including high-fiber diet, increased fluid intake, increased exercise, and use of bulk-forming medications—instead of managing constipation with laxatives and enemas which frequently result in diarrhea.	Gastrointestinal motility decreases with age and may be aggravated by medications, decrease in activity, and dietary alterations resulting in constipation, which is frequently treated by laxatives or enemas. Chronic use of laxatives and enemas is not recommended because of long-term side effects on the bowel.
Initiate appropriate referrals to mental health professionals or eating disorder programs when chronic diarrhea is associated with laxative abuse and eating disorders.	The diarrhea in chronic laxative abuse associated with eating disorders will be treated by managing the underlying psychological disorder.
Community Health/ Home Care Evaluate the new onset of diarrhea for degree of severity, possible cause, and necessity for referral to a physician for diagnostic evaluation and treatment.	Severe diarrhea can quickly result in dehydration.
Assess for perianal irritation and evaluate for potential perianal skin breakdown and infection.	Immunocompromised clients (AIDS, cancer) are at risk for perianal skin breakdown and infection because of impaired healing ability.

INTERVENTIONS	**R**ATIONALE
Provide instructions on maintaining oral hydration and monitoring signs and symptoms to prevent dehydration.	Maintain hydration with clear liquids such as broth, tea, jello, juice, non-cola soft drinks, Gatorade, other sport supplements, or Pedialyte rehydration fluid to minimize irritation to the bowel during the course of the diarrhea. Many of these liquids also provide electrolytes that are lost with the diarrhea.
Instruct on the advancement of the diet when the diarrhea has subsided to include soft, low-fiber, and low-lactose foods.	High-fiber foods may cause irritation and stimulation of the bowel, exacerbating the diarrhea.
Provide instructions on the proper cleansing of tube-feeding equipment and handling of the formula.	Bacterial contamination of the equipment or inadequate rinsing after cleaning, leaving a soap residue, can cause diarrhea. Bacterial contamination of formulas may occur during preparation, with improper storage, or if left hanging in the tube-feeding bag for greater than six hours.
Instruct clients in rural areas in methods to prevent and observe for potential contaminants of home-canned products.	Botulism may result from contaminated home-canned products.
Instruct clients in areas of natural disasters or power failures in methods to ensure safety of food and water.	Products without the proper refrigeration may be contaminated with bacteria that will cause diarrhea. Water may also be contaminated and require boiling before use.
Instruct clients with infectious diarrhea to prevent spread to other members of the household by careful handwashing, proper cleaning of the bathroom facilities, not sharing eating utensils or toothbrushes, and not allowing the infected person to prepare food.	Infectious diarrheas are spread through the fecal-oral contamination route. Good handwashing and proper food handling will minimize exposure to others.

REFERENCES/BIBLIOGRAPHY

Basch, A. (1987). Changes in elimination. **Seminars in Oncology Nursing, 3,** 287–292.

DiJohn, D., & Levine, M.M. (1988). Treatment of diarrhea. **Infectious Disease Clinics of North America, 2,** 719–745.

Edes, T.E., Walk, B.E., & Austin, J.L. (1990). Diarrhea in tube-fed patients: Feeding formula not necessarily the cause. **American Journal of Medicine, 88,** 911–93.

Fine, K.D., Krejs, G.J., & Fordtran, J.S. (1989) Diarrhea. In Sleisinger, M.H., & Fordtran, J.S. (Eds.). **Gastrointestinal Disease**. Philadelphia: Saunders.

Hahn, K. (1987). Think twice about diarrhea. **Nursing, 87** (9), 78–80.

* Hartfield, M., Cason, C. (1981) Effect of information on emotional response during barium enema. **Nursing Research, 30,** 151–155.

* Horsely, J.A., Crane, J., & Haller, K.B. (1981). **Reducing diarrhea in tube-fed patients**. New York: Grune & Stratton.

Johansen, J.F., & Sonnenberg, A. (1990). Efficient management of diarrhea in the Acquired Immunodeficiency Syndrome (AIDS). **Annals of Internal Medicine, 112,** 942–948.

Maresca, J.G., & Strinari, S. (1986). Assessment and management of acute diarrhea illness in adults. **Nurse Practitioner, 11,** 15–28.

National Institutes of Health. (1985). Traveler's diarrhea. **National Institutes of Health, Consensus Development Conference Statement, 5** (8).

North American Nursing Diagnosis Association. (1990). **Taxonomy I** (Rev. 1990). St. Louis: NANDA.

* Smith, C.E., et al. (1990). Diarrhea associated with tube feeding in mechanically ventilated critically ill patients. **Nursing Research, 39** (3), 148–152.

Strauss, A.L. (1975). **Chronic illness and the quality of life**. St. Louis: Mosby.

In addition to the above references, the following client education materials are available:

Janowitz, H.D. (1987). **Your gut feelings**. New York: Oxford.

National Digestive Diseases Information Clearinghouse. 1255 23rd St. NW, Suite 275; Washington, D.C. 20037. Fact sheets available include: Lactose intolerance; Diarrhea: infectious and other causes; Inflammatory bowel disease; What is irritable bowel syndrome?; IBD and IBS: Two very different problems.

National Foundation for Ileitis and Colitis, 444 Park Ave. South, New York, NY 10016. Pamphlets available.

Disuse Syndrome: Risk

A state in which an individual is at risk for deterioration of body systems as the result of prescribed or unavoidable musculoskeletal inactivity (NANDA, 1990, p. 44). (Also see Physical Mobility: Impaired.)

Brenda S. Nichols, R.N., D.N.Sc.

RISK FACTORS

Pathophysiological

Altered level of consciousness
(e.g. Alzheimer's disease, cerebrovascular accident, coma)
Amputation
Arthritis
Brain tumor
Cerebral palsy

Immobilization of a body part
Neuromuscular disorders (e.g. Spina bifida, spinal cord injury)
Paralysis
Prescribed bedrest
Severe pain
Terminal diseases (particularly cancer)
Trauma

Psychosociobehavioral

Hopelessness
Ineffective coping

Powerlessness
Severe depression

EXPECTED OUTCOMES

Client will experience no complications of immobility.
Circulatory system:
Pulses (pedal and radial) are normal.
No edema is present in feet and/or legs.

No evidence of venous thrombosis is present. No pain in calves, thighs or in thoracic region.
No falls due to orthostatic hypotension (no dizziness, etc., upon ambulation) are experienced.
Gastrointestinal system:
   Normal bowel pattern, sounds, formed semiformed stools (at least every third day) is maintained.
   Normal appetite and adequate dietary intake are achieved.
   No weight is gained due to decreased energy expenditure.
Genitourinary system:
   An adequate urinary output is maintained.
   No urinary tract retention or infection is experienced.
   Adequate hydration is maintained.
   No renal calculi develop.
Integumentary system:
   Intact skin is maintained with no reddened areas.
   Skin turgor is normal.
Musculoskeletal system:
   Muscle strength and tone are maintained.
   Joint mobility and flexibility are maintained.
   There are no contractures.
Neurological system:
   No changes in level of consciousness are experienced.
   A sense of hopelessness is not developed or maintained.
Respiratory system:
   Normal chest expansion is maintained.
   Auscultation of the chest reveals no rales or rhonchi.
   No pulmonary embolism develop.
   Adequate oxygenation is maintained to peripheral tissues.
   Emotional, intellectual and social functioning are maintained.
   Effective coping strategies are used.

INTERVENTIONS

RATIONALE

Universal

Assess and document the following:

- Muscle strength, range of motion of joints
- Signs of thrombosis—e.g. calf pain (positive Homan's sign), warmth, swelling, tenderness and/or redness in the extremity
- Skin condition (redness, irritation, dryness, pressure points— heels, elbows, buttocks, etc.), peripheral pulses and presence/absence of edema

Baseline data provide information for accurate interpretation and prompt intervention, which are essential to avoid further complications.

INTERVENTIONS	**R**ATIONALE
• Bowel elimination pattern • Urinary elimination (e.g., daily output, time and amount of voiding, bladder distention before and after voiding, color, odor, or cloudiness) • Coping mechanisms and psychosocial functioning • Chest excursion, rate and rhythm, use of accessory muscles	
Avoid straining when defecating or moving.	The Valsalva maneuver can increase cardiac workload.
Assist with frequent position changes—e.g., sidelying, back, Fowler's.	Position changes promote venous circulation and prevent venous stasis.
Perform active and passive range-of-motion activities.	Exercises promote circulation in legs, prevent venous stasis, and inhibit the formation of thrombus in extremities.
Use anti-embolism stockings (obtain order if indicated).	Stockings promote the return of blood to the heart, preventing venous stasis. However, external pressure on veins can totally or partially occlude circulation in the extremities.
Ambulate after changing position gradually (from supine position to a Fowler's position to dangling on the side of the bed prior to ambulation).	Changing position prior to ambulation allows the circulatory system to adjust and avoids orthostatic hypotension.
Plan activities to provide periods of rest as well as a gradual increase in daily activity level.	The body requires alternating periods of rest and activity. Increasing the activity level enhances muscle tone and prevents muscle weakness.
Encourage client to yawn several times per day. (Note: If you yawn, the client will also yawn.)	A yawn encourages a deep breath and expands the lungs. Yawning also relaxes smooth muscles.

INTERVENTIONS	RATIONALE
Encourage fluids of choice to total 2000 cc/day. (Contraindications: cardiac and renal/liver insufficiencies or failure, preeclampsia, eclampsia, actual or risk for increased intracranial pressure, or other fluid restrictions.)	Adequate fluids ensure adequate hydration for moist respirations, renal clearance and aids in the prevention of constipation.
Provide well-balanced diet high in protein, fiber, and calories and low in calcium. (Note: Within normal dietary restrictions.)	Proteins are needed due to the negative nitrogen balance being experienced. High-fiber content in the diet aids in maintaining normal bowel elimination. Avoid additional calcium intake due to the increased risk of renal calculi.
Serve small frequent meals in a pleasant environment.	Anorexia is common for the immobile; serving small portions of foods in a pleasant environment may encourage better eating.
Provide privacy and proper positioning to facilitate elimination. Administer stool softeners, suppositories, or laxatives as ordered and indicated.	Each individual has a different bowel elimination pattern. Stool softeners, suppositories, and laxatives aid in elimination.
Apply lotion to red or irritated areas.	Lotion and massage deter breakdown of the skin.
Use heel and elbow protectors. Use pressure-reducing or equalizing beds.	Pressure beds, etc. relieve venous stasis and prevent skin breakdown.
Provide frequent social interactions with staff and family.	Socialization helps prevent depression and a sense of hopelessness.
Encourage diversional activities—magazines, television, handicrafts, cards, or other games.	Activities are designed to help cope with immobility.
Teach client and significant other range-of-motion, leg exercises, and quadricep setting exercises (if capable).	Exercise encourages blood flow to extremities and promotes muscle tone.
Teach client and significant other to turn, cough, deep	These activities (coughing, deep breathing, and use of the incentive spirometer) clear the airway

INTERVENTIONS

RATIONALE

INTERVENTIONS	RATIONALE
breathe, and use of an incentive spirometer.	and provide for chest expansion, which prevents pulmonary complications.
Inpatient Monitor clotting times.	Accelerated clotting time encourages thrombus formation.
Avoid use of knee gatch on bed.	Total or partial occlusion of the vessels is caused by external pressure on the veins.
Administer anticoagulants as ordered.	Therapeutic action of an anticoagulant is to prevent or resolve thrombus formation.
Community Health/ Home Health Teach family/significant other NEVER to rub legs if complaints of pain or aching are present.	Pain may indicate thrombus formation and friction could cause an embolism to be released.
Teach client to report chest pain, any temperature change, leg cramps, productive cough or urinary frequency, burning or flank pain to the physician.	These signs and symptoms can indicate thrombus, emboli, or urinary problems.

REFERENCES/BIBLIOGRAPHY

Beare, P.G., & Myers, J.L. (1990). **Principles and practices of adult health nursing.** St. Louis: Mosby.

Carpenito, L.J. (1987). **Nursing diagnosis: Application to clinical practice.** (2nd ed.). Philadelphia: Lippincott.

Gordon, M. (1987). **Nursing diagnosis: Application and process.** (2nd ed.). New York: McGraw-Hill.

Guyton, A.C. (1981). **Textbook of medical physiology.** (6th ed.). Philadelphia: Saunders.

Jennings, M.C. (1988). **Nursing care planning guides for home health care.** Baltimore: Williams & Wilkins.

Lentz, M. (1981). Selected aspects of deconditioning secondary to immobilization. **Nursing Clinics of North America, 16,** 729–737.

McKenry, L.M., & Salerno, E. (1989). **Mosby's pharmacology in nursing.** (17th ed.). St. Louis: Mosby.

North American Nursing Diagnosis Association. (1990). **Taxonomy I** (Rev. 1990). St. Louis: NANDA.

Olson, E.V. (1967). The hazards of immobility. **American Journal of Nursing, 67** (4), 780–797.

Sundberg, M.C. (1989). **Fundamentals of nursing.** (2nd ed.). Boston: Jones & Bartlett.

Taylor, C., Lillis, C., & LeMone, P. (1989). **Fundamentals of nursing.** Philadelphia: Lippincott.

Weinberg, L.K. (1989). Potential for disuse syndrome. In McFarland, G.K., & McFarlane, E.A. **Nursing diagnosis and intervention: Planning for patient care.** St. Louis: Mosby.

Diversional Activity Deficit

A state in which an individual experiences a decreased stimulation from or interest or engagement in recreational or leisure activities (NANDA, 1990, p. 76).

Marilyn J. Rantz, R.N., M.S.N., N.H.A.

• • • • • • • • • • • • • •

DEFINING CHARACTERISTICS

Disinterested in surroundings
Fatigues easily, limited energy to participate
        in group activities offered
Frequent daytime napping
Isolates self in room

Perception of time passing slowly
Refuses to go to therapeutic activities offered
Statements regarding: boredom, wish there
        was something to do, usual
        hobbies cannot be undertaken

CONTRIBUTING FACTORS

Pathophysiological

Impaired mobility
Long–term illness
Loss of physical ability to perform preferred activities
Sensory deficit

Psychosociobehavioral

Depression
Environmental lack of diversional activity,
        as in long-term hospitalization,
        frequent lengthy treatments

Fatigue
Former lifestyle
Personal preference

EXPECTED OUTCOMES

Client will actively participate in a therapeutic recreational activity of choice at least (frequency) per week.

Simple, one-step directions in activities are followed.

Conversation regarding therapeutic recreational activities is initiated.

Schedule of therapeutic activities is reviewed regularly.

INTERVENTIONS	RATIONALE
Universal	
Obtain a comprehensive activity assessment, e.g., past hobbies, view of current activity level, likes, dislikes, and hobbies which can be continued at this time and later.	Information from a comprehensive assessment can guide selection of activities which the client is more likely to engage in.
Assist to recognize the need for diversional activity.	Unless a need is recognized, participation in an activity is unlikely.
Assist in selection of an activity that is seen as having value and importance.	Valued activities support motivation toward accomplishing them. Activity may then invoke feelings of productivity.
Assist in selection of an activity in which physical engagement is possible.	Physical limitations and endurance must be considered for activity to be possible.
Inpatient	
Assess activity tolerance and previous activities that can be considered within the level of tolerance, e.g., passive activities such as radio, talking, books, reading, puzzles, and television as low-energy options. Encourage family or significant other to bring in appropriate hobbies from home.	Continuing "normal" hobbies assists in reinforcing "recovery" and/or "normal" perspectives of self and self-worth.

Interventions	Rationale
• Provide volunteer visitor for long-staying clients with limited family, significant other, or community support system • Invite and encourage attendance in scheduled therapeutic recreation activities of interest • Conduct 1:1 staff visits each week to encourage involvement in activities of choice • Use kind, firm approach to encourage time in day area after meals • Offer reminders regarding regularly scheduled activities • Provide assistance to and from activities for clients with low energy	Visitors, whether staff, volunteers, or other clients, provide social interaction, which aids overall mental/physical condition.
Encourage interaction with pets in long-term care facility.	Involvement in pet care can encourage feelings of responsibility and productivity. Developing a relationship with a pet can improve communication and involvement with other clients, staff, and family members.
Encourage outdoor walks or assist in wheelchair for outdoor activities.	Outdoor activities increase feelings of well-being and normalcy.
Respect the right to choose to refuse activities.	Activities need to be personally meaningful to derive the most enjoyment from them.
Encourage reminiscence.	Reflecting upon past experiences and successes validates self-worth and feelings of adequacy and value.
Encourage conversation about current events.	Discussing current events facilitates involvement in issues outside the immediate health care environment, which encourages feelings of normalcy and/or recovery.

INTERVENTIONS	**R**ATIONALE
Encourage to pace activities to tolerance.	Bodily requirement for alternating periods of rest and activity is heightened during periods of illness.
Community Health/ Home Care Assess environmental constraints to resuming activities of interest.	Minor modifications may provide access to prior activities of interest.
Consult occupational therapy as appropriate to assist in resuming activities of interest.	Professional consultation can provide guidance in activity selection and modifications necessary for resuming activities of interest.
Facilitate referral for volunteer visitor for clients with limited family or community support system.	Visitors provide social interaction and stimulate client mentally/physically to improve overall condition.

REFERENCES/BIBLIOGRAPHY

Baker, N. (July 1985). Reminiscing in group therapy for self-worth. **Journal of Gerontological Nursing, 11** (7), 21–24.

Beck, P. (1982). Two successful interventions in nursing homes: The therapeutic effects of cognitive activity. **The Gerontologist, 22** (4), 378–383.

Bulechek, G., & McCloskey, J. (1985). **Nursing interventions: Treatments for nursing diagnoses**. Philadelphia: Saunders.

Cook, J. (1984). Reminiscing: How it can help confused nursing home residents. **Social Casework, 65** (2), 90–93.

Cusack, D., & Smith, E. (1984). **Pets and the elderly—The therapeutic bond**. New York: Hawthorne.

Ebersole, P., & Hess, P. (1981). **Toward healthy aging human needs and nursing response**. St. Louis: Mosby.

Gettrust, K.V., Ryan, S.C., & Engelman, D.S. (1985). **Applied nursing diagnosis: Guides for comprehensive care planning**. Albany, NY: Delmar.

Goodwin, D. (1985). Innovative "resident volunteer" programming. **Activities Adaptation and Aging, 6** (3), 69–71.

North American Nursing Diagnosis Association. (1990). **Taxonomy I** (Rev. 1990). St. Louis: NANDA.

Rantz, M. (1986). Unpublished data of Diversional activity deficit care plans prepared for geriatric patients from 1983–1986 in a 328-bed midwestern long-term care facility. Elkhorn, WI.

Dressing/Grooming Deficit

A state in which an individual experiences an impaired ability to perform or complete dressing and grooming activities independently (NANDA, 1990, p. 84).

Suellyn Ellerbe, R.N., M.N.
Carol Dickel, R.N.
Rosemary J. McKeighen, R.N., Ph.D., F.A.A.N.
Peg. A. Mehmert, R.N., C., M.S.N.
Dianne C. Kolb, R.N., B.A.

DEFINING CHARACTERISTICS

Impaired ability to put on or take off items of clothing

Impaired ability to obtain or replace articles of clothing

Impaired ability to secure clothing

Inability to maintain personally satisfying appearance

CONTRIBUTING FACTORS

Pathophysiological

Activity intolerance
Altered strength and endurance
Discomfort
Mobility impairment

Musculoskeletal impairment
Neuromuscular impairment
Pain

Psychosociobehavioral

Anxiety, severe
Depression

Perceptual or cognitive impairment:
    Lack of cognitive awareness of affected body parts
    Impaired vision

EXPECTED OUTCOMES

Client will achieve personally satisfying, optimum functional level in dressing/grooming activities in a manner which is both safe and effective.

Maximum level of independence in performing total dressing/grooming activities is demonstrated.

Maximum level of independence in performing partial dressing/grooming activities is demonstrated.

Acceptance of limitations in performing dressing/grooming activities is stated.

Correct use of adaptive device(s) to assist with each dressing/grooming activity is demonstrated—(Specify device(s)).

Measures are described that provide safety during dressing/grooming activity.

INTERVENTIONS / RATIONALE

INTERVENTIONS	RATIONALE
Universal	
Assess current functional ability for independence in dressing/grooming activities.	Alterations in activity tolerance, mobility, strength and endurance, vision, and/or pain and discomfort may inhibit ability to dress/groom independently.
Establish maximum level of independence for performing dressing/grooming activities with or without adaptive devices.	Alleviation/stabilization of health problem may increase functional ability. Use of adaptive devices may enable independence in performing activities.
Monitor and document progress toward independently performing dressing/grooming activity.	Documentation provides a measurement level for evaluation of achievement of expected outcome(s) and a legal record of results of nursing intervention.
Monitor for feelings of anger, depression, fatigue, frustration, and intolerance of limitations. Provide opportunity for discussion of feelings.	The opportunity for discussion of negative feelings is allowed. Provision of positive input may decrease negative feelings.
Involve client/significant other(s) in setting goals for achieving independence in dressing/grooming.	Mutual planning enhances motivation for participation in activity and achievement of outcomes.

INTERVENTIONS	**R**ATIONALE
Establish schedule with client for dressing/grooming activity that is congruent with personal needs and preferences.	Self-control is increased, thus feelings of powerlessness are decreased and the ethical principle of autonomy is promoted. Structured schedule with expectations promotes participation in individuals with decreased motivation.
Provide positive reinforcement for efforts and/or advancement in performance of dressing/grooming activities.	Self-esteem and self-confidence are reinforced, and motivation towards achievement of maximum level of independence is promoted.
Schedule and perform dressing/grooming activities following periods of rest.	Rest restores energy for activity and prevents excessive physical fatigue.
Use consistent language for verbal prompts when encouraging/monitoring independence in dressing/grooming.	Uniform directives promote comprehension in the presence of decreased cognition.
Place clothing/assistive devices/grooming tools in consistent, convenient location.	Uniform placement enhances independence in the presence of decreased visual acuity and/or mobility restrictions.
Medicate with analgesic prior to initiating activity, when required.	Pain associated with activity is decreased, which optimizes functional ability.
Assist client in assuming safe and comfortable position to perform dressing/grooming.	Risk of injury from physical exertion/strain and environmental hazards is reduced.
Provide partial or total assistance with dressing/grooming activities in a private environment.	Personal needs for satisfaction in appearance are met and individual's right to privacy is respected.
Collaborate with physician on need for occupational therapy referral.	Interdisciplinary interventions may be required to achieve maximum functional level.

INTERVENTIONS	RATIONALE
Initiate teaching regarding self-care activity when client demonstrates capability and readiness to learn.	Acute and/or exacerbations of chronic health problems may inhibit ability and/or interest in learning independent self-care activity.
Instruct on: • Use of energy conservation techniques • Use of adaptive device(s) • Use of dressing techniques (specify) • Use of safety/supportive measures to provide self and/or environmental stability during dressing/grooming activities • Use of larger sizes/velcro closures/frontal closures	Strength and endurance are preserved throughout period of activity. Devices enhance independence and facilitate manual dexterity in dressing/grooming activity. Techniques specific for hemiplegia, paraplegia, etc. enhance independence. Risk of injury is decreased. Ease in dressing is facilitated which decreases energy expenditure.
Inpatient	None
Community Health/ Home Care	None

REFERENCES/BIBLIOGRAPHY

See Bibliography for "Feeding Deficit." (pp. 234–235).

Dysreflexia

A state in which an individual with a spinal cord injury at T_7 or above experiences or is at risk of experiencing a life threatening uninhibited sympathetic response of the nervous system to a noxious stimulus (NANDA, 1990, p. 18).

Judith K. Sands, R.N., Ed.D.

• • • • • • • • • • • •

DEFINING CHARACTERISTICS

Individual with a spinal cord injury at T_7 or above with the following:

Blurred vision

Bradycardia or tachycardia (pulse rate of less than 60 or over 100 beats per minute).

Chest pain

Chilling (shivering accompanied by the sensation of coldness or pallor)

Conjunctival congestion (excessive blood or tissue fluid in the conjunctivae)

Diaphoresis (above the level of the injury)

Headache (diffuse pain in different portions of the head and not confined to any nerve distribution)

Horner's syndrome (miosis of the pupil, partial ptosis of the eyelid, enophthalmos (sunken eyes), and facial anhidrosis (loss of sweating)

Metallic taste in the mouth

Nausea

Pallor (below the level of the injury)

Paraesthesia (abnormal sensation such as numbness, prickling, tingling, or increased sensitivity)

Paroxysmal hypertension (sudden periodic elevated blood pressure where the systolic pressure is over 140 mm Hg and the diastolic pressure is above 90 mm Hg)

Pilomotor reflex (gooseflesh when the skin is cooled)

Seizures if untreated

CONTRIBUTING FACTORS

Pathophysiological

Abdominal distention

211

Disease processes with visceral symptoms, i.e., abdominal injury; gallbladder or pancreatic disease
Injury present for three months or longer
Skin pressure or irritation, i.e., abrasions, burns, or decubitus ulcers
Skin stimulation to the abdomen or thighs
Visceral stretching or irritation:
    Urinary: bladder distention, urinary calculi, infection, blocked or clogged drainage
        equipment
    Bowel: constipation or impaction
    Menstrual cramping or pain
    Sexual intercourse

Psychosociobehavioral

Excess fluid intake
Inadequate turning or pressure relief schedule
Lack of knowledge of the client or caregiver
Noncompliance with the treatment regimen
Restrictive clothing
Unregulated bladder program
Unregulated bowel program

EXPECTED OUTCOMES

Client will remain free of episodes of dysreflexia or recover from episodes without residual damage.
    The factors that can trigger dysreflexia are correctly identified.
    A stable blood pressure within normal limits is maintained.
    A regulated bowel program is followed and bowel distention is not present.
    A regulated catheterization program is followed and bladder distention is not present.
    A regular turning and pressure release program is followed and the skin is free of pressure
        and irritation.
    Appropriate treatment measures for dysreflexia are accurately described.

INTERVENTIONS	RATIONALE
Universal	
(Note: The universal interventions are initiated when an episode of dysreflexia is present or strongly suspected.)	
Determine an initial blood pressure and continue to monitor the pressure every two to five minutes until it returns to baseline.	A systolic pressure that is 20 points higher than the baseline is a probable sign of dysreflexia. The blood pressure typically continues to rise rapidly to a life-threatening level. A return to baseline is an excellent indication that the episode has ended.

INTERVENTIONS	RATIONALE
Assess for bladder fullness, the patency of the urinary drainage, and symptoms of infection.	Bladder distention causes stretching of the nerves and initiates massive sympathetic stimulation. It causes dysreflexia in over 75% of cases. As little as 200 cc in the bladder may trigger dysreflexia.
Assess for impaction or the presence of stool in the rectum after first inserting one half to one ounce of Nupercainal (dibucaine) or Xylocaine ointment and waiting for it to take effect.	The presence of stool in the rectum stretches the rectal fibers and stimulates firing of the pelvic nerves. It is the second most common cause of dysreflexia. If the nerve endings have not been numbed prior to insertion of the fingers, the digital stimulation can dramatically worsen the dysreflexia.
Assess for other sources of irritation, pressure, or skin breakdown.	Any irritating or painful stimulus can trigger dysreflexia from stimulation of the cutaneous nerves. Skin breakdown is the third most common cause of dysreflexia and is a frequent problem with spinal cord injury.
Assist to an upright sitting posture if possible.	The vasomotor instability of spinal cord injury (SCI) causes the blood pressure to drop almost immediately with postural changes. This action alone may reverse the dysreflexia or prevent it from worsening while definitive treatment is instituted.
Call for assistance and remain at the bedside.	The process of dysreflexia occurs very rapidly and is extremely frightening. The nurse's presence at the bedside provides reassurance and support and allows for constant monitoring.
Ensure patency of the urinary drainage system, empty the drainage bag, catheterize if indicated, or gently irrigate the catheter if obstructed. Send a urine sample to the lab if infection is suspected.	Obstruction of urinary drainage quickly results in bladder over-distention. Reestablishing urinary drainage and emptying the bladder relieve the bladder stretch stimuli.
Administer rectal suppository, enema, or gently remove stool from the rectum once anesthetic ointment has taken effect.	Emptying the rectum of stool removes the rectal stretch stimuli triggering dysreflexia. Local anesthesia is used to prevent further stimulation from digital stimulation.

INTERVENTIONS	RATIONALE
Eliminate sources of skin pressure or irritation if identifiable.	Cutaneous stimulation or irritation causes firing of the peripheral nerves. Decubiti are frequent stimuli, but twisted linens, constrictive clothing, and foreign objects in the bed linens are other irritating sources.
Notify the physician if standard interventions do not promptly reverse the episode of dysreflexia.	Dysreflexia is a potentially life-threatening situation which may require massive pharmacologic interventions if the primary cause cannot be promptly identified and eliminated.
Ensure intravenous access and administer prescribed medications which may include: hydralazine (Apresoline)—fast acting diazoxide (Hyperstat)—fast acting nifedipine (Procardia)—can be given sublingually without IV access	These medications all act promptly to reduce the blood pressure from life-threatening levels. The most commonly used drugs require intravenous access. Nifedipine use allows for management in the home setting.
Inpatient (Note: The remaining interventions are applicable to clients at risk for dysreflexia) Monitor intake and output balance and utilize data in teaching.	Careful monitoring of intake and output provides data about bladder capacity at various times of day. This information is useful for planning the distribution of daily fluid intake to provide sufficient fluids to prevent constipation and yet prevent bladder overdistention.
Administer medications as needed for pain, particularly abdominal or menstrual.	Abdominal discomfort and pain are potential secondary sources of dysreflexia from visceral stretching within the abdomen. The risk exists even when sensory losses are present. Discomfort can be overlooked in dealing with SCI.

INTERVENTIONS	RATIONALE
Assist to develop an individualized bladder-emptying program and evaluate for effectiveness, modifying as needed.	A successful bladder program involves the use of an indwelling catheter or an intermittent catherization regimen. It prevents bladder over-stretching and nerve stimulation. The program is modified over time in response to ongoing assessment of effectiveness in preventing dysreflexia.
Assist to develop an individualized bowel program that establishes a regular pattern of bowel elimination and prevents constipation and impaction.	A successful bowel program involves use of diet modification, stool softeners, bulk formers, digital stimulation, suppositories, or enemas. These strategies are designed to prevent hard stool from initiating rectal nerve stimuli.
Teach about the appropriate use of fluids and dietary fiber to augment the bowel program.	Adequate fiber and fluids keep the stool soft and ensure regular elimination from the rectum. They prevent rectal stretching from initiating nerve stimuli.
Teach the pathology of dysreflexia.	There is massive sympathetic nerve outflow from the spinal cord in the region above T_6. Injuries in this area disconnect the sympathetic system from the normal autonomic balance and leave it vulnerable to uncontrolled firing, which produces dysreflexia. Injuries lower in the spinal cord do not result in dysreflexia.
Teach warning signs of dysreflexia and the importance of immediate intervention.	Headache, palpitations, and diaphoresis are primary warning signs. Prompt intervention is essential, as failure to reverse dysreflexia can result in seizures, stroke, or death.
Community Health/ Home Care	
Assess knowledge of the symptoms of dysreflexia and prior experience with its management.	Clients who have never or infrequently experienced dysreflexia may require reteaching about the seriousness of the pathology and the warning signs.
Assist to reduce risks and prevent future episodes of dysreflexia.	Diet, fluids, bladder and bowel regimens, and skin care are under tight control in the inpatient setting. The home setting is less structured and more under the client's control. The risk of dysreflexia is dramatically increased by nonadherence to the overall regimen.

Interventions	Rationale
Teach to avoid extremes of temperature.	The ability to adjust to changes in temperature is compromised by SCI and this stressor can precipitate dysreflexia by initiating skin nerve responses. Temperature variations are unusual in inpatient settings but common in the community.
Teach about medications such as phenoxybenzamine (Dibenzyline) and prazosin (Minipress) which may be used to reduce the incidence of bladder distention.	These medications relax the bladder neck and promote full bladder emptying, which may be an important adjunct to the regimen to reduce the risk of bladder distention.

REFERENCES/BIBLIOGRAPHY

Finocchiaro, D.N., & Herzfeld, S.T. (1990). Understanding autonomic dysreflexia. **American Journal of Nursing, 90** (9), 56–59.

Hickey, J. (1986). **The clinical practice of neurological-neurosurgical nursing.** (2nd ed.). Philadelphia: Lippincott.

Mandjdak-McCanon, K. (1988). Rehabilitation of the patient with spinal cord injury. **Trauma Quarterly, 4** (3), 45-49.

Manson, R. (1981). Autonomic dysreflexia: A nursing challenge. **Rehabilitation Nursing, 6,** 18–22.

McCagg, C. (1986). Postoperative management and acute rehabilitation of patients with spinal cord injury. **Orthopedic Clinics of North America, 17,** 171–178.

Nikas, D.L.C. (1988). Pathophysiology and nursing interventions in acute spinal cord injury. **Trauma Quarterly, 4** (3), 23–28.

North America Nursing Diagnosis Association. (1990). **Taxonomy I** (Rev. 1990). St. Louis: NANDA.

Verduyn, W.H. (1986). Spinal cord injured women, pregnancy and delivery. **Paraplegia, 24,** 231–240.

Family Processes, Altered

A state in which a family that normally functions effectively experiences a dysfunction (NANDA, 1990, p. 57).

Patricia Danaher-Dunn, R.N., M.S.

DEFINING CHARACTERISTICS

Blurred hierarchical system
Failure to send and receive clear messages
Family disengagement
Family failing to accomplish current/past developmental task
Family not demonstrating respect for individuality and autonomy of its members
Family system unable to meet the emotional needs of its members
Family system unable to meet the physical needs of its members
Family system unable to meet the spiritual needs of its members
Family unable to adapt to change/deal with traumatic experience constructively
Family unable to meet security needs of its members
Family uninvolved in community activities
Fixed triangulation
Impaired communication
Inability of the family members to relate to each other for mutual growth and maturation
Inability to accept/receive help appropriately
Inability to express or accept a wide range of feelings
Inability to express or accept the feelings of other family members
Inappropriate boundary maintenance
Inappropriate level and direction of energy
Inappropriate or poorly communicated family rules, rituals, symbols
Members who use distance to maintain homeostasis
Parents who do not demonstrate respect for each other's views on child-rearing practices
Parents who do not respect childrens' age-appropriate abilities
Physical or sexual abuse

Rigidity in function, roles, and rules
Substance abuse of family members
Unexamined family myths
Unhealthy decision-making process
Use of member scapegoating

CONTRIBUTING FACTORS
Pathophysiological

Effects of chronic illness
Hospitalization
Loss of body part or function

Mental retardation
Surgery
Trauma

Psychosociobehavioral

Absent or ineffective family role models
Breach of trust between members
Change in a family member's ability to
    function
Conflict or change in family role
Disaster
Intrapsychic conflicts
Large number of family members
Learned patterns of behavior

Loss or gain of significant member
Multigenerational family
Reduced income
Relocation
Single-parent family
Situational or developmental transitions
    and/or crises
Social deviance by a family member
Unemployment

EXPECTED OUTCOMES

Family members will develop effective, open communication.
    Thoughts and feelings related to the crisis and its effects upon themselves as individuals
        as well as relationships within the family are verbalized.
    Conflict among members is resolved and individual coping needs are respected.
    A desire to work together to resolve the crisis is expressed.
Family will achieve effective problem solving and decision making.
    All aspects of the problem are explored together to develop mutual understanding.
    Goals are identified consistent with role relationships and which focus on crisis resolution.
    Realistic time frames for achieving goals are identified.
    Inhibiting factors are anticipated and strategies are developed for coping with them.
Family will achieve new state of equilibrium with enhanced coping and problem-solving abilities. Crisis will be resolved.
    Energy is directed toward crisis resolution.
    Mutual support and cohesion are experienced.
    Basic emotional and physical needs of one another are met.

Family will promote nurturance and growth of its members.
   Role relationships are clarified.
   Enhanced understanding and support for one another are experienced.
   Individual developmental agendas are addressed.

INTERVENTIONS

RATIONALE

Universal

Interventions	Rationale
Create a supportive environment which provides safety, protects privacy, supports trust, and promotes the comfort of the family.	Family members must feel comforted and basic needs must be met before they can engage in crisis resolution.
Facilitate a shared exploration of the presenting problem, its effects upon individual family members, and the family system as a whole. Include feelings and interpretations of each member.	A shared definition of the problem promotes a sense of unity and combined purpose among family members. Exploring effects of the problem upon individual members facilitates sensitivity and respect for the unique needs of that individual.
Assess family structural, behavioral, and interactive patterns including: boundaries, developmental stages, coping skills, role expectations, overt and covert rules, and energy output. Identify areas of strength and areas to strengthen or develop.	Careful examination of the family system reveals the existing resources available for crisis resolution and highlights areas to strengthen.
Engage family members in the problem-solving process, including setting realistic goals, and identifying clear behavioral objectives, as well as anticipating possible barriers to crisis resolution.	Positive outcomes more likely result when family members identify their own shared goals and objectives. Anticipation of potential barriers and contingency plans reinforces a sense of empowerment among family members.

INTERVENTIONS	RATIONALE
Rally additional formal and informal supports to assist the family move toward crisis resolution. May include: teaching stress reduction and coping skills, use of extended family, referral to family therapy, social support agencies, self-help groups, financial assistance, and church affiliated supports, as appropriate.	Additional supports may reduce stress and ease the burden of concern over a variety of issues until the family is again able to cope effectively.
Once crisis is resolved, positively reinforce adaptive family behaviors.	Positive feedback empowers the family and reinforces newly learned behavior.
Inpatient Provide for the physical and emotional comfort of the family throughout the hospitalization. Provide liberal visitation, orientation to important areas of the unit/hospital, adequate space for family privacy, overnights as appropriate, and emotional support as needed.	This legitimizes the roles of family as significant others and begins to establish an alliance with the inpatient staff.
Seek out family. Provide empathy and support for their feelings and dilemmas. Assess and acknowledge their needs. Identify family strengths.	Assessment of the needs and strengths of the family provides direction for further intervention.
Provide basic information about the nature of the illness, dispel erroneous notions, and discuss strategies for managing symptoms.	Anxiety may be reduced as family members develop understanding of the illness.

INTERVENTIONS	RATIONALE
Teach family members how to apply what is learned and engage in problem solving about how to work through potential problems that might arise following discharge.	This engages the family in partnership with the staff and provides some sense of control over management of problems.
Develop a discharge plan that includes referral to appropriate community supports.	Additional support at home can help the family cope with a new care-giving role.
If death occurs, respond quickly to family members' immediate emotional needs. Rally extended family or clergy as appropriate. Refer to a bereavement group when the family is ready.	Loss of a loved one is a crisis requiring immediate intervention.
Community Health/ Home Care Obtain information about the family, including demographics of each member, the environmental context in which they live, family structure and function, the developmental stage of each member, and the current health and illness concerns. Seek only information which is relevant to the concerns at hand.	Decisions regarding intervention approaches are grounded in a reliable information base. Probing for irrelevant information may violate the privacy of the family.
Assist in identifying problems and establish goals for crisis resolution.	Goals must be based upon family needs, definition of problems, and beliefs about what constitutes the appropriate remedy.
Assume appropriate role(s) when intervening with families in crisis. Consider among the following: support, education and guidance, role modeling, monitoring, facilitating, advocacy, and referral.	A variety of roles and functions may be appropriate for use by the community health nurse in working with families.

INTERVENTIONS	**R**ATIONALE
Explore community resources available to assist the family to resolve the immediate crisis or to cope more effectively with the crisis. Consider: self-help groups, advocacy groups, home health agencies, family therapy, financial assistance.	Additional supports may reduce stress and ease the burden of concern over a variety of issues until the family is again coping effectively.

REFERENCES/BIBLIOGRAPHY

Alexander, J., & Parsons, B.V. (1982). **Functional family therapy**. Monterey, CA: Brooks/Cole.

Carpenito, L.G. (1989). **Nursing diagnosis: Application to clinical practice**. Philadelphia: Lippincott.

Dimond, M., & Jones, S.L. (1983). **Chronic illness across the life span**. Norwalk, CT: Appleton-Century-Crofts.

Getty, C., & Humphries, W.G. (1990). Family assessment: A basis for nursing practice. In B. Bullough, & V. Bullough. (Eds.). **Nursing in the community.** (pp. 244–271). St. Louis: Mosby.

Hatfield, A.B. (1987). Coping and adaptation: A conceptual framework for understanding families. In A.B. Hatfield, & H.P. Lefley. (Eds.). **Families of the mentally ill: Coping and adaptation.** (pp. 60-84). New York: Guilford.

Lomax, J.I., & Van Servellen, G.M. (1989). Family therapy. In L. M. Birckhead. (Ed.). **Psychiatric mental health nursing: The therapeutic use of self.** (pp. 207–227). Philadelphia: Lippincott.

McFarland, G.K., & McFarlane, E.A. (1989). **Nursing diagnosis and intervention**. St. Louis: Mosby.

McLane, A.M. (1987). **Classification of nursing diagnosis: Proceedings of the seventh conference**. St. Louis: Mosby.

Minuchin, S., Fishman, H.C. (1981). **Family therapy techniques**. Cambridge: Harvard Press.

North American Nursing Diagnosis Association. (1990). **Taxonomy I** (Rev. 1990). St. Louis: NANDA.

Schwartz, M.F. (1989). Altered family processes. In J.M. Thompson, G.K. McFarland, J.E. Hirsch, S.M. Tucker, & A.C. Bowers. (Eds.). **Mosby's manual of clinical nursing.** (pp. 1770–1772). St. Louis: Mosby.

Terkelson, K.G. (1980). Toward a theory of the family life cycle. In E.A. Carter, & M. McGoldrick. (Eds.). **The family life cycle: A framework for family therapy.** (pp. 21–52). New York: Gardner.

Whall, A.L. (1986). **Family therapy for nursing: Four approaches**. Norwalk, CT: Appleton-Century-Crofts.

Zipple, A.M., & Spanoil, L. (1987). Current educational and supportive models of family intervention. In A.B. Hatfield, & H.P. Lefley. (Eds.). **Families of the mentally ill: Coping and adaptation.** (pp. 167–190). New York: Guilford.

Fatigue

A state in which there is a sustained subjective sensation reflected by aversion to physical and mental activity, which may include a sense of personal inadequacy and futility and be unrelieved by rest.

Julia D. Emblen, R.N., Ph.D.

DEFINING CHARACTERISTICS

General:

Decreased mental and physical performance, speed, and capability

Impatience

Inaccuracy and increase in errors

Irritability

Listlessness

Loss of libido

Nervousness

Passivity

Tearfulness

Yawning

Mental effects:

Confusion

Decreased attention

Decreased motivation

Difficulty concentrating

Drowsiness

Forgetfulness

Headache

Impaired thinking

Slowed and impaired perception

Muscle effects:

Clumsy motions

Diminished muscle tone

Eyelid spasms

Eyestrain

Heaviness throughout body, first manifested in legs

Inability to straighten posture

Tremor in limbs

Unsteadiness in standing

Sleep related:

Disturbance in or diminished sleep pattern

223

CONTRIBUTING FACTORS

Pathophysiological

Dietary inadequacies
Illness, i.e., infections, anemia, chemo-
   therapy, or chronic disease
Lack of sleep

Metabolic disorders
Neuromuscular diseases
Obesity
Pain

Psychosociobehavioral

Emotional factors, i.e., worries, conflict
Emotional pain
Environmental surroundings, i.e., light,
   temperature, noise

Long and intense manual or mental
   work
Monotonous repetition of activities
Stress due to excess physical, mental,
   emotional, or spiritual demands

EXPECTED OUTCOMES

Client will experience an increase in energy and activity levels.
   There is greater alertness and strength.
   There is improved self-image and zest for life.
   Identification of essential activities of daily living (ADL), scheduling the day with periods
      of rest and activity, and identification of ways to delegate some activities occurs.
   Nonessential activities are eliminated.

INTERVENTIONS

RATIONALE

INTERVENTIONS	RATIONALE
Universal Assess perception of fatigue.	Fatigue is a subjective experience.
Assess physiological fatigue and endurance during physical activities.	Fatigue is an expected response to physical activity, but when strength is not sufficient to complete usual ADL, fatigue is problematic.
Assess psychosocial perception of fatigue.	Fatigue is a subjective experience which may be present even when there is no physical evidence of it.
Provide specific treatments designated for illness-related effects, e.g., medication for pain relief, iron supplements for anemia.	Fatigue may have a specific pathological cause.

INTERVENTIONS	RATIONALE
Provide palliative and supportive care as required.	Exhaustion interferes with the management of ADL, and supportive assistance provides an increase in strength.
Encourage physical exercise outdoors when possible.	Research indicates that contrary to the popular notion that tired people need to rest, activity is essential to decrease fatigue.
Improve general metabolism by glucose, vitamin, mineral, and oxygen supplements.	When metabolic processes are improved, there is less build-up of metabolic acids which tend to produce fatigue symptoms.
Assist with scheduling activities to wisely utilize available energies.	Realistic schedules that are compatible with available energies decrease the feeling of failure which accompanies fatigue. Though there may be no physical evidence of fatigue, the client may feel fatigue.
Provide time to listen, which allows the ventilation of feelings and thoughts regarding life experiences that have been painful and stressful.	Holding in traumatic experiences requires high amounts of emotional energy which depletes reserves required for daily living tasks.
Encourage expression of emotional conflicts.	Conflicts require inordinate energy expenditures.
Assist with motivating to take steps to make life-style changes.	Intrinsic motivation is diminished by depression and discouragement requiring external assistance with change.
Explore for things which are restful.	Work-oriented persons often need help to plan restful and /or leisure activities which allow personal pleasures to restore esthetic and spiritual needs.
Provide opportunities for engagement in things which are viewed as restorative of energy.	Weariness adds to the fatigue cycle by causing abandonment of all activities.
Provide guidance for obesity control.	If weight is within normal limits fatigue will decrease.

INTERVENTIONS	RATIONALE
Inpatient (Note: Inpatient care is usually only provided when hospitalization is needed to correct some major pathophysiological imbalance, e.g., raise life-threatening hemoglobin level.)	
Community Health/ Home Care Assess physiological and psychosocial levels of fatigue.	Fatigue responses change in accord with specific activities, and when typical environment and normal ADL are resumed, the sensation of fatigue may increase.
Provide opportunities to vary daily routines.	Strict adherence to a pattern of activities leads to boredom and an inability to recognize alternatives.
Introduce changes to provide incentive and improve personal outlook on life.	Variations can elminate monotony, which for some personalities is fatiguing.
Suggest literature that describes seasonal and calendar changes.	Recognizing changes in nature and in years may afford greater perspective with respect to changes which are needed for human beings to survive.
Modify surroundings to ensure proper lighting, temperature, and sound levels.	Environmental aspects which are outside of the normal parameters can deplete energy.
Suggest modification of intensity and length of activities.	For prolonged activities, short breaks allow for muscle restoration. Sometimes experts suggest that completion of the hardest task first makes it easier to do the less difficult tasks.
Encourage reading and/or attendance at workshops that focus on topics which as time management and energizing.	Self-help books and seminars can provide effective resources. Fatigue, especially chronic fatigue, is common for young, educated adult women. They are often able to profit from educational options.

INTERVENTIONS	**R**ATIONALE
Identify support groups which might be of use to persons in learning to manage fatigue.	Exploring ways to deal with fatigue with others who have found effective approaches may be instructive for clients with chronic fatigue without a specific identifiable illness cause.

REFERENCES/BIBLIOGRAPHY

Bartley, H.S. (1965). **Fatigue mechanism and management**. Springfield, IL: Thomas.

Dranov, P. (1989). "Am I sick or am I tired?" **Ladies Home Journal, 106,** 120–126.

Elias, S. (Ed.). (1987). Coping with chronic fatigue syndrome. **Patient Care, 21,** 79–82.

Grandjean, E. (1968). Fatigue: Its physiological and psychological significance. **Ergonomics, 11,** 427–436.

* Gueldner, S.H., & Spradley, J. (1988). Outdoor walking lowers fatigue. **Journal of Gerontological Nursing, 14,** 6–12.

Haslam, P. (1970). Noise in hospital: Its effect on the patient. **Nursing Clinics of North America, 5,** 715–724.

Narrow, B.W. (1967). Rest is...**American Journal of Nursing, 67,** 1646–1649.

* Piper, B.F., et al. (1989). Recent advances in the management of biotherapy-related side effects: Fatigue. **Oncology Nursing Forum, 16,** Supplement, 27–34.

* Potempa, K., Lopez, M., Reid, C., & Lawson L. (1986). Chronic fatigue. **Image, 18,** 165–169.

Rhodes, V.A., Watson, P.M., & Hanson, B.M. (1988). Patients' descriptions of the influence of tiredness and weakness on self-care abilities. **Cancer Nursing, 11,** 186–194.

Tierney, L.M. (1989). Chronic fatigue syndrome. **Consultant, 29,** 25–32.

Tournier, P. (1965). **Fatigue in modern society**. Richmond, VA: Knox.

Weir, M.S. (1991). **Wear and tear or hints for the overworked**. (5th ed.). Philadelphia: Lippincott.

* Woods, N.F., & Falk, S.A. (1974). Noise stimuli in the acute care area. **Nursing Research, 23,** 144–150.

Fear

A state in which an individual (or aggregate) exhibits a complex emotional reaction to feelings which have origins in identifiable, concrete, extremely threatening external circumstances in the present or imminent future.

Marga S. Coler, R.N., Ed.D., C.S., C.T.N.

DEFINING CHARACTERISTICS (Culture-bound; in Western culture)

Ability to identify the object of fear
Apprehension
Avoidance behavior
Escape behavior
Guilt
Heightened imagination

Intelligent, intentional action toward object of fear
Psychophysiological changes (i.e., tremors, diaphoresis, hypervigilance, palpitations, hyperventilation, etc.)
Shame

CONTRIBUTING FACTORS (Culture-bound; in Western culture)

Pathophysiological

Death
Disease
Physiological changes (i.e., tachycardia, loss of vision, loss of hearing, loss of limb, paralysis, etc.)

Psychosociobehavioral

Abandonment
Attack
Dangerous, threatening objects
(The) Dark

Disaster
Incarceration
Incongruity
Supernatural

228

EXPECTED OUTCOMES

Client will put object of fear into the proper perspective.
>Object of fear is identified.
>Significance of object of fear is identified to self and life's goals.

Client will utilize appropriate coping skills.
>Past coping mechanisms are identified that will be appropriate in dealing with object of fear.
>New coping mechanisms are learned that will be appropriate in dealing with the object of fear.

Client will link up with support systems.
>Past and present supports are identified that can be utilized in dealing with object of fear.
>Object-of-fear-specific support group is joined if available in the community.
>Client is protagonist in instituting new support systems.

INTERVENTIONS	RATIONALE
Universal	
Examine the significance of the object of fear.	The significance of the object will help to gain insight regarding the perceptive reality. Frequently, the greater the significance, the greater the distortion.
Identify the mechanisms by which the fear is expressed.	The response to fear may be rational and/or irrational. It is important to identify both rational and irrational responses to mobilize appropriate coping mechanisms.
Assess the intensity of fears relative to age, sex, class, and ethnicity.	Responses to an object of fear may be determined by age, sex, class, and ethnicity.
Determine extent of victimization by fear production and/or management strategies.	Fear-inducing techniques are frequently employed as part of conscious attempts to muster commitment to groups or causes; or to create divisiveness.
Aid in the separation of emotional, cognitive, perceptual, and behavioral responses to fear.	The separation of response components helps in coping with object of fear in a rational manner.
Aid in separating *beliefs about* the object of fear from the actual object of fear.	Undesirable emotional consequences can often be traced to irrational beliefs.

INTERVENTIONS	**RATIONALE**
Assist in channeling fear-producing energy into creative fear-resolution strategies.	Maladaptive behavior can be channeled into creativity through the use of insight and education.
Relate cultural concepts to conditions under which fear arises.	The origin of a fear may be culturally different from one individual to another. In order to respond to the object of fear appropriately, the insights must be culturally appropriate.
Teach the physiological response reactions to fear.	Knowledge about the mechanisms of physiological responses helps to maintain control over them.
Teach how fear is expressed and communicated through symbols and public media within a culture.	Knowledge of the mechanisms of fear, and their effect on the human organism, will provide insight into irrational emotions, feelings, and behaviors toward the object of fear.
Inpatient	None
Community Health/ Home Care	None

REFERENCES/BIBLIOGRAPHY

Aguilera, D. (1990). **Crisis intervention: Theory and methodology**. St. Louis: Mosby.

Carpenito, L. (1983). **Nursing diagnosis: Application to clinical practice**. Philadelphia: Lippincott.

Corisini, R. (1984). **Current psychotherapies**. Itasca, IL: Peacock.

Hoff, L. (1989). **People in crisis: Understanding and helping.** (3rd ed.). Redwood City, CA: Addison-Wesley.

Kim, M.J., McFarland, G., & McLane, A. (1984). **Pocket guide to nursing diagnoses**. St. Louis: Mosby.

North American Nursing Diagnosis Association. (1990). **Taxonomy I** (Rev. 1990). St. Louis: NANDA.

Rachman, S.J. (1978). **Fear and courage**. San Francisco: Freeman.

Sluckin, W. (1979). **Fear in animals and man**. New York: Van Nostrand Reinhold.

Scruton, D. (1986). **Sociophobics**. London: Westview.

Tuan, Y. (1979). **Landscapes of fear**. New York: Pantheon.

Feeding Deficit

A state in which an individual experiences an impaired ability to perform or complete feeding activities independently (NANDA, 1990, p. 79).

Carol Dickel, R.N.
Suellyn Ellerbe, R.N., M.N.
Rosemary J. McKeighen, R.N., Ph.D., F.A.A.N.
Peg A. Mehmert, R.N., C., M.S.N.
Diane C. Kolb, R.N., B.A.

DEFINING CHARACTERISTICS

Inability to bring food from a receptacle to mouth

CONTRIBUTING FACTORS

Pathophysiological

Activity intolerance
Decreased strength and endurance
Discomfort

Musculoskeletal impairment
Neuromuscular impairment
Pain

Psychosociobehavioral

Anxiety, severe
Depression
Perceptual or cognitive impairment

EXPECTED OUTCOMES

Client will achieve personally satisfying, maximum functional level in self-feeding with dietary intake meeting minimum nutritional daily requirements.
Desire to eat and self-feed is expressed.
Ability to bring finger foods to mouth is demonstrated.
Foods are inserted into oral cavity.
Ability to manipulate tableware and bring food from utensil to mouth is demonstrated.
Satisfaction is stated with level of independence achieved in self-feeding.

INTERVENTIONS	RATIONALE
Universal	
Assess current functional ability for self-feeding.	Alterations in activity tolerance, neuromuscular or musculoskeletal status, strength and endurance, vision and/or pain and discomfort may impair ability to bring hand to mouth.
Assess availability of significant other for support/assistance as necessary.	Significant other support provides resources for clients, not achieving/maintaining maximum functional level.
Monitor for feelings of anger, depression, fatigue, frustration, and intolerance of limitations. Provide for discussion of feelings.	The opportunity for a nonjudgmental discussion may decrease negative feelings.
Monitor and document progress towards independence in feeding activity.	Documentation provides a measurement level for evaluation of achievement of expected outcomes(s) and a legal record of results of nursing intervention.
Involve client/significant others in setting goals for achieving independence in feeding.	Mutual planning of nurse and client enhances motivation for participation in activity and achievement of outcomes.
Establish schedule for meals with client (to the extent possible within organizational structure) that is congruent with their personal needs and preferences.	Self-control is increased, thus decreasing feelings of powerlessness; and the ethical principle of autonomy is promoted.
Establish maximum level of independence with/without adaptive devices.	Alleviation/stabilization of current health problem may increase functional ability. Adaptive devices (e.g., plate guards, scooper bowls, hand splints) may enable independence.
Provide positive reinforcement for advancement of self-feeding functional ability.	Reinforcement enhances self-esteem, self confidence, and provides motivation towards achievement of maximum level of independence.

INTERVENTIONS	RATIONALE
Provide periods of rest prior to scheduled meals.	Rest restores the energy level required for self-feeding activity and digestion.
Use consistent language for verbal prompts when encouraging/monitoring independence in self-feeding.	Uniform directives enhance comprehension in the presence of decreased cognition.
Place food in clockwise rotation and communicate location of food.	Uniform placement enhances independence in the presence of decreased visual acuity.
Assist in assuming safe and comfortable position for meals.	Physical comfort facilitates hand-to-mouth motion.
Provide partial or total assistance with feeding.	Nutritional needs are met when unable to self-feed.
Collaborate with physician on need for occupational therapy referral.	Interdisciplinary interventions may be required to achieve maximum functional level.
Initiate teaching regarding self-feeding, when capability and readiness to learn are demonstrated.	Decreased cognition and/or musculoskeletal status may impinge on ability to learn.
Instruct on: • Use of adaptive device(s) • Use of safety/supportive measures to provide self and/or environmental stability during feeding • Pacing self-feeding activities	 Devices enhance independence and facilitate manual dexterity in feeding. Hand to mouth motion is facilitated and risk of injury is reduced. Energy level to complete self-feeding activity and digestion is sustained.
Inpatient	None
Community Health/ Home Care	None

REFERENCES/BIBLIOGRAPHY

* Baer, C.A., Delorey, M., & Fitzmaurice, J.B. (1984). A study to evaluate the validity of the rating system for self-care deficit. In M.J. Kim, G.K. McFarland, & A.M. McLane. **Classification of nursing diagnoses: Proceedings of the Fifth National Conference.** (pp. 185–191). St. Louis: Mosby.

Carpenito, L.J. (1989). **Nursing diagnosis: Application to clinical practice.** (3rd ed.). Philadelphia: Lippincott.

* Chang, B.L., Hirsch, M., Brazal-Villanueva, E., & Ray Iverson, K.W. (1990). Self-care deficit with etiologies: Reliability of measurement. **Nursing Diagnosis, 1** (1), 31–36.

* Fensler, J. (1986). A comparison of patient and nurse perceptions of patients' self-care deficits associated with cancer chemotherapy. **Cancer Nursing, 9,** 50–57.

Gettrust, K.V., Ryan, S.C., & Engelman, D.S. (1985). **Applied nursing diagnosis: Guides for comprehensive care planning.** Albany, NY: Delmar.

Goldstein, N., et al. (1983). Self-care: A framework for the future. In P.L. Chinn. (Ed.). **Advances in nursing theory development.** Rockville, MD: Aspen.

Gordon, M. (1987). **Manual of nursing diagnosis: 1986–1987.** New York: McGraw-Hill.

Gordon, M. (1976). Assessing activity tolerance. **American Journal of Nursing, 76** (1), 72–75.

Gulanick, M., Klopp, A., Galanes, S., Gradishar, D., & Puzas, M.K. (1990). **Nursing care plans: Nursing diagnosis & intervention.** (2nd ed.). St. Louis: Mosby.

Kim, M.J., McFarland, G.K., & McLane, A.M. (1989). **Pocket guide to nursing diagnoses.** (3rd ed.). St. Louis: Mosby.

* Levin, R.F., Krainovitch, B.C., Bahrenburg, E., & Mitchell, C.A. (1989). Diagnostic content validity of nursing diagnoses. **IMAGE: Journal of Nursing Scholarship, 21** (1), 40–44.

Logue, P.A. (1984). Brothers/keepers: Ethical implications of the self-care deficit nursing diagnosis. In M.J. Kim, G.K. McFarland, & A.M. McLane. **Classification of nursing diagnoses: Proceedings of the Fifth National Conference.** (pp. 336–342). St. Louis: Mosby.

McFarland, G.K., & McFarlane, E.A. (1989). **Nursing diagnosis & intervention: Planning for patient care.** St. Louis: Mosby.

* McKeighen, R.J., Mehmert, P.A., & Dickel, C.A. (in press). Bathing/hygiene self care deficit: Defining characteristics and related factors across age groups and Diagnosis Related Groups in an acute care setting. **Nursing Diagnosis.**

Mercy Continuing Care. (1990). **Nursing diagnoses and standards for home health-care.** Unpublished content. Davenport, IA: Author.

Mercy Hospital-Division of Nursing. (1990). Computerized nursing diagnosis care planning pathway. Unpublished content. Davenport, IA: Author.

* Metzger, K.L., & Hiltunen, E.F. (1987). Diagnostic content validation of ten frequently reported nursing diagnoses. In A.M. McLane. (Ed.). **Classification of nursing diagnoses: Proceedings of the Seventh Conference.** (pp. 144–152). St. Louis: Mosby.

North American Nursing Diagnosis Association. (1990). **Taxonomy I** (Rev. 1990). St. Louis: NANDA.

* Parsons, L.C., Peard, A.L., & Page, M.C. (1985). The effects of hygiene interventions on the cerebrovascular status of severe closed head injured persons. **Research in Nursing and Health, 8,** 173–181.

Piper, B. (1986). Fatigue. In V. Carriert, A. Lindsey, & C. West. (Eds.). **Pathophysiological**

phenomena in nursing: Human responses to illness. Philadelphia: Saunders.

* Rhodes, V.A., Watson, P.M., & Hanson, B.M. (1988). Patients' descriptions of the influence of tiredness and weakness on self-care abilities. **Cancer Nursing, 11** (3), 186–194.

Richmond, T.S. (1990). Spinal cord injury. **Nursing Clinics of North America, 25** (1), 57–69.

Taylor, S.G. (1988). Nursing theory and nursing process: Orem's theory in practice. **Nursing Science Quarterly, 1** (3), 111–119.

Thompson, J., McFarland, G., Hirsch, J., Tucker, S., & Bowers, A. (1989). **Clinical nursing.** (2nd ed.). St. Louis: Mosby.

* Tracy, C.A. (1989). Etiologies of the nursing diagnosis of self-care deficit. In R. Carroll-Johnson. (Ed.). **Classification of nursing diagnoses: Proceedings of the Eighth National Conference.** (pp. 349–351). Philadelphia: Lippincott.

Wesorik, B. (1990). **Standards of nursing care: A model for clinical practice**. Philadelphia: Lippincott.

* Winslow, E.H., Lane, L.D., & Gaffney, F.A. (1985). Oxygen uptake and cardiovascular reponses in control adults and acute myocardial infarction patients during bathing. **Nursing Research, 34** (3), 164–169.

Fluid Volume Deficit

A state in which an individual experiences a decrease in circulating fluid volume related to decreased intake or increased loss of fluid, volume shifts within body fluid compartments, or a combination thereof.

S. Jill Ley, R.N., M.S., C.C.R.N.

. . . .

DEFINING CHARACTERISTICS

Subjective

Dizziness
Lethargy

Thirst
Weakness

Physical Findings

Confusion and disorientation
Decreased cardiac output
Decreased central venous pressure
Decreased pulmonary capillary wedge
      pressure
Decreased urine output
Delayed capillary refill
Diaphoresis
Dry mucous membranes
Dry skin

Hyperthermia
Hypotension
Narrow pulse pressure
Negative intake and output
Poor skin turgor
Postural vital sign changes
Tachycardia
Tachypnea
Thready pulse
Weight loss

Laboratory Findings

Decreased urine sodium
Increased blood urea nitrogen
Increased hematocrit
Increased serum osmolality

Increased serum sodium
Increased urine osmolality
Increased urine specific gravity

236

CONTRIBUTING FACTORS

Pathophysiological

Decreased intake:
    anorexia
    malabsorption syndromes
    nausea
External fluid loss:
    diaphoresis
    diarrhea
    diuresis
    draining wounds
    emesis
    fistulas
    hemorrhage

    nasogastric drainage
    surgery
Internal fluid loss/shifts:
    anaphylaxis
    ascites
    blunt trauma
    burns
    capillary leak syndromes
    hemothorax
    intestinal obstruction
    sepsis
    vasodilation

Psychosociobehavioral

Age extremes
Altered level of consciousness
Eating disorders

Nothing by mouth (NPO) status
Psychologic disorders

EXPECTED OUTCOMES

Client will have central nervous system (CNS) symptoms resolved.
    Fatigue, dizziness, and confusion are denied.
    Level of consciousness returns to baseline.
Client will develop a net fluid gain.
    Fluid intake exceeds output.
    Body weight increases.
Client will have no physical findings of hypovolemia.
    Capillary refill is within normal limits.
    Skin is warm and dry with normal turgor.
    Urine output equals or exceeds 50 cc/H or 1500 cc/d.
    Vital signs return to client's baseline values.
    Abnormal laboratory findings resolve.
    Central venous pressure is 2–6 mmHg.
    Pulmonary capillary wedge pressure is 6–10 mmHg.
    Cardiac output is 4–8 L/min.
    Heart rate (HR) is $\leq$ 100 beats/min.
    Pulse pressure is $\geq$ 30 mmHg.
    Systolic blood pressure (SBP) is $\geq$ 90 mmHg.

INTERVENTIONS	RATIONALE
Universal	
Ascertain the cause(s) of the fluid disturbance via history and physical examination.	Definitive treatment for fluid status abnormalities relies on identification and correction of ongoing fluid losses.
Assess the degree of hypovolemia present, noting the potential for progression towards hypovolemic shock: • Assess vital signs • Assess neurologic status • Note evidence of ongoing fluid loss • Summon emergency medical assistance if signs of shock are present.	Up to 20% of the circulating blood volume may be lost before overt symptoms of hypovolemia develop. Progression to life-threatening shock can occur rapidly.
Assess the appropriate method of rehydration to restore fluid balance in a timely manner: • Assess the degree of hypovolemia present and the need for oral versus intravenous fluid therapy • Assess ability to ingest oral fluids • Assess ability to understand and comply with the fluid regimen	Oral hydration is indicated for mild degrees of hypovolemia, if the client can tolerate oral fluids, while intravenous (IV) therapy is indicated for more severe fluid deficits.
Provide comfort measures as indicated for clients experiencing signs of dehydration: • Apply lip balm to lips • Apply moisture drops to eyes • Apply body lotion to skin • Add oil to bath water • Offer lozenges to moisten mouth	Local measures which restore body fluids to the skin, mucous membranes, and respiratory tract are effective in decreasing the discomfort associated with dehydration.

INTERVENTIONS	**R**ATIONALE
• Provide frequent oral care • Place humidifier in room • Humidify supplemental oxygen	
Increase fluid intake to achieve a positive fluid balance. • Increase oral intake as tolerated by offering a variety of fluids at frequent intervals, in small amounts, and between meals; and offer assistance as needed • Calculate baseline fluid requirements according to the following formula: 100 cc/kg for first 10 kg/body weight, plus 50 cc/kg for next 10 kg/body weight, plus 20 cc/kg for additional body weight	This will yield the 24-hour fluid requirement; (total divided by 24 equals hourly IV infusion rate). Fluid intake must meet at least the baseline requirements to counteract decreased intake or excess loss. Oral methods pose less risk of fluid overload and relieve symptoms of thirst.
Teach about interventions to maintain fluid balance: • Increase fluid intake during periods of increased fluid loss • Notify physician of illnesses leading to prolonged decrease in oral intake or excessive fluid loss	Hypovolemia may be avoided if prevention or early intervention is available.

INTERVENTIONS	**R**ATIONALE
Inpatient	
Monitor vital signs (including orthostatic changes), intake and output, body weight, skin and mucous membranes, mentation, laboratory values, cardiac output, and filling pressure measurements.	A variety of clinical indicators is necessary to accurately assess fluid status. Resolution of abnormal findings should occur with restoration of fluid balance.
• After changing from supine to upright or sitting position, a systolic blood pressure (SBP) decrease ≥ 20 mmHg associated with a heart rate (HR) increase ≥ 10 beats/min indicates hypovolemia, when present one minute after position change	
• A change in body weight of one kg corresponds to a net change in fluid balance of one L	
Monitor for signs of fluid overload during rehydration therapy. (See "Fluid Volume Excess" care planning guide.)	Clients with decreased cardiac and renal function have limited ability to respond to an increased fluid load. Rapid IV infusion rates may also contribute to fluid overload during fluid rehydration therapy.
Administer rapid IV fluid boluses if signs of shock are present including: SBP < 90 mmHg, HR > 100, UO < 20 cc/hr.	Rapid restoration of the circulating fluid volume is necessary to reverse life-threatening shock. Colloid solutions remain in the vascular compartment to a greater degree than crystalloids, therefore less fluid and time will be required to restore fluid balance.
• Infuse 100–250 cc aliquots of fluid over 15–30 min., then reassess fluid status. (Note: Specific type, amount, and infusion rate to be ordered by physician.)	

INTERVENTIONS	RATIONALE
• Colloid solutions (blood, albumin, dextran, hetastarch) may be indicated, as they will restore the circulating fluid volume faster than crystalloids (normal saline, lactated Ringer's)	
Community Health/ Home Care Monitor vital signs (including orthostatic changes), daily body weight, skin and mucous membranes, and mentation. • Weight loss exceeding one kg/day is related to a net fluid loss • Instruct to obtain daily weight at same time, on same scale, with similar clothing to promote accuracy	Orthostatic changes indicate the presence of a severe fluid deficit, warranting immediate intervention. Assessment of a variety of clinical indicators is necessary to accurately assess fluid status. Resolution of abnormal findings should occur with restoration of fluid balance.

REFERENCES/BIBLIOGRAPHY

* Gershan, J.A., et al. (1990). Fluid volume deficit: Validating the indicators. **Heart & Lung, 19,** 152–156.

Gettrust, K.V., Ryan, S.C., & Engelman, D.S. (1985). Nursing diagnosis: Fluid volume deficit. In **Applied nursing diagnosis: Guides for comprehensive care planning**. Albany, NY: Delmar.

Gomella, L.G. (1989). **Clinician's pocket reference.** (6th ed.). Norwalk, CT: Appleton & Lange.

Ley, S.J. (1988). Fluid therapy following intracardiac operation. **Critical Care Nurse, 8** (1), 26–36.

* Ley, S.J., Miller, K., Skov, P., Preisig, P. (1990). Crystalloid versus colloid fluid therapy after cardiac surgery. **Heart & Lung, 19,** 31–40.

Thelan, L.A., Davie, J.K., & Urden, L.D. (1990). Renal and fluid care plans: Theoretical basis and management. In **Textbook of critical care nursing: Diagnosis and management.** (pp. 664–671). St. Louis: Mosby.

Fluid Volume Deficit: Risk

A state in which an individual is at risk for the development of a decrease in circulating fluid volume related to decreased intake or increased loss of fluid, volume shifts within body fluid compartments, or a combination thereof.

S. Jill Ley, R.N., M.S., C.C.R.N.

. . . .

RISK FACTORS

Pathophysiological

Age extremes
Alcohol use
Altered level of consciousness
Altered sensory perception
      (i.e., decreased smell, taste)
Anaphylaxis
Anorexia
Ascites
Burns
Capillary leak syndromes
Coma
Confusion
Diaphoresis
Diarrhea
Diuretic use
Draining wounds
Emesis
Fatigue
Fever

Fistulas
Fluid-restricted diet
Hemorrhage
Hemothorax
Hypermetabolic states
Hyperventilation
Immobility
Infection
Intestinal obstruction
Malabsorption syndromes
Nasogastric drainage
Nausea
Pleural effusion
Polyuria
Sepsis
Surgery
Trauma
Vasodilation
Visual impairment

Psychosociobehavioral

Climate exposure
Depression or other psychological disorder
Knowledge deficit (e.g., fluid balance)

EXPECTED OUTCOMES

Client will maintain an equal or positive fluid balance.
    Fluid intake equals or exceeds output.
    Body weight increases or remains unchanged.
Client will have no physical findings of hypovolemia.
    Capillary refill is within normal limits.
    Skin is warm and dry with normal turgor.
    Urine output equals or exceeds 50 cc/H or 1500 cc/d.
    Vital signs remain at client's baseline.
    Laboratory findings are within normal limits.
Client and/or family will verbalize understanding of fluid maintenance strategies.
    Potential sources of fluid loss are stated.
    Strategies to maintain intake are identified.
    Signs and symptoms warranting notification of physician are listed.

INTERVENTIONS	RATIONALE
Universal	
Assess for the presence of risk factors which may contribute to a fluid deficit, via history and physical examination.	A fluid deficit may be prevented by careful ongoing assessment and implementation of appropriate interventions.
Assess current strategies being utilized to maintain a positive fluid balance. • Calculate baseline fluid requirements according to the following formula: 100 cc/kg for first 10 kg body weight, plus 50 cc/kg for next 10 kg body weight, plus 20 cc/kg for additional body weight, yields 24-hour fluid requirement	Fluid intake must meet at least baseline requirements to counteract decreased intake or increased loss. Oral methods pose less risk of fluid overload and relieve symptoms of thirst.

INTERVENTIONS	**R**ATIONALE
• Assess ability to maintain base-line fluid intake via current oral, nasogastric (NG), and/or intravenous (IV) regimen	
Teach about interventions to maintain fluid balance: • Increase fluid intake during periods of increased fluid loss • Notify physician of illnesses leading to prolonged decrease in oral intake or excessive fluid loss	A fluid deficit may be avoided if prevention or early intervention is available.
Inpatient Monitor vital signs (including orthostatic changes), intake and output, body weight, skin and mucous membranes, mentation, laboratory values, cardiac output, and filling pressure measurements. • After changing from supine to upright or sitting position, a systolic blood pressure (SBP) decrease $\geq$ 20 mmHg associated with a heart rate (HR) increase $\geq$ 10 beats/min indicates hypovolemia, when present one min after position change • A change in body weight of one kg corresponds to a net change in fluid balance of one L	A variety of clinical indicators is necessary to accurately assess fluid status. Resolution of abnormal findings should occur with restoration of fluid balance.

INTERVENTIONS	RATIONALE
Increase fluid intake to achieve a positive or equal fluid balance. • Increase oral intake as tolerated by offering a variety of fluids at frequent intervals, in small amounts, and between meals; and offer assistance as needed • Increase IV/NG (intravenous/nasogastric) fluids as ordered, if oral intake is insufficient to meet baseline fluid requirements	Fluid intake must meet at least baseline requirements to counteract decreased intake or excess loss. Oral methods pose less risk of fluid overload and relieve symptoms of thirst.
Community Health/ Home Care Monitor vital signs (including orthostatic changes), daily body weight, skin and mucous membranes, and mentation. • Weight loss exceeding 1 kg/d is related to a net fluid loss • Instruct to obtain daily weight at same time, on same scale, with similar clothing to promote accuracy • Orthostatic changes indicate the presence of a severe fluid deficit warranting immediate intervention	Assessment of a variety of clinical indicators is necessary to accurately assess fluid status. Resolution of abnormal findings should occur with restoration of fluid balance.
Increase fluid intake to achieve a positive or equal fluid balance. • Increase oral intake by offering frequent fluids, in small amounts, a variety of hot and cold fluids; and offer assistance as needed	Oral fluid intake must meet at least baseline requirements to counteract decreased intake or increased loss of fluid.

REFERENCES/BIBLIOGRAPHY

* Gershan, J.A., et al. (1990). Fluid volume deficit: Validating the indicators. **Heart & Lung, 19,** 152–156.

Gettrust, K.V., Ryon, S.C., & Engelman, D.S. (1985). Nursing diagnosis: Potential fluid volume deficit. In **Applied nursing diagnosis: Guides for comprehensive care planning.** Albany, NY: Delmar.

Gomella, L.G. (1989). **Clinician's pocket reference.** (6th ed.). Norwalk, CT: Appleton & Lange.

Ley, S.J. (1988). Fluid therapy following intracardiac operation. **Critical Care Nurse, 8** (1), 26–36.

North American Nursing Diagnosis Association. (1990). **Taxonomy I** (Rev. 1990). St. Louis: NANDA.

Thelan, L.A., Davie, J.K., & Urden, L.D. (1990). Renal and fluids care plans: Theoretical basis and management. In **Textbook of critical care nursing: Diagnosis and management.** (pp. 664–671). St. Louis: Mosby.

Fluid Volume Excess

A state in which an individual experiences an increase in fluid volume related to increased intake or decreased loss of fluid, volume shifts within body fluid compartments, or a combination thereof.

S. Jill Ley, R.N., M.S., C.C.R.N.

• • • • • • • • • • • • • •

DEFINING CHARACTERISTICS

Subjective

Anxiety
Dyspnea
Restlessness

Physical Findings

Abnormal breath sounds (crackles)
Altered mentation
Anasarca
Bounding pulses
Edema
Hypertension
Increased central venous pressure
Increased pulmonary capillary wedge
       pressure
Jugular venous distention

Oliguria
Orthopnea
Pleural effusion
Positive hepatojugular reflex
Positive intake and output
Pulmonary congestion on chest x-ray
S3 gallop
Tachycardia
Tachypnea
Weight gain

Laboratory Findings

Decreased blood urea nitrogen
Decreased hematocrit
Decreased PaO_2
Decreased SaO_2

Decreased serum osmolality
Decreased serum sodium
Decreased urine osmolality
Decreased urine specific gravity

CONTRIBUTING FACTORS
Pathophysiological

Increased intake of fluid or sodium:
   Administration of IV fluids or blood products
   Administration of radiopaque dye
   Administration of sodium bicarbonate
   Oral ingestion of large amounts of salty foods
   Oral ingestion of large volumes of fluid
Decreased excretion of fluid or sodium:
   Congestive heart failure
   Hyperaldosteronism
   Renal insufficiency
   Severe stress
   Steroid therapy

Psychosociobehavioral

Age extremes
Cultural: high intake of soy sauce and/or monosodium glutamate (MSG)
Psychological disorders

EXPECTED OUTCOMES

Client will develop a net fluid loss.
   Fluid output exceeds intake.
   Body weight decreases.
Client will have no physical findings of hypervolemia.
   Vital signs return to client's baseline.
   Pulmonary congestion is absent on auscultation and chest x-ray.
   Edema resolves.
   Jugular venous distension and S3 gallop are absent.
   Abnormal laboratory findings resolve.
   Central venous pressure is 2–6 mmHg.
   Pulmonary capillary wedge pressure is 6–10 mmHg.
   Heart rate is ≤ 100 beats/min.

INTERVENTIONS	RATIONALE
Universal	
Ascertain the cause(s) of the fluid disturbance via history and physical examination.	Definitive treatment for fluid status abnormalities relies on identification and correction of ongoing fluid status changes.
Institute appropriate skin care measures for clients with edema: • Assess dependent areas (ankles or sacrum) for edema formation • Assist with repositioning every two hours, as needed • Apply antiembolic stockings to lower extremities prior to arising to minimize fluid accumulation when upright	Edema fluid can contribute to the development of skin breakdown.
Teach about interventions to maintain fluid balance: • Dietary instruction regarding sodium content of foods • Guidelines for fluid restriction if chronic illness is present • Notify physician of early signs of fluid overload	Hypervolemia may be avoided if prevention or early intervention is available.
Inpatient	
Monitor vital signs, intake and output, body weight, breath sounds, skin integrity, laboratory values, and filling pressure measurements. (A change in body weight of one kg corresponds to a net change in fluid balance of one L.)	A variety of clinical indicators is necessary to accurately assess fluid status. Resolution of abnormal findings should occur with restoration of fluid balance.

INTERVENTIONS	RATIONALE
Restrict fluid intake via oral and IV routes: • Implement an appropriate dietary fluid restriction; instruct client and family about fluid allotment and need to monitor all oral intake • Offer hard candies and frequent oral care to moisten dry mouth associated with fluid restriction • Notify pharmacy that IV fluids and medications should be maximally concentrated • Administer IV fluids via infusion pump to maintain precise infusion rate • Discontinue nonessential IV fluids; heparin lock IV lines to maintain patency	Restriction of fluid intake is necessary to restore fluid balance. Education of client and family is necessary to promote compliance with regimen.
Administer diuretics as ordered, to promote a net fluid loss: • Administer as early in the day as possible • Assess need for indwelling catheter	Early administration may avoid sleep loss due to frequent nocturnal voiding. An indwelling urinary Foley catheter is indicated during vigorous diuretic therapy when hourly intake and output assessment is necessary.
Monitor for signs of hypovolemia during diuretic therapy (see "Fluid Volume Deficit" care planning guide). • Notify physician if signs of hypovolemia develop to avoid unnecessary diuresis and a severe fluid deficit	The response to diuretics varies. Some experience an exaggerated response to initial therapy, leaving a predisposition to a fluid deficit. Clients with impaired cardiac function may develop a significant decrease in contractility during diuretic therapy.
Monitor for electrolyte and acid-base imbalances during diuretic therapy.	In addition to fluid and sodium loss, diuretics promote the excretion of potassium, magnesium, calcium, hydrogen, and bicarbonate ions in variable amounts.

INTERVENTIONS

RATIONALE

Implement resuscitative measures as indicated if signs of pulmonary edema are present, including severe dyspnea, pink frothy sputum, severe hypoxemia, bilateral crackles throughout lung fields.

- Assist with intubation or administration of high flow oxygen therapy
- Administer IV diuretics and vasodilators (morphine, nitroglycerine) as ordered
- Administer IV inotropes if hypoperfusion is present

Pulmonary edema is a condition where there is abnormal extravascular water accumulation in the lungs, producing rales, productive cough, cyanosis, and possibly signs and symptoms of respiratory distress and/or arrest.

Community Health/ Home Care

Monitor vital signs, daily body weight, heart and lung sounds, and mentation.

- Weight gain exceeding one kg/d is related to a net fluid gain
- Instruct to obtain daily weight at same time, on same scale, with similar clothing to promote accuracy
- Dyspnea associated with pulmonary crackles indicates pulmonary congestion and warrants prompt therapy

Assessment of a variety of clinical indicators is necessary to accurately assess fluid status. Resolution of abnormal findings should occur with restoration of fluid balance.

INTERVENTIONS	**R**ATIONALE
Decrease fluid intake to achieve a negative fluid balance. • Provide a written fluid restriction program that allows greatest fluids during daytime hours, with a 24-hour fluid limit of 1000–1800-cc/d • Instruct client and family about rationale for fluid restriction and how to measure fluid sources using household measurements	Education of client and family is necessary to ensure compliance with regimen. Intake must be less than output to achieve a negative fluid balance.

REFERENCES/BIBLIOGRAPHY

Holloway, N.M. (1989). **Critical care plans**. Springhouse, PA: Springhouse.

McKinney, M.R., Packa, D.R., & Dunbar, S.B. (1988). **AACN's clinical reference for critical care nursing.** (2nd ed.). New York: McGraw-Hill.

North American Nursing Diagnosis Association. (1990). **Taxonomy I** (Rev. 1990). St. Louis: NANDA.

*Pierson, M.G., & Funk, M. (1989). Technology versus clinical evaluation for fluid management decisions in CABG patients. **Image, 21** (4), 192–195.

Thelan, L.A., Davie, J.K., & Urden L.D. (1990). Renal and fluids care plans: Theoretical basis and management. In **Textbook of critical care nursing: Diagnosis and management.** (pp. 664–671). St. Louis: Mosby.

Gas Exchange, Impaired

A state in which an individual experiences a decreased passage of oxygen and/or carbon dioxide across the alveolar capillary membrane.

Claudia M. West, R.N., M.S.

DEFINING CHARACTERISTICS

Agitation
Arrhythmias
Bradycardia
Bradypnea
Central cyanosis
Clubbing
Confusion
Decreased ability to calculate numbers
Decreased oxygen saturation
Depression
Dyspnea
Fatigue
Forgetfulness
Hypercapnia
Hypoxemia

Increased hematocrit
Increased or decreased blood pressure
Increased or decreased cardiac output or index
Increased or decreased systemic vascular resistance
Increased pulmonary artery resistance and pressure
Irritation
Restlessness
Somnolence
Stupor
Tachycardia
Tachypnea

CONTRIBUTING FACTORS

Pathophysiological

Decreased mixed venous oxygen saturation, e.g., decreased cardiac output as in cardiogenic or septic shock
Diffusion defects, e.g., pulmonary fibrosis, emphysema
High altitude
Hypoventilation, e.g., emphysema, bronchitis, respiratory depression
Intrapulmonary or intracardiac shunting, e.g., atelectasis, pulmonary edema
Ventilation-perfusion mismatch, e.g., emphysema, pneumonia

253

Psychosociobehavioral

None

EXPECTED OUTCOMES

Client will have normal or baseline gas exchange at rest and with exercise.

> PaO_2 is $\geq$ 60 mmHg.
>
> Oxygen saturation is $\geq$ 90%.
>
> $PaCO_2$ returns to normal or baseline.
>
> Respiratory and heart rates return to normal or baseline.
>
> Client is alert, oriented, and displays no agitation or somnolence.
>
> Color of skin and mucous membranes are usual color.

Client will have normal or baseline hemodynamic parameters.

> Pulmonary artery pressure is systolic 20–30 mmHg and diastolic 10–20 mmHg or baseline.
>
> Pulmonary vascular resistance is 100–300 dynes · sec · cm^{-5} or baseline.
>
> Cardiac output is 4–81/min or cardiac index is 2.5–41/min/m² or baseline.
>
> Systemic vascular resistance is 770–1500 dynes · sec · cm^{-5} or baseline.

Client will have improved activity level with little or no oxygen desaturation.

> Walking distance (6 or 12 minutes) increases.
>
> Performance of activities of daily living increases.
>
> Strategies for conserving energy are identified.

Client will have improved neuropsychological status.

> Improved short-term memory is reported.
>
> Measures of short-term memory show improvement (e.g., mini-mental state).
>
> Ability to calculate (e.g., balance a checkbook) improves.
>
> Less depression is reported.

Client will demonstrate correct use of all prescribed respiratory therapy and equipment.

> Postural drainage and percussion, coughing, and incentive spirometry are performed correctly.
>
> Aerosol nebulizer is used accurately.
>
> Oxygen therapy is administered safely and effectively.
>
> Mechanical ventilator is operated correctly.

INTERVENTIONS

RATIONALE

Universal

Monitor the following:

INTERVENTIONS	RATIONALE
• Arterial blood gases and/or oxygen saturation via oximetry at rest and/or with exercise	PaO_2, $PaCO_2$, and SaO_2 are the most important indicators of gas exchange. Exercise may cause worsening oxygenation, although oxygenation may be acceptable at rest. Knowing this will assist in the oxygen prescription and promote optimal functional status.

INTERVENTIONS	RATIONALE
• Vital signs	Hypercapnia and hypoxemia stimulate ventilation and the sympathetic nervous system, resulting in tachypnea, tachycardia and sometimes increased blood pressure. Bradycardia and hypotension may result if hypoxemia is severe or prolonged. Severe or prolonged hypercapnia may cause respiratory depression and bradypnea. Arrhythmias may also occur secondary to the effect of hypoxemia on the cardiac conduction system. Monitoring temperature is important to determine the presence of atelectasis or a respiratory infection. In addition, changes in the breathing pattern may result in impaired gas exchange. For instance, a rapid, shallow breathing pattern without periods of deep breathing will result in atelectasis.
• Color of skin, nailbeds, and mucous membranes of the mouth	The presence of cyanosis in these areas indicates significant oxygen desaturation (< 75%). Cyanosis of the mucous membranes is a more reliable indicator than that of the skin or nailbeds since skin pigmentation can alter perception of cyanosis, and vasoconstriction can produce a peripheral cyanosis that is not necessarily associated with impaired oxygenation.
• Mental status	Acute hypoxemia results in cerebral hypoxia as evidenced by restlessness and agitation and progressing to confusion, stupor, and coma. Chronic hypoxemia is evidenced by memory loss, impaired ability to calculate, and depression. Hypercapnia causes somnolence and lethargy progressing to stupor and coma.
• Presence of dyspnea and fatigue	Respiratory distress may indicate impaired gas exchange. This assists in establishing a baseline against which to measure improvement or deterioration in functional status as a response to changes in gas exchange. The presence of worsening dyspnea or fatigue with activity reflects the increased ventilatory demand resulting from the increased oxygen requirements and carbon dioxide production. The oxygen prescription may need to be altered as a result.

INTERVENTIONS	RATIONALE
• Physical findings, such as the presence of chest pain, decreased or asymmetrical thoracic expansion, dullness or hyperresonance, diminished or absent breath sounds, or adventitious breath sounds	These are important indicators of respiratory or cardiac problems that may be responsible for impaired gas exchange.
• Hematocrit	If thrombocytosis is present, long-term oxygen therapy (several weeks) may lower the hematocrit.
• Response to oxygen therapy	In clients who are hypercapnic, raising the PaO_2 may result in further hypoventilation and hypercapnia. The nurse should assess alertness and arousability as oxygen therapy is begun or increased.
• Areas where nasal cannula or face mask cause pressure	Nasal cannula rub and press inside the nares, under the nose, and superiorly between the ears and skull. The face mask can cause pressure across the nose and cheeks. Areas of skin breakdown can occur in these areas causing pain and, possibly, unacceptance of the therapy. Skin breakdown also will provide a source of infection.
Assess understanding of the effects of cigarette smoking on pulmonary or cardiac disease.	Cigarette smoking is the most important risk factor for the development of obstructive lung disease, lung cancer, and coronary artery disease. The nurse must know what the client's understanding of this relationship is so that a teaching plan to address the issue can be developed.
Ascertain the presence of cigarette smoke in the home or work place and the response to it.	Passive smoking in the non-smoker has been shown to greatly increase the risk of emphysema and myocardial infarction. It also may be a trigger of bronchospasm in asthmatics. Knowledge of the client's environment and how the issue of passive smoking is dealt with would help the nurse explore various coping strategies.

INTERVENTIONS	RATIONALE
Assess for correct self-administration of medication and use of metered-dose inhalers.	Some clients take their medications sporadically and adjust the dose according to their symptoms. Hypoxemia also may cause forgetfulness, and medications may not be taken correctly. During acute dyspnea or wheezing, anxiety may cause incorrect use of the metered-dose inhaler, causing delivery of too much or too little medication.
Explore with the asthmatic what triggers acute exacerbations.	This knowledge allows the nurse to help the client identify approaches to eliminating or minimizing the triggers.
Discuss self-care strategies the client usually employs to manage acute episodes of dyspnea and their effectiveness.	Many individuals with acute or chronic dyspnea have learned coping strategies to help them manage this symptom and its associated distress. Knowledge of these helps the nurse evaluate how well the client is coping and whether additional strategies may be of help.
Assess respiratory response to narcotic analgesia.	Morphine in therapeutic doses and, presumably, other opioids can result in diminished or absent sighing reflex because of their action on the respiratory center in the medulla. Large doses can result in slowed, shallow breathing and, eventually, respiratory arrest.
Administer oxygen at the prescribed dose and with the prescribed delivery system.	Most hypoxemia is easily treated with supplemental oxygen. The primary goals of oxygen therapy are to reduce work of breathing and cardiac work and to provide adequate tissue oxygenation. The dose should be enough to meet these goals, while minimizing the hazards of oxygen such as hypoventilation and oxygen toxicity. Research has shown that continuous administration of oxygen for up to 15 hours or more per day in those who require it results in significantly decreased pulmonary artery pressure, improved neuropsychological function, and increased survival. Therefore, it is vital that clients understand the importance of adhering to their oxygen prescription. The method of administration must be suitable to the FiO_2 desired, the client's ventilatory pattern, and comfort.

INTERVENTIONS	RATIONALE
Make sure oxygen mask or nasal cannula is correctly placed and fits properly.	This will assure delivery of the correct FiO_2 and minimize discomfort. The cannula should be directed toward the back of the nose rather than upward toward the frontal sinuses.
Provide humidification of oxygen if giving over 2 L or > 30% concentration.	Dry oxygen over these amounts will result in dehydration of the mucous blanket in the airways, dried mucus and plugging, non-motile cilia, inflammation, and infection.
Provide aerosolization of oxygen if prescribed and monitor response to it.	Aerosolization delivers water in small droplets and is useful for hydrating the mucous blanket, liquefying viscous secretions, and promoting expectoration. Complications of aerosolization include bronchospasm, swelling of secretions and airway obstruction, and water retention— a particular danger for persons with heart disease. Observation during the initiation of therapy, auscultation for secretions, and production of cough are necessary in preventing these complications.
Encourage coughing or huffing if secretions are present. [1]	Coughing when performed with several initial deep breaths allows air to enter the airways distal to the secretions. The force generated by the chest wall assists in pushing the secretions up to the pharynx where they can be expelled. Huffing is a forced expiration while the glottis remains open. Usually after a series of deep breaths, two to three huffs are performed from a complete inspiration. This technique is useful for persons with copious secretions or who cannot generate a large vital capacity.
Encourage deep breathing with sustained inspiratory hold or use of an incentive spirometer.	Hourly performance of these maneuvers may prevent atelectasis and respiratory infection, particularly in those at high risk for respiratory complications, e.g., heavy smokers and those breathing at low lung volumes.

[1] Coughing may cause airways to collapse, worsening bronchospasm, and dyspnea and hypoxemia, and should be performed only when secretions are present.

INTERVENTIONS	RATIONALE
Change humidifier or nebulizer and water every 24 hours.	This minimizes contamination by microorganisms and their delivery to the respiratory tract.
Empty water from respiratory tubing as needed, allowing water to drain out away from the client and into a receptacle (not the humidifier).	Accumulated water in the corrugated tubing is a medium for growth of organisms and also increases resistance to the gas flow, possibly resulting in decreased delivery of oxygen.
Help splint the chest or abdomen with a pillow or blanket if deep breathing or coughing is painful.	Splinting helps to support the painful area so that less pressure is transmitted to the area and less pain is felt. Deep breathing and coughing then can be more effective.
Perform chest physical therapy if secretions are present and coughing is ineffective.	Accumulated secretions can obstruct the airways and decrease ventilation, resulting in impaired oxygenation. Percussion helps loosen secretions from the walls of airways, and postural drainage allows gravity to help propel secretions toward the large central airways. From there, they can be more easily expectorated or removed by suctioning. Chest physical therapy, however, can cause bronchospasm and oxygen desaturation, and the head-down position is contraindicated in a variety of conditions. Therefore, the need for chest physical therapy must be carefully weighed.
Provide or assist with mouth and/or nose care as needed if receiving oxygen.	Even humidified oxygen can be drying to the mouth or nose if delivered at high flow rates. In addition, the client may experience an unpleasant taste in the mouth that can be eliminated with a mouth wash and brushing.
Provide long tubing or a portable oxygen delivery system if ambulatory.	This will promote independence and increase activity level, which are critical for improving ventilation, functional status, and overall well-being. Long tubing can be a hazard for tripping, however, so a portable oxygen system is preferable in relatively active individuals.
Encourage or assist with changing position in bed, sitting in a chair, or ambulating.	These activities encourage clearance of secretions, increase lung volumes and ventilation, and prevent the effects of immobility. Also, early

INTERVENTIONS	RATIONALE
	mobilization after surgery results in fewer respiratory complications.
Position with "bad" lung up if unilateral lung disease is present, unless prescribed otherwise.	This position increases blood flow to normal lung and maximizes ventilation-perfusion matching and gas exchange. Positioning with the "bad" lung down worsens intrapulmonary shunting by increasing blood flow to the lung that is not ventilating. Gas exchange, therefore, is further impaired.
Alter position according to optimal oxygenation (i.e., oxygen saturation on oximetry) if diffuse bilateral disease exists.	Studies have shown that rotating position from side to side or from supine to prone can significantly impair or enhance gas exchange, even in persons with diffuse or bilateral lung disease. As above, position changes ventilation-perfusion relationships, which the nurse must be aware of and apply accordingly.
Perform endotracheal suctioning as needed to remove secretions. Use intermittent suction for no longer than 10–15 sec.	Suctioning removes secretions that may be obstructing large airways and decreasing distal ventilation, and thus improves gas exchange. Prolonged suctioning, however, removes oxygen from the airways, causing decreased alveolar oxygen, atelectasis, and hypoxemia. Therefore, suctioning should be performed only when secretions are auscultated or suspected and coughing is ineffective.
Obtain a dietary consult regarding nutritional requirements and strategies for optimizing intake.	Protein-calorie malnutrition results in decreased respiratory muscle mass, strength, and endurance and places the client at risk for respiratory infection. Acute exacerbations of disease and chronic respiratory or cardiac disease increase respiratory work and caloric needs. Anorexia and early satiety are common and also interfere with nutritional intake.
Provide small, frequent feedings high in protein with remaining calories equally distributed between fat and carbohydrates.	Small feedings result in less energy demand, bloating, and dyspnea than large meals. Meals high in carbohydrates or greatly in excess of energy needs should be avoided, since carbon dioxide production and ventilatory demand may increase significantly.

INTERVENTIONS	RATIONALE
Reduce fever if present.	Elevated body temperature causes increased oxygen consumption and carbon dioxide production, thus increasing ventilatory demand.
Treat pain.	Pain, acute or chronic, causes increased muscle tension, which will increase oxygen consumption and carbon dioxide production. Pain in the chest wall or upper abdomen will cause shallow tidal volumes and will increase the risk of atelectasis and pneumonia.
Suggest that the physician make a referral to a local pulmonary rehabilitation program.	The combination of education and progressive exercise in a safe environment promotes self-care and increased functional status. Although gas exchange generally is not improved by such a program, there is improved aerobic efficiency so that exercising muscles extract less oxygen and produce less carbon dioxide for a given work load. As a result, ventilatory demand is reduced and dyspnea decreases. Pulmonary rehabilitation programs also have been shown to significantly reduce hospital days per year, improve survival, and increase quality of life.

Inpatient

INTERVENTIONS	RATIONALE
Monitor the respiratory response to epidural narcotics.	Epidural narcotics can result in significant respiratory depression and respiratory arrest. Respiratory rate and depth should be assessed hourly. Narcan should be available at the bedside for rapid administration.
Assess the client's resources and home situation with regard to the management of long-term mechanical ventilation, i.e., finances, accessibility of follow-up care, space in the home, etc.	These data are essential in determining the suitability of managing long-term mechanical ventilation in the home or in choosing an alternate care setting.
Help the client to participate in decision making regarding long-term mechanical ventilation or alternatives, such as a rocking bed, pneumobelt, or diaphragm pacing.	The client must have complete information about the risks and benefits of long-term ventilation in order to evaluate its appropriateness. The need for continued community resources, and the financial and emotional cost of mechanical ventilation in the home or a chronic care setting are very great.

INTERVENTIONS	RATIONALE
Support the client's decision to withdraw mechanical ventilation when there is no hope for recovery.	This decision is very painful for families and loved ones, as well as the client if conscious. The ability to express feelings of loss and guilt in the presence of a concerned and nonjudgmental person will help to facilitate this decision.
Teach regarding use and maintenance of the ventilator. Provide several days of practice for the primary and alternate care givers before discharge, using the actual ventilator to be sent home with the client.	This provides the opportunity to learn the care of the client and the ventilator in a safe environment. Reinforcement, support, and correction can be provided until the client is ready for discharge.
Assist in notifying the local fire department, emergency medical service, or power company before discharge home on mechanical ventilation.	The fire department or emergency medical service may wish to arrange for a home visit to visualize the layout of the house, the client's condition, and equipment needs. This will assist them in the future in case of an emergency. The power company can, in case of a power failure, arrange for priority service such as a portable generator.
Instruct in the correct use of prescribed respiratory therapy and equipment, including side effects and hazards.	This will enhance therapeutic effects of the therapy and minimize hazards.
Refer to appropriate community resources such as community health nursing, home care agency, respiratory home care, etc.	These will assure adequate follow-up in the home and promote consistency of care.

Community Health/ Home Care

Assess for correct use and cleaning of respiratory therapy equipment such as nebulizers, oxygen delivery system, suction, ventilators, cuirass, and CPAP system.	Correct use enhances therapeutic effects and reduces the hazards of the equipment. Proper cleaning prevents transmission of organisms and respiratory infections (see care planning guide for "Airway Clearance, Impaired").

INTERVENTIONS	**R**ATIONALE
Follow up in the home as frequently as seems necessary.	This serves as a means of assessing the client's respiratory status as well as the dynamics of the client-care giver interaction. Needed reassurance and additional teaching can be done also.
Provide additional support services as needed, such as home health aid, care-giver respite, etc.	These services will assist in maintaining client independence in the home, while minimizing costly hospitalizations.

REFERENCES/BIBLIOGRAPHY

Chang, S.C., Shiao, G.M., & Perng, R.P. (1989). Postural effect on gas exchange in patients with unilateral pleural effusions. **Chest, 96** (1), 60–63.

Egbert, L.D., & Bendixen, H.H. (1964). Effect of morphine on breathing pattern. **JAMA, 188** (6), 485–488.

Hodgkin, J.E. (1990). Pulmonary rehabilitation. **Clinics in Chest Medicine, 11** (3), 447–454.

Kersten, L.D. (1989). **Comprehensive respiratory nursing**. Philadelphia: Saunders.

* Kohlman-Carrieri, V., & Janson-Bjerklie, S. (1986). Strategies patients use to manage the sensation of dyspnea. **Western Journal of Nursing Research, 8** (3), 284–305.

Lucas, J., Golish, J.A., Sleeper, G., & O'Ryan, J.A. (1988). **Home respiratory care**. Norwalk, CT: Appleton & Lange.

Make, B.J., & Gilmartin, M.E. (1990). Mechanical ventilation in the home. **Critical Care Clinics, 6** (3), 785–796.

Nelson, L.D., & Anderson, H.B. (1989). Physiological effects of steep positioning in the surgical intensive care unit. **Archives of Surgery, 124,** 352–355.

North American Nursing Diagnosis Association. (1990). **Taxonomy I** (Rev. 1990). St. Louis: NANDA.

Piehl, M.A., & Brown, R.S. (1976). Use of extreme position changes in acute respiratory failure. **Critical Care Medicine, 4** (1), 13–14.

Shapiro, B.A., Kacmarek, R.M., Cane, R.D., Peruzzi, W.T., & Hauptman, D. (1991). **Clinical applications of respiratory care.** (4th ed.). St. Louis: Mosby.

Spearing, C., & Cornell, D.J. (1987). Incentive spirometry: Inspiring your patient to breathe deeply. **Nursing '87, 17** (9), 50–51.

Stock, M.C., Downs, J.B., Gauer, J.K., Alster, J.M., & Imrey, P.B. (1985). Prevention of postoperative pulmonary complications with CPAP, incentive spirometry, and conservative therapy. **Chest, 87** (2), 151–157.

Tiep, B.L. (1990). Long-term home oxygen therapy. **Clinics in Chest Medicine, 11** (3), 505–521.

Grieving, Anticipatory

A sequence of subjective states in which there is the expectation of, or actual, loss of life, bodily function, cherished experience, activity, or thing.

Julia D. Emblen, R.N., Ph.D.

DEFINING CHARACTERISTICS

Absentmindedness
Acceptance
Anger
Attempt to hold onto person by doing
    everything according to person's
    wishes, doing every treatment,
    behaving like person one is losing
Bargaining
Change in eating habits
Change in energy level which may
    increase or decrease, and which
    may include any extreme
    changes in ADL
Change in interpersonal responses
Change in sleep patterns
Confusion

Despondence
Endurance
Expression of pain regarding potential loss
Fantasizing about lost person, experience,
    activity, or thing
Free discussion about the possibility/
    reality of loss
Guilt
Passivity
Personal preoccupation
Questioning
Searching for meaning and purpose of
    loss occurrence, help, and comfort
Sense of emptiness
Sorrow

CONTRIBUTING FACTORS

Pathophysiological

Expectation of biological loss, body part, or function, i.e., chronic disease, paralysis, amputation,
    sexual functioning
Expectation of loss due to aging, i.e., decreased joint mobility

Psychosociobehavioral

Expectation of emotional loss, i.e., friendship, love
Expectation of object loss, i.e., home, jewelry
Expectation of personal loss, i.e., spouse, child, parent, friend, pet
Expectation of social loss, i.e., independence, job

EXPECTED OUTCOMES

Client will adjust and/or adapt to expected loss and reinvest energy and activities in living a
       productive, meaningful, and useful life.
    Normal ADL are resumed.
    Emotional communication occurs within normal limits.
    Social service and activities are resumed.
    Work or work substitute is found if income or meaningful activity is needed.

INTERVENTIONS	RATIONALE
Universal	
Assess physiological function to determine deficiencies.	Normal homeostasis may be disturbed, and imbalances can affect all body systems. Insomnia, head, joint, or abdominal pain; GI disturbances; and autoimmune deficiencies are most common symptoms occurring as a result of imbalances.
Assess emotional (affective) patterns for excessive or diminished responses of crying, talking, depression, etc.	Anger, anxiety, aggression, bargaining, crying, confusion, denial, passivity, and questioning are typical responses to anticipatory grief.
Assess support network.	The feeling of aloneness heightens grief.
Assess coping skills.	Successful use of coping skills facilitates management of stressors. Coping skills may need to be reinforced as new challenges emerge.
Assist in the identification of strengths.	Marshalling personal resources promotes integrity of self.
Provide specific care to maintain homeostatic levels.	Maintaining physiological function is essential to support life and to prevent negative stress-related socioemotional responses such as bursts of anger.
Provide for rehearsal of outcomes.	Mental rehearsal of the loss before it actually occurs facilitates adjustment when it occurs.

INTERVENTIONS	**R**ATIONALE
	Rehearsal of outcomes is a technique by which one can practice behaviors that anticipate the loss, thereby facilitating adjustment.
Encourage detachment behaviors.	Detachment behaviors distance self from the source of loss.
Allow to experience the pain of the expected loss.	Some experience of loss before it actually occurs facilitates the adjustment to it.
Provide opportunity to ventilate feelings.	Ventilation of feelings releases body energy which could otherwise be turned inward to cause negative physical symptoms.
Encourage the expression of feelings by directed/reflective questioning.	Directed questioning, e.g., "Do you sometimes feel angry?" provides an opportunity to express negative thoughts or emotions.
Reassure that some physical symptoms are a normal part of grief.	The knowledge that one's symptoms of insomnia, lack of appetite, chest tightness, etc. are not unlike the experience of others in similar situations can be comforting.
Provide opportunity for venting freely.	Open-ended questions provide for verbalizing divergent responses, e.g., "Could you describe your thoughts and feelings so that I can more clearly understand what is distressing you?"
Provide privacy when behaviors are such that embarrassment may occur.	Hyperactivity, excessive emotional response such as continuous crying, and extreme passivity may be the only response which can be mustered at a given point in time; but these responses may add the anxiety of embarrassment if they occur in public.
Suggest ways to lighten the grief work by planning a variation in activities, e.g., watching TV, reading, talking about specific things unrelated to grief experiences.	Constant preoccupation with pain creates potentially life-threatening responses.
Reassure that some physical and emotional symptoms are a normal part of grief.	The knowledge that one's symptoms of insomnia, lack of appetite, chest tightness, sadness, lethargy, etc. are not unlike the experience of others in similar situations can be comforting.

INTERVENTIONS	**R**ATIONALE
Inpatient	
Assess responses to distinguish those which relate to physical illness and those which relate to anticipatory loss.	In illness the anticipatory grief and physical symptoms tend to merge.
Provide opportunity for talking with person who has successfully adjusted following a similar anticipated loss.	Seeing someone who has adjusted provides hope that it is possible to survive and adjust to live without a body part, or even a loved one.
Discuss adjustments which may be made in a way that presents a positive challenge.	Meeting a challenge can become a source of physical and emotional energy.
Provide educational materials which describe the normal process persons go through in adjusting to the loss.	Knowledge of normal events decreases apprehension and uncertainty regarding the unknown and dispels negative imaginary fears.
Community Health/ Home Care	
Assess adjustment to changes in life-style and role resulting from expectation of loss.	Planning for undesired change may be difficult to incorporate into life-style.
Indicate a time pattern for focusing on the loss.	In the home setting it is too easy to think constantly about the anticipated loss. It is helpful if that focus is limited. Spending an hour reminiscing and then an hour when thoughts are directed to another area may be helpful for some grievers.
Encourage the griever to focus on specific small tasks or details.	The experience of the whole may become overwhelming. When ideas, emotions, etc. can be sorted and broken down into smaller portions, they can be managed more easily.
Provide a list of support groups which would be appropriate.	For some, especially extroverted personalities, it is helpful to share feelings with others who have experienced similar losses.

INTERVENTIONS	RATIONALE
Reassure that there are many different responses to grief, and that experiences may not follow the popular patterns written about in the literature.	Because grief work is so universal, much has been written about what to expect and patterns which occur. Individual clients may have very different responses because of their own personalities, values, support systems, and internal strengths. They need to know that there is no exact pattern.
Indicate that the initial sensations and desperate feelings of grief do decrease with time.	Reassurance of this relieves some of the emotional pressure.
Encourage the engagement in a variety of activities with time for quiet introspection when that is comfortably manageable.	Recovery from grief is enhanced by the knowledge that changes in ADLs which include both quiet and active times, result in increased coping.
Suggest finding a person to contact every day to listen to feelings.	Daily contact with a caring person helps adjust to the loss experience.
Provide instruction in journaling to express feelings.	Putting negative painful feelings into this written form releases emotional energy, thereby averting negative physiological responses.

REFERENCES/BIBLIOGRAPHY

Bowlby, J. (1980). **Loss, sadness and depression**. New York: Basic Books.
Bowlby, J. (1961). Process of mourning. **International Journal of Psychoanalysis, 42**, 317–340.
* Carter, S.L. (1989). Themes of grief. **Nursing Research, 38**, 354–358.
Engel, G.L. (1964). Grief and grieving. **American Journal of Nursing, 64**, 93–98.
Gifford, B.J. (1990). Supporting the bereaved. **American Journal of Nursing, 90**, 50–53.
* Hainsworth, M. (1987–1988). Women in grief. **Perspectives in Psychiatric Care, 24**, 85–90.
Kizilos, P. J. (1990). Grief groups for children. **Journal of Christian Nursing, 7**, 10–14.
Laliberte, S. (1988). Loss. In J.M. Flynn, & P.B. Heffron. (Eds.). **Nursing from concept to practice.** (2nd ed.). (pp. 559–579). Palo Alto, CA: Appleton & Lange.
Lindemann, E. (1944). Symptomatology and management of acute grief. **American Journal of Psychiatry, 101**, 141–148.
Paterson, G.W. (1987). Managing grief and bereavement, **Primary Care, 14**, 403–415.
Sanders, C.M., Mauger, P.A., & Strong, P.N. (1985). **A manual for the grief experience inventory**. Palo Alto, CA: Consulting Psychologists Press.
Werner-Beland, J.A. (1980). **Grief responses to long-term illness and disability**. Reston, VA: Reston Publishing.

Grieving, Dysfunctional

A state in which an individual experiences prolonged abnormal or impaired responses which accompany the loss of life, bodily function, cherished experience, activity, or thing.

Julia D. Emblen, R.N., Ph.D.

. . . .

DEFINING CHARACTERISTICS: (All of these are prefaced with **prolonged** time intervals. Grief experiences are highly individualized, and normal grief work may include short periods of all the characteristics identified as dysfunctional.)

Continuous questioning regarding
    reason for loss
Development of symptoms similar to
    those of deceased loved one
Excessive guilt
Inability to recognize loss
Incessant talking of loss
Increased hostility toward persons/groups

Lack of affective response to loss
Major disruption in ADL, i.e., insomnia,
    over- or under-eating to 20
    pounds plus or minus
Marked social isolation
Suicidal comments, thoughts, or attempts
Total denial of reality of loss

CONTRIBUTING FACTORS

Pathophysiological

Chronic disease: myasthenia gravis, stroke
Experience of biological loss, body part or function
Experience of loss due to aging: e. g., decreased hearing acuity
Sexuality: mastectomy, prostatectomy

Psychosociobehavioral

Experience of emotional loss: friendship, love
Experience of object loss: home, jewelry

269

Experience of personal loss: spouse, child, parent, friend, pet
Experience of social loss: independence, job

EXPECTED OUTCOMES

Client will adjust and/or adapt to changes occurring due to loss and reinvest energy and
activities in living a productive, meaningful, and useful life.
Reengagement in normal ADL is evident.
Emotional communication exists within normal bounds.
Social service and other activities are resumed.
Suitable work and/or work substitute is found if income and meaningful activities
are needed.

INTERVENTIONS / RATIONALE

Interventions	Rationale
Universal	
Assess physiological function to determine deficiencies.	Homeostasis must be maintained for life to be sustained. Insomnia and GI changes are commonly occurring symptoms which may become life-threatening.
Assess emotional responses for excesses or absent responses.	Hostility, isolation, denial, and guilt are typical responses in dysfunctional grief.
Assess support network.	The sense of isolation and aloneness perpetuates negative grief responses.
Assess coping patterns.	Patterns of response to stresses may need to be altered if they fail to facilitate coping with new challenges.
Assess needs in the spiritual dimension.	The spiritual dimension provides a means of identifying a new purpose and meaning in life.
Identify personal resources and strengths.	Family members, friends, financial means, and such sources may be used to reestablish normal functioning.
Establish optimal nutritional intake.	While working to overcome dysfunctional grieving, a strenuous dietary modification should not be introduced, but binge patterns or cessation of eating requires intervention to reestablish a nutritionally adequate diet that maintains desired weight.

INTERVENTIONS	RATIONALE
Maintain/reestablish normal sleep-rest patterns.	Abnormal or inadequate sleep-rest patterns increase dysfunctional grieving.
Establish normal affective responses and seek support during crying.	Tears stimulate the immune system to release toxic enzymes, which build up when crying becomes excessive.
Suggest private places, i.e., bathroom, car, or chapel where tears can be managed.	Perception of private and public behaviors will require reestablishment.
Support tears, but discourage constant crying in every setting.	Public places are not socially acceptable for displaying personal emotions.
Allow expression of other emotional responses, i.e., shock, numbness, denial, anger, depression, apathy, lack of emotional response to any event, jealousy, panic, insecurity, fear of continuing with life and of dying.	Expression of emotional pain provides catharsis and decreases the symptoms resulting from the stress of trying to hold in the pain.
Provide support for displaying bizarre behavior, but indicate which are appropriate for place and time.	Affective expressions of grief can become so pervasive that feedback is needed as to how constant venting and/or display of feelings is affecting one's life and the lives of others.
Establish a pattern allowing for venting of feelings with some time limitations.	Grief work requires timely but not all-consuming expression.
Reestablish social dimensions such as friendly relationships with members of both sexes.	Encouragement in social relationships which highlight the change of social status, e.g., husband to widower, enhances adjustment.
Encourage use of past tense with regard to any permanent loss.	Persistence in denial, by continuing to refer to loss in present or future tense, interferes with overcoming grief.
Allow time to tell the story of the loss and to reminisce about the meaning.	Initially, verbalization of details facilitates healing; however, the constant reiteration of the story should be discouraged because such fixation creates a pathologic response.

INTERVENTIONS

RATIONALE

INTERVENTIONS	RATIONALE
Discourage social withdrawal.	Opening the curtain of one's home allows old and new friends to reenter lives.
Plan ways to celebrate holidays and other special events, such as birthdays and anniversaries, so they do not become personally devastating.	Losses alter previous patterns of celebration which require the establishment of new satisfying occasions.
Allow expression of questions regarding the loss and about the effect the loss has on the belief system, faith, and trust.	Freedom to express transcendent issues which loss experiences raise, provides opportunity to discuss new levels of understanding of the meaning of beliefs and values.
Provide opportunity for expression of guilt.	Expression, both in conversation and in writing, vents the sense of personal responsibility for the loss.
Discourage constant preoccupation with death.	The experience of major personal or bodily loss sometimes exhibits itself in the expression of a preference for dying, e.g., "I'm just waiting for the undertaker." Such a view reinforces personal apathy and interferes with reengagement in life activities.
Discourage hallucinations/fantasies and other unrealistic thoughts regarding the presence of the lost person, body part, or experience.	The experience of flashbacks triggered by almost anything, such as shoes or a smile, is common. Constant thoughts on what is lost prevent focus and concentration on present details.
Encourage a sense of hope that there will be some good experiences yet to come in life, despite the loss experience.	A hopeless view of the future leads to negative thinking and eventual suicide of ideas and/ or life.
(Any of the interventions identified under the "Universal" category may be instituted and continued until the assessed need is satisfactorily met.)	Dysfunctional grief may curtail any normal functioning, e.g., sleeping, eating, urinating, etc.

INTERVENTIONS	RATIONALE
Inpatient	
Assess physiological functioning level.	Homeostasis may be disturbed during dysfunctional grieving, and body systems may be affected.
Identify affective responses.	Abnormal emotional responses must be identified before planning intervening care.
Institute a plan of normal physiological function.	A normal schedule must be maintained, even in illness when the grief incapacitates and/or reduces the client to an infantile state.
Intervene selectively according to need to reestablish normal affective responses.	Dysfunctional grief impedes and/or eliminates normal emotional responses. Selective interventions need to be instituted.
Community Health/ Home Care	
Assess adjustment to change in life-style and role resulting from loss experience.	Change is very difficult for some people to incorporate into their lives.
Allow verbalization of concerns related to new roles.	If a spouse or child dies, the client has to adjust to major changes in personal status.
Encourage expressions of intimate issues related to sexual relationships.	Some losses require major adjustments for sexual functioning, but talking about sexual problems is generally not socially accepted.
Provide assistance with managing physical aspects, such as clothes and other articles which are no longer needed as a result of the loss of a person or experience.	In dysfunctional grieving there is often difficulty getting rid of the personal effects of the deceased person, in an effort to deny the loss.
Suggest resources to use to replace lost articles, pets, etc.	Environmental concerns such as housing, furniture, and clothes may be issues a dysfunctional griever cannot consider.

INTERVENTIONS	**R**ATIONALE
Suggest ideas for visiting a place of memorial or establishing a memorial if the loss was the death of a person.	Grief work is often relieved when remembrances and other memorials are established.
Provide assistance with suggestions on changing life-style habits and residence.	Help with reestablishing lives after a loss is needed. Some grievers want to move, while others desire to escape through excessive dependence on drugs, alcohol, or selected people. Counseling regarding advisability and suitability of possible alternatives for adaptation to loss provides movement toward positive changes and away from negative life-styles and dependency.
Suggest resources which might be helpful in coping with loss. Consider the use of booklets or pamphlets.	The gathering of resources provides a sense of control and a source of information for dealing with this and future crises.
Call an appropriate group to initiate contact.	Dysfunctional grieving decreases energy necessary for initiating activity. Making connections and gathering resources, i.e., support groups, written material, crisis centers appropriate to the type of loss decreases the feeling of aloneness and increases feelings of empowerment.
Provide options so that the grieving person does not replace one dysfunctional pattern with another, e.g., overdependence on a support person.	Intervention by a caring, supportive person enhances grief work, and appropriate and timely withdrawal of that support does not permit overdependence.
Suggest new sources to use to cope with grief.	Humor, self-help books, work, hobbies, and a host of other things may be used to help adjust to grief, but one must be selective with suggestions which are specifically helpful for the particular needs of the one grieving.
Provide for resources which will protect from suicidal thoughts and/or actions.	Suicide may preoccupy thinking in dysfunctional grieving and lead to action unless precautions are taken.

INTERVENTIONS	**R**ATIONALE
Facilitate actions which will lead to a degree of resolution of loss and reintegration in life.	Planning ADL which involve the person in satisfying experiences will help movement to a satisfactory level of adjustment to the changes in living that result from the loss experience.

REFERENCES/BIBLIOGRAPHY

Bowlby, J. (1980). **Loss, sadness and depression**. New York: Basic Books.

Bowlby, J. (1961). Process of mourning. **International Journal of Psychoanalysis, 42,** 317–340.

*Carter, S. (1989). Themes of grief. **Nursing Research, 38,** 354–358.

Engel, G.L. (1964). Grief and grieving. **American Journal of Nursing, 64,** 93–98.

Fowler, M. (1989). Weal and woe: On the loss of lament. **Heart & Lung, 18,** 640–641.

Gifford, B.J. (1990). Supporting the bereaved. **American Journal of Nursing, 90,** 50–53.

Gyulay, J.E. (1989). **Issues in Comprehensive Pediatric Nursing, 12,** 1–31.

Houseman, C., & Pheifer, W.G. (1988). Potential for unresolved grief in survivors of persons with AIDS. **Archives of Psychiatric Nursing, 2,** 296–301.

Kizilos, P.J. (1990). Grief groups for children. **Journal of Christian Nursing, 7,** 10–14.

Laliberte, S. (1988). Loss. In J.M. Flynn, & P. B. Heffron. (Eds.). **Nursing from concept to practice.** (2nd ed.). (pp. 559–579). Palo Alto, CA: Appleton & Lange.

Leliaert, R.M. (1989). Spiritual side of 'good grief': What happened to holy saturday? **Death Studies, 13,** 103–117.

Lindemann, E. (1944). Symptomatology and management of acute grief. **American Journal of Psychiatry, 101,** 141–148.

*Matthiesen, V. (1989). Guilt & grief when daughters place mothers in nursing homes. **Journal of Gerontological Nursing, 15,** 11–15.

Paterson, G.W., (1987). Managing grief and bereavement. **Primary Care, 14,** 403–415 .

Romond, J.L. (1990). "It's sad & you hurt a lot": Letters from bereaved brothers & sisters. **Journal of Christian Nursing, 7,** 4–8.

Sanders, C.M., Mauger, P.A., & Strong, P.N. (1985). **A Manual for the grief experience inventory**. Palo Alto, CA: Consulting Psychologists Press.

Simpson, K. (1989). Understanding mourning. **Nursing Times, 85,** 43–45.

Werner-Beland, J.A. (1980). **Grief responses to long-term illness and disability**. Reston, VA: Reston Publishing.

Health Maintenance, Altered

A state in which an individual is unable to identify, manage, and/or seek out help to maintain health (NANDA, 1990, p. 78).

Marilyn Frenn, R.N., Ph.D.
Helena Lee, R.N., M.S.N.

DEFINING CHARACTERISTICS

Age-related preventive measures
    not taken
Expressed health concerns
Limited adaptive behaviors to internal/
    environmental changes
Regular and unmitigated exposure to
    health hazards:
    Abuse
    Ageism

Crime
Pollution
Poverty
Racism
Sexism
Regular practice of behaviors that:
    Increase risk of illness
    Limit optimal function
    Limit recovery from illness or disability

CONTRIBUTING FACTORS

Pathophysiological

Responses to illness or disability that inhibit health behaviors, e.g., fatigue, impaired mobility, inability to concentrate, pain, perceptual deficits

Psychosociobehavioral

ENVIRONMENTAL
Cultural barriers to use of health care system
Health advice incongruent with beliefs (cultural, health, religious)
Lack of environmental resources:
    Acceptable and affordable health care
    Equipment
    Finances

276

Food
Health care providers/systems that promote health
Health resources—e.g., food nutrients not labeled, healthy foods expensive or not
    available, lack of safe place to exercise
Housing
Transportation
Limited social support for health:
    Dysfunctional family system
    Lack of meaningful and supportive relationships
    Peer modeling and support of unhealthy behaviors
Public or workplace policies that do not promote health
Societal support of unhealthy products and behaviors

INDIVIDUAL
Depression
Dysfunctional grieving
Illiteracy
Lack of information regarding:
    Age-appropriate screening and self-care
    Community resources
    Health hazards
    Health promotion services
    Personal health status
Lack of personal requisites:
    Goals or purpose
    Motivation
    Perceived control over health
    Perceived responsibility for health behaviors
    Previous health-promoting life-style
    Self-efficacy
Lack of skills in:
    Communication
    Individual coping
    Learning
    Stress management
    Time management
Perceived barriers outweigh benefits
Spiritual distress
Unachieved developmental tasks

Expected Outcomes

Client will be able to pursue chosen health-seeking behaviors.
  Participation in monitoring of baseline patterns and changes in health is reported.
  Required health maintenance services are accessible.
Client will state a realistic plan for pursuing health behaviors within limitations.
  Responses to illness or disability are controlled as much as possible.

Interventions	Rationale

Universal
 	
Assess current practice of age-appropriate health maintenance. (Base age-appropriate health maintenance schedules according to most recent Center for Disease Control (CDC), National Screening Council, and other national association guidelines, e.g., American Heart Association). General guidelines are as follows:
 	
YOUNG ADULTS (20–39 YEARS)
Assess need for health education/counseling:
  Creating a healthy environment
  Disease-prevention measures
  Exercise
  Nutrition and weight management
  Parenting skills
  Safety
  Stress management
  Substance use
Dental hygiene: every 6–12 months
Immunizations:
  Tetanus—every 10 years
  Rubella for women with zero antibodies—once
	Assessment reinforces the need for ongoing practice and provides data for specific teaching or referral.

Interventions

Screenings:

Blood cholesterol—once; rescreen if high-risk client—every 4 years

Complete physical—every 5–6 years

Skin and other cancer screening—every 3 years

Substance use screening—every 5–6 years

Male:

Testicular self exam—every month

Female:

Breast self exam—every month

Pap smear—every 1–3 years

Mammography—baseline (once)

High-risk young adults:

Females with breast cancer or immediate family history—mammography every year

History of abnormal Pap smears, multiple partners, or early age of first intercourse—Pap smear every year

Family history of colorectal cancer—stool guiac, digital exam, sigmoidoscopy every year

Exposure to tuberculosis—PPD once (chest x-ray for previous positive PPD reading)

Rationale

Assessment reinforces the need for ongoing practice and provides data for specific teaching or referral.

INTERVENTIONS

RATIONALE

*MIDDLE AGED ADULT
(40–59 YEARS)*
Continue previous assessment
and add the following:
  Assess need for health
  education/counseling:
  Adjustment to grandparent-
  hood
  Caring for aged loved ones
  Empty nest syndrome
  Midlife changes
  Preparing for retirement
Immunizations for those with
chronic illness:
  Influenza—every year
  Pneumoccocal—every year
Screening:
  Blood pressure—every 3–5
  years
Schiotz tonometry (for
glaucoma)—every 3–5 years
Sigmoidoscopy—every 4 years
after age 50
Stool guiac—every year after
age 50
Female:
  Mammography—every year

OLDER ADULT (60–74)
Continue previous assessment
and add the following:
Assess need for health educa-
tion/counseling:
  Age-related changes
  Bowel and bladder function
  Nutrition and weight
  management

Assessment reinforces the need for ongoing
practice and provides data for specific teaching
or referral.

INTERVENTIONS	RATIONALE

Sleep pattern
Vision and hearing acuity
Coping with chronic illness
Coping with loss
Fall prevention
Home care options in caring for other(s)
Options for developing and maintaining activity, relationships, and societal contributions
 	
Screenings:
  Blood pressure—every year
  Complete physical exam—every year
  Depression and suicide—every visit
 	
OLD OLD ADULT
(75 YEARS AND OVER)
Continue previous assessment and add the following:
Assess need for health education/counseling:
  Community resources for home maintenance
 	
Immunizations:
  Influenza—every year
  Pneumoccocal—every year
 	
Death and dying:
  Long-term care/supportive living options
  Reminiscence
	Assessment reinforces the need for ongoing practice and provides data for specific teaching or referral.

Develop written health maintenance contract that is specific, time-dated, rewardable, and evaluated.	Contract enables effective performance and evaluation.

INTERVENTIONS	RATIONALE
Incorporate age-appropriate health maintenance schedules into standardized/computerized care plan.	A busy staff is more likely to use a health maintenance schedule which has been included in the plan of care.
Plan individual health promotion activities considering responses to illness or disability.	Plans that incorporate symptom management are more likely to be effective.
Provide health maintenance services that client/family are unable to accomplish.	Preventive health actions aid overall recovery and maintenance.
Reinforce age-appropriate health maintenance.	Health information changes and accuracy are needed regarding specific risks, appropriate screening, and self-care activities.
Review existing health care resources.	The complexity and change in health care systems may prevent usage of existing resources.
Work with health care systems, employers, and policy makers to create healthy public policy.	Major barriers to health maintenance are societal in origin.
Work with professional organizations to reduce environmental threats to health, e.g., poverty, pollution, crime, and abuse.	Organized nursing effort can produce positive change.

Inpatient

INTERVENTIONS	RATIONALE
Collaborate with other disciplines in creating an institutional health promotion program for staff and clients.	Those who practice health promotion may be more effective role models. Organized approaches to health promotion enable access to services in a cost-effective manner and maintain relationships with health care providers after discharge.
Send written materials home and set up referrals for health maintenance prior to discharge.	Eighty percent of those who begin life-style change return to previous life-style behaviors. Follow-up care can aid in maintaining changed behaviors.

Interventions	Rationale
Community Health/ Home Care	
Continue previous health maintenance programs in the home as needed.	Continuity of care fosters health outcomes.
Develop consumer health advocacy programs.	Cost-effective health maintenance and referral can be accomplished by trained volunteers.
Develop programs that can be offered to employers and others seeking to provide health maintenance services.	Services provided where people work, learn, and play may improve access and utilization.
Develop specific screening and risk-reduction programs based on national and regional health goals.	Those at risk will have health services available to them.
Distribute health information updates to health providers and consumer groups.	Misinformation may result from lack of knowledge or changes in health information.
Provide advocacy services for groups with limited access to health maintenance services.	Underserved groups are at high risk for health problems.
Provide health screening and referral services at regular intervals.	Convenience may enhance utilization by those at high risk for health problems.
Reevaluate need for individual and group health maintenance programs as client/family skills are acquired.	Services can be provided to those most in need.

REFERENCES/BIBLIOGRAPHY

Albert, M. (1987). Health screening to promote health for the elderly. **Nurse Practitioner, 12** (5), 42–58.

American Nurses Association. (1980). **A Social Policy Statement.** Kansas City, MO: ANA.

* Frenn, M., Borgeson, D., Lee, H., & Simandl, G. (1989). Lifestyle changes in a cardiac rehabilitation program: The client perspective. **Journal of Cardiovascular Nursing, 3** (2), 43–55.

* Haan, M., Kaplan, G.A., & Camacho, T. (1987). Poverty and health: Prospective evidence from the Alameda County study. **American Journal of Epidemiology, 125,** 989–998.

Houldin, A.D., Saltstein, S.W., & Ganley, K.M. (1987). **Nursing diagnoses for wellness: Supporting strengths.** Philadelphia: Lippincott.

Lindberg, S.C. (1987). Adult preventive health screening: 1987 update. **Nurse Practitioner, 12,** 19–41.

Maglacas, A.M. (1988). Health for all: Nursing's role. **Nursing Outlook, 36** (2), 66–71.

North American Nursing Diagnosis Association. (1990). **Taxonomy I** (Rev. 1990). St. Louis: NANDA.

Office of Disease Prevention and Health Promotion, Department of Health Education and Human Services, (1990). **Healthy people 2000.** Washington D.C.: Government Printing Office.

* Stuifbergen, A.K., Becker, H.A., Ingalsbe, K., & Sands, D. (1990). Perceptions of health among adults with disabilities. **Health Values, 14** (2), 19–26.

* Wierenga, M.E., Browning, J.M., & Mahn, J.L. (1990). A descriptive study of how clients make lifestyle changes. **The Diabetes Educator, 16** (6), 469–473.

Health Seeking Behaviors (Specify)

A state in which an individual in stable
health is actively seeking ways to alter
personal health habits and/or the environment in order to move toward a higher
level of health (NANDA, 1990, p. 70).

Helena Lee, R.N., M.S.N.
Marilyn Frenn, R.N., Ph.D.

DEFINING CHARACTERISTICS

Desire for increased control of health practice
Desire to seek a higher level of wellness
Evidence of stable health with movement toward higher level of wellness
Legislation and/or workplace policies promoting safety and health behaviors
Observed consequences of unhealthy behaviors of others
Perceived control of health
Pursuit or seeking of health promotion information
Response to health-seeking and role-modeling behaviors of others
Sense of personal efficacy and self-confidence
Situational/maturational event precipitating concern about current health status

CONTRIBUTING FACTORS

Pathophysiological

Aging and its related physical changes
Altered health status

Psychosociobehavioral

Absence of interpersonal support
Cultural factors that inhibit health behaviors
Health values inconsistent with personal goals
Inadequate knowledge/skills for promoting health in a specific way
Lack of awareness/concern about environmental hazards affecting personal health

285

Lack of knowledge in health promotion behaviors
Limited availability of health care resources
Presence of specific environmental health hazards
Unfamiliarity with wellness community resources
Unhealthy living situation characterized by abuse, crime, overcrowding, pollution, poverty, stress

EXPECTED OUTCOMES

Client will engage in specific desired behavior(s) and will express satisfaction with changes.
>   Desire to make specific life style changes is expressed.
>   Information is used to plan for desired changes.
>   Motivation and personal competence to pursue behavioral changes is expressed.
>   Available community resources are sought to assist with planned changes.
Client will identify/take action toward necessary environmental changes to promote healthier life style.
>   Awareness of related environmental issues is demonstrated.

INTERVENTIONS	RATIONALE
Universal	
Assess specific life-style concerns.	Beginning a life-style program with focus on perceived needs enhances a successful outcome.
Determine facilitators and barriers to change (i.e., motivation, affective response, interpersonal support, stressors, knowledge, skills, resources).	Incorporating known assets and limitations to achieve goal(s) helps define scope and dimension of change to be made.
Identify time management and/or values conflicts.	Unresolved value conflicts about proposed changes or skill deficits in time management will interfere with goal achievement.
Promote development of a realistic plan for change.	Assuring successes in early stages of life-style change programs increases self-confidence and motivation.
Include outcome measures in plan for change.	Specific outcome measures allow immediate and individualized evaluation of progress.
Encourage participation of family/significant others in proposed changes.	Family involvement may enhance overall adaptation to change.

INTERVENTIONS	RATIONALE
Identify appropriate resources in the community.	Use referrals to individuals and agencies that will enhance the learning and mastery of specific behaviors.
Select appropriate role models for reinforcement.	Role modeling stimulates belief in the possibility of change and awareness of how change can occur.
Arrange for reevaluation of progress toward specific goal(s) after appropriate period of time with revision of plan, as necessary.	Awareness of future evaluation/reinforcement may promote adherence to original plan with modifications as necessary.
Provide support for learning about environmental issues that relate to specific health promotion change being addressed.	Environmental and social issues that remain unaddressed may have a negative impact on successful life-style change as well as reinforce unhealthy life-styles for others.
Instruct in specific health promotion behaviors using a variety of teaching methods.	Learning is promoted when it addresses expressed needs and when various approaches reinforce the material taught.
Inpatient	None
Community Health/ Home Care	None

REFERENCES/BIBLIOGRAPHY

* Brown, J.S., & McCreedy, M. (1986). The hale elderly: Health behavior and its correlates. **Research in Nursing and Health, 9,** 317–329.

Brubacher, B.H. (1983). Health promotion: A linguistic analysis. **Advances in Nursing Science, 5** (3), 1–14.

Clark, C.C. (1986). **Wellness nursing: Concepts theory, research and practice**. New York: Springer.

Hannah, T.E. (1987). Health behavior: The role of health as a personal life concern. **Canadian Journal of Public Health, 78,** 165–167.

Houldin, A.D., Saltstein, S.W., & Ganley, K.M. (1987). **Nursing diagnoses for wellness: Supporting strengths**. Philadelphia: Lippincott.

Lee, H.A., & Frenn, M.D. (1987). The use of nursing diagnoses for health promotion in community practice. **Nursing Clinics of North America, 22** (4), 981–986.

Norman, R. (1986). Health behavior: The implications of research. **Health Promotion, 25,** (1,2), 2–9.

North American Nursing Diagnosis Association. **Taxonomy I** (Rev. 1990). St. Louis: NANDA.

Pender, N.J. (1987). Health promotion and illness prevention. In H.H. Werley, & J.J. Fitzpatrick. (Eds.). **Annual review of nursing research.** (Vol. 2.). New York: Springer.

Pender, N.J. (1987). **Health promotion in nursing practice**. Norwalk, CT: Appleton & Lange.

Rakowski, W. (1986). Personal health practices, health status and expected control over future health. **Journal of Community Health, 11** (3), 189–203.

* Walker, S.N., Volkan, K., Sechrist, K.R., & Pender, N.J. (1988). Health-promoting life-styles of older adults: Comparisons with young and middle-aged adults, correlates and patterns. **Advances in Nursing Science, 11** (1), 76–90.

* Weitzel, M.H., & Waller, P.R. (1990). Predictive factors for health-promotive behaviors in white, Hispanic, and black blue-collar workers. **Family & Community Health, 13** (1), 23–34.

ome Maintenance Management, Impaired

A state in which an individual is unable or could be unable to maintain self or family in a safe home environment.

Joan Randall, R.N., M.S.

DEFINING CHARACTERISTICS

Describes outstanding debt or financial crisis
Disorderly surroundings
Expresses inability to cope at home
Expressions of difficulty in "managing at home"
Impaired care giver: overtaxed, anxious, lack of knowledge
Lack of necessary equipment or aids

Poor hygienic practices:
    Accumulation of dirt and wastes
    Inappropriate household temperature
    Infections
    Infestations
    Offensive odors
    Unwashed cooking/eating utensils
Presence of vermin or rodents
Requests assistance with home maintenance
Unavailable support systems

CONTRIBUTING FACTORS

Pathophysiological

Chronic debilitating disease
Impaired mental status
Injury

Substance abuse
Surgery

Psychosociobehavioral

Inadequate support systems
Insufficient family planning or organization

Insufficient finances
Lack of knowledge

EXPECTED OUTCOMES

Client will establish specific plan for home maintenance management.
 Understanding of disease process and its effects on the home situation is verbalized.
 Ability to manage care needs is demonstrated.
 Financial planning is initiated.
 Knowledge about community resources is articulated.
 Necessary equipment or aids are available.

INTERVENTIONS	RATIONALE
Universal Assess individual functioning in the areas of: Communication Hearing Mental status Mobility Vision Assess ability to manage: home maintenance (housekeeping) personal safety self-care self-medication	Evaluation of capabilities for self-care will provide a framework for necessary components of the discharge plan. Individual functioning will predict self-care capabilities.
Assess support systems.	Relatives, friends, neighbors, community groups may need to be activated to provide support and assistance to enable client to manage at home. Availability and accessibility of emergency services will further support management at home.
Assess community resources.	Knowledge of community resources and how to access these resources will provide needed support to manage at home. Community agencies may provide the support necessary to allow the client to remain at home. Provide written information on available community resources with program descriptions and telephone numbers.

INTERVENTIONS	**R**ATIONALE
Assess need for social worker.	Social worker can provide support, guidance, and information to strengthen capabilities to manage at home through establishment of realistic home management plan.
Assess family's ability to care for family member at home.	Care giver's physical and psychological ability to care for client must be carefully evaluated for successful home management. Inability to physically care for client will result in stressful, unsafe environment. Illness of other family members may affect home maintenance management.
Assess client/family's knowledge and skills of treatments, medications, personal care, nutritional needs, emergency procedures, awareness of available personnel.	Assessment of current knowledge will identify necessary learning needs. Lack of knowledge or understanding may result in unwarranted anxiety, fear of the unknown.
Assess emotional response of family/caretaker.	Caretakers may be too overwhelmed, anxious, or unwilling to provide client care. Time and energy demands on care givers may conflict with other roles, e.g., occupation, parenting, spouse.
Assess financial constraints.	Determining financial status will determine appropriate resource referral and planning and arranging for care needs after discharge. Anxiety over finances and lack of knowledge about available resources may impede home maintenance management.
Assess home environment.	Client/care giver's report of home environment and ability to accommodate needs of client is necessary for initiation of discharge plan. Safety of home environment and environmental barriers must be assessed. Assist in identifying obstacles that may impede home maintenance management.
Assess access to transportation.	Public transportation or arranged transportation may be necessary for follow-up treatment. City and county transit districts or area community service organizations may provide needed transportation. Accessibility to transportation, assistance provided, and costs should be assessed.

INTERVENTIONS	**R**ATIONALE
Initiate discharge planning.	Determining anticipated needs after discharge will allow for establishment of appropriate discharge plan. Discharge planning will facilitate transition to self-care.
Initiate referrals to other members of the health care team.	Based on assessment and evaluation of needs, referrals to appropriate resources will provide direction, guidance, and assistance needed to manage at home.
Inpatient Initiate teaching of care needs. Include the following: 1. Encourage active participation in the learning process 2. Allow frequent feedback to determine understanding and learning 3. Repeat information as repetition strengthens learning 4. Observe repeat demonstrations of skills to assess accurate learning and ability to perform skill in home environment 5. Provide written information to strengthen the learning process	Knowledge of the disease process, implications for the home situation, and available community resources are necessary to allay fears and provide for a safe home environment.
Evaluate ability to perform learned skills.	Return demonstrations will validate understanding of needs and ability to manage at home. Demonstrations of learned skills enhance learning and reinforce retention.

Community Health/ Home Care
 	
Assess home environment for the following:
 	
    Access (in and out of home)
    Accommodations for client/family
	Adequate home environment is necessary to enable home maintenance management. Assessment will reveal modifications or additional supports necessary for home management.

INTERVENTIONS	RATIONALE
Appearance Furnishings Garbage disposal Heating Lighting Sewage Type Ventilation Water supply	
Assess for safety: Adequate illumination Disaster/emergency exit plan Fire alarms Furniture height Grab bars Handrails secured Night lights Non-skid mats, rugs Proper storage of poisonous/ hazardous materials Removal of electrical cords Routine maintenance of gas/ electrical appliances Telephone	Safety hazards need to be corrected. Indoor and outdoor hazards need to be identified. Environmental climatic factors may contribute to safety hazards, e.g., snow, ice, rain, temperature.
Assess learning needs.	Appropriate interventions can only be initiated after a careful assessment of learning needs has been obtained.
Accept and support without judgment the realities of the living conditions.	A nonjudgmental attitude toward the home situation will minimize defensiveness and resistance to change.
Assist to develop plan for maintaining a clean, healthful environment.	Providing information about the relationship between unsanitary conditions/structural defects and health and establishing a realistic plan involving the client/family will increase the chances of compliance.

INTERVENTIONS	**R**ATIONALE
Initiate improvements to home environment deficits.	Adaptations to home environment or correction of hazards need to be made to support home maintenance management.

REFERENCES/BIBLIOGRAPHY

Carpenito, L.J. (1987). **Nursing Diagnosis Application to Clinical Practice** (2nd ed.). Philadelphia: Lippincott.

Harrell, J.S., McConnell, E.S., Wildman, D.S., & Samsa, G.P. (1989). Do nursing diagnoses affect functional status? **Journal of Gerontological Nursing, 15**(10), 13–19.

Schlapman, N. (1990). Elderly women and falls in the home. **Home Healthcare Nurse, (8)**, 20–24.

Hopelessness

A subjective state in which an individual sees limited or no alternatives or personal choices available and is unable to mobilize energy on own behalf (NANDA, 1990, p. 94).

Lynda Slimmer, R.N., Ph.D.

DEFINING CHARACTERISTICS

Altered sleep pattern (increased or decreased)
Decreased affect
Decreased appetite
Decreased response to stimuli
Decreased verbalization
Lack of initiative and future orientation
Lack of involvement in care/passively allowing care
Lack of involvement /interest in significant others

Noncompliance with treatment regimen
Nonverbal communication indicating social withdrawal, e.g., closing eyes, turning away from speaker, shrugging in response to speaker
Passivity
Psychosomatic complaints
Verbal cues indicating despondency, e.g., "I can't," sighing, suicidal ideations
Withdrawal

CONTRIBUTING FACTORS

Pathophysiological

Failing or deteriorating health status (actual)

Psychosociobehavioral

Abandonment (actual or perceived)
Failing or deteriorating health status (perceived)
Long-term stress

Lost belief in transcendent values/God
Prolonged activity restriction creating isolation

EXPECTED OUTCOMES

Client will be involved in self-care activities.
>   ADLs are performed according to physical ability.
>   Decisions are made about self-care.
>   Questions are asked and informed decisions are made about therapeutic regimen.
>   Therapeutic regimen is followed.

Client will maintain relationships with significant others and a social network.
>   Role responsibilities are performed.
>   Diversional activities are included in ADLs.
>   Satisfaction is reported in relationships with others.

Client will express feelings/concerns.
>   Feelings are identified.
>   Verbal and nonverbal communications are congruent.
>   Affect is appropriate to situations.
>   Psychosomatic complaints decrease.
>   Despondent verbalizations decrease.
>   No suicidal ideations are present.

Client will demonstrate control and influence over self and the environment.
>   Realistic, future-oriented goals are set.
>   Goals are revised as necessary.
>   Initiation for action to achieve goals comes from client.
>   Appropriate problem-solving skills and coping mechanisms are present.

INTERVENTIONS

RATIONALE

Universal	
Assess for signs of suicidal ideation.	The avoidance of a suicidal attempt is dependent upon recognition of the intent which can be expressed in verbal or nonverbal ways.
Assess ability to provide therapeutic and self-care activities.	The setting of goals which are appropriate to capabilities is dependent upon an accurate assessment of physical ability.
Assess past coping skills, both effective and ineffective.	The planning of interventions to improve present coping abilities is dependent upon an accurate assessment of past coping styles.
Assess what relationships are or have been important.	When emerging from a self-imposed isolation, it is most comfortable to relate to those perceived as having been supportive in the past.
Assess past enjoyed diversional activities.	The planning of activities designed to decrease isolation is dependent upon the accurate assessment of past diversional activities.

INTERVENTIONS	RATIONALE
Establish a therapeutic/ facilitative relationship.	To emerge from withdrawal, a safe environment in which to disclose concerns and to feel understood is necessary.
Facilitate expression of feelings by active listening and therapeutic communication, e.g., open-ended questions, reflection, paraphrasing.	Expression of feelings releases tension that contributes to behaviors associated with hopelessness, e.g., psychosomatic complaints.
Provide opportunities to express feelings in nonverbal ways, e.g., writing, drawing, physical exercise.	When there is a difficulty expressing feelings in words, a release of tension can be obtained through nonverbal means.
Convey an empathetic understanding of feelings.	Empathetic expression demonstrates care and concern while maintaining enough objectivity not to identify with the hopelessness.
Clarify and modify reality misperceptions (negative cognitions).	The perception of hopelessness and negative cognitions (verbal cues indicating despondency) is decreased by countering the cognition with an example of how that cognition is not always true.
Provide feedback on the appropriateness of goals.	Goals set beyond ability cause frustration and increase the perception of hopelessness, while goals set below ability slow progress toward increased control and independence.
Encourage risk-taking situations in which success can be experienced.	Reaching beyond a minimal level of achievement increases self-confidence and decreases the perception of hopelessness.
Seek input in decisions about care.	When alternatives and personal choices are available, the perception of hopelessness decreases.
Modify the environment to facilitate an active role in care.	While feeling hopeless there is an assumption that an internal, personal limitation is responsible for the inability to perform care activities. Modification of the environment demonstrates that the problem may be external and increases the perception of self-abilities.

INTERVENTIONS	RATIONALE
Involve client in care, gradually adding new activities.	Hopelessness is exhibited by a lack of initiative to be independent or to attempt new behaviors. The demonstration that self-care abilities are present is helpful.
Provide positive feedback for successful attempts at self-care.	Positive feedback reinforces the behavior, increases self-confidence, and decreases feelings of hopelessness.
Provide care that client is unable to perform.	Provision of care that the client is unable to perform decreases the frustration of striving for an unachievable goal and assists in the recognition that accepting some assistance does not necessitate total dependency.
Stimulate curiosity about different aspects of care, especially those involved in a new treatment regimen.	Curiosity is one indicator of readiness to learn.
Discuss options for increasing the social network.	Information about available social activities encourages decision making about which activities are most appropriate, and planning involvement increases initiative and problem-solving skills.
Provide supportive counseling to family members.	Hopeless behavior may confuse and frustrate family members. Counseling about causes leads to understanding and support.
Teach alternative ways to provide for therapeutic and self-care.	Demonstrating that alternatives and personal choices are available decreases the perception of hopelessness.
Teach how to discriminate between controllable and uncontrollable situations.	The recognition that some situations are intrinsically and universally outside control decreases the perception of personal weakness.
Teach stress-reduction techniques.	Inability to cope with stress is a contributing factor in the development of hopelessness.
Teach decision-making/problem-solving/coping skills.	Adding to the repertoire of health-promoting behaviors decreases the possibility of the return to a hopeless state.

INTERVENTIONS	RATIONALE
Inpatient	
Encourage visits by significant others.	Concern and support of significant others stimulates involvement and interest outside of self and decreases the perception of isolation.
Community Health/ Home Care	
Encourage family members to allow independent role activities within the client's abilities.	In an attempt to be caring, families may foster dependence which serves to decrease self-confidence and increase the perception of hopelessness.

REFERENCES/BIBLIOGRAPHY

Abramson, L., Seligman, M., & Teasdale, J. (1978). Learned helplessness in humans: Critique and reformulation. **Journal of Abnormal Psychology, 87**(1), 49–74.

Doenges, M., & Moorhouse, M. (1988). **Nursing diagnoses with interventions** (2nd ed.). Philadelphia: Davis.

Kim, M., McFarland, G., & McLane, A. (1989). **Pocket guide to nursing diagnoses** (3rd ed.). St. Louis: Mosby.

McFarland, G., & McFarlane, E. (1989). **Nursing diagnosis and intervention: Planning for patient care**. St. Louis: Mosby.

North American Nursing Diagnosis Association. (1990). **Taxonomy I** (Rev. 1990). St. Louis: NANDA.

*Slimmer, L., Lopez, M., LeSage, J., & Ellor, J. (1987). Perceptions of learned helplessness. **Journal of Gerontological Nursing, 13**(5), 33–37.

Stuart, G., & Sundeen, S. (1987). **Principles and practice of psychiatric nursing** (3rd ed.). St. Louis: Mosby.

Hyperthermia

A state in which an individual's core body temperature is elevated above 38.0° C (100.2°F); elderly clients may become symptomatic at temperatures 1.0° less.

Sharon Summers, R.N., Ph.D.

DEFINING CHARACTERISTICS

Confusion
Decreased perspiration
Decreased sodium and potassium levels
Headache
Hot/dry skin
Increased core temperature

Increased thirst
Malaise
Seizures
Shivering
Tachypnea

CONTRIBUTING FACTORS

Pathophysiological: Accidental

Cardiovascular disease
Dehydration
Elderly
Exposure to ambient temperatures
        ≥ 32.2° C (90.0 ° F)
Exposure to high humidity

Exposure to the sun
Heatstroke
Infection
Intraoperative medications
Overactivity
Overweight

Psychosociobehavioral: Accidental

Alcoholism
Inappropriate clothing for the temperature
Living in insecure neighborhoods

Low income/poverty
Poor ventilation in housing
Senility/dementia

Pathophysiological: Inadvertent

Genetic predisposition combined with general anesthesia

Psychosociobehavioral: Inadvertent

None

Pathophysiological: Intentional

Malignancy or HIV positive diagnosis

Psychosociobehavioral: Intentional

None

EXPECTED OUTCOMES

Client will be normothermic for age.
    Appropriate clothing is worn for ambient temperatures.
    Artificial ventilation equipment is obtained for home use.
    Cool shelters are sought if needed.
    Genetic predisposition for inadvertent hyperthermia is known.
    Support is received when undergoing intentional hyperthermia.

INTERVENTIONS   RATIONALE

ACCIDENTAL HYPERTHERMIA Universal	
Monitor core temperatures using age-specific criteria.	High core temperatures are incompatible with cellular life. Specific criteria need to be used for determination, as they vary with age.
Monitor fluid replacement.	Intravenous fluids and electrolyte replacements should be given with care to avoid fluid overload. Fluid overload may cause alterations in cardiopulmonary status.
Monitor neurological status.	Seizures and confusion may occur as a result of thermal stress.
Move to cool facility.	Lower ambient temperatures will help reduce core temperature by conduction.

INTERVENTIONS	RATIONALE
Give oral fluids that contain electrolytes.	Dehydration contributes to increased temperature. Electrolytes are lost in prolonged production of perspiration.
Give sponge bath with cool water while avoiding shivering.	External applications of coolants will reduce core temperature by conduction where heat is transferred from concentrations of heat to concentrations of cold. Shivering is a result of skeletal muscle contractions and may increase heat production by 60%.
Provide calm, cool environment.	Thermal stress results in overstimulation of the autonomic nervous system and, thus, conditions that are conducive to adaptation need to be achieved.
Inpatient	
Monitor for cardiac arrhythmias.	Electrolyte disturbances may precipitate arrhythmias.
Monitor external cooling blanket.	Shivering may result in heat generation, thus causing temperature elevation.
Community Health/ Home Care	
Evaluate for potential development of hyperthermia.	Primary prevention of hyperthermia will help to decrease thermal stress responses.
Assess security and safety of the home/neighborhood.	Fears about safety and security may prevent opening doors and windows for ventilation.
Monitor medication regimen.	Certain drug therapies may exacerbate thermal stress. For example: diuretics, anticholinergics, phenothiazines, tricyclic antidepressants, butyrophenones, antihistamines, amphetamines, thyroid replacements, hallucinogens, beta blockers, methyldopa, propylthiouracil, salicylates in high doses, MAO inhibitors, succinylcholine, glutethimide, and barbiturates.

INTERVENTIONS	**RATIONALE**
Refer those susceptible to community centers during heat alerts.	Cool community centers are frequently provided during periods of high heat and humidity when cooling resources are lacking.
Establish neighborhood networks to check on susceptible clients during heat alerts.	Neighborhood networks can check on the elderly and disabled and notify the nurse of clients in need.
Obtain cooling equipment.	Community resources are usually available to loan fans or window air conditioners in hot weather.
Teach about reducing physical activity during hot weather.	During periods of high heat and high humidity, physical activity should be decreased since skeletal muscle is a primary source of body heat production.
Teach about fluid and food intake during hot weather.	Consumption of fluids to replace water and electrolyte losses is necessary since heat loss by evaporation may approximate 1.5 liters per hour and precipitate dehydration. Instruct to avoid overeating during hot weather since overeating may contribute to heat production.
INADVERTENT HYPERTHERMIA **Universal** None	
Inpatient Evaluate susceptibility to malignant hyperthermia by taking a careful family history.	Malignant hyperthermia is a pharmacogenetic disorder that may occur as a result of intra-operative medications. Medications may include halothane, enflurane, isoflurane, succinylcholine, tubocurarine, gallamine, and may be exacerbated in the presence of physical and emotional stress.
Monitor core temperature postoperatively.	Malignant hyperthermia may occur intra-operatively or several hours postoperative, and temperatures may range from 38.8° C–42.2° C (102° F–108° F).

INTERVENTIONS	RATIONALE
Evaluate changes in physical status.	Elevated temperature is frequently accompanied by muscle rigidity related to elevated calcium concentrations in the muscle.
Implement treatment protocol for malignant hyperthermia.	Malignant hyperthermia must be treated as an emergency situation, since survival is dependent on rapid treatment with usual emergency medications. Cooling the client is combined with relieving muscle contractions, as a source of heat production, using dantrolene sodium as the primary drug of choice.
Community Health/ Home Care None	
INTENTIONAL HYPERTHERMIA **Universal** None	
Inpatient Provide emotional support.	Hyperthermia is an adjunct to chemotherapy for malignancy and HIV-positive diagnoses. Fear of the unknown may occur regarding the use of heat ranging from 41° C–45° C (106° F–112° F) for whole body and regional and local sites.
Provide teaching about the rationale for the treatment.	Heating of tumors potentiates the action of chemotherapeutics, since dividing cells respond to various modes during various stages of cell division.
Instruct about the modes of hyperthermia.	Tissue heating may be accomplished by radio frequency waves, microwaves, and ultrasound. Understanding of these various modes increases feelings of control and promotes compliance.
Community Health/ Home Care None	

REFERENCES/BIBLIOGRAPHY

Abbott, C.A. (1990). Planning for unexpected outcomes. In J.C. Rothrock (Ed.). **Perioperative nursing care planning** (pp. 476–495). St. Louis: Mosby.

Burnside, I. (1990). **Nursing and the aged: A self-care approach**. St. Louis: McGraw-Hill.

Carpenito, L.J. (1989). **Nursing diagnosis application to clinical practice**. Philadelphia: Lippincott.

Caruso, C., & Posey, V. (July/August, 1985). Heat waves threaten the old. **Geriatric Nursing, 6**(4), 209–212.

Drain, C.B., & Christoph, S.S. (1987). **The recovery room: A critical care approach to post anesthesia nursing**. Philadelphia: Saunders.

Frederick, C., Rosemann, D., & Austin, M.J. (1990). Malignant hyperthermia: Nursing diagnosis and care. **Journal of Post Anesthesia Nursing, 5**(1), 29–32.

Ganong, W.F. (1989). **Review of medical physiology**. Norwalk, CT: Appleton & Lange.

Hahn, G.M. (1982). **Hyperthermia and cancer**. New York: Plenum.

Lydon, J., McDonald-Lynch, A., Marshall, I., & Villnaueva, W. Patient teaching about hyperthermia (1989). **Oncology Nursing Forum, 16**(6), 856–860.

McFarland, G.K., & McFarlane, E.A. (1989). **Nursing diagnosis & intervention**. St. Louis: Mosby.

Newberry, J.E. (1990). Malignant hyperthermia in the postanesthesia care unit: A review of current etiology, diagnosis, and treatment. **Journal of Post Anesthesia Nursing, 5**(1), 25–28.

North American Nursing Diagnosis Association. (1990). **Taxonomy I** (Rev. 1990). St. Louis: NANDA.

Nursing '85 Books. (1985). **Nurse's reference library: emergencies**. Springhouse, PA: Springhouse Corp.

Reed, G., & Anderson, R.J. (August, 1986). Emergency: heatstroke. **Hospital Medicine, 22**(8), 19–21, 25, 29–30, 36.

* Summers, S. (in progress). **Concept analysis of hyperthermia**.

Hypothermia

A state in which an individual's core body temperature is reduced ≤ 36° C (96.8°F).

Sharon Summers, R.N., Ph.D.

. . . .

DEFINING CHARACTERISTICS

Bradycardia
Cardiac arrhythmias
Confusion
Cyanotic nail beds
Decreased core temperature
Decreased surface temperature
Drowsiness
Hypertension

Hypotension
Hypoventilation
Pallor
Piloerection
Restlessness
Shivering
Slow capillary refill
Slurred speech

CONTRIBUTING FACTORS

Pathophysiological: Accidental

Advanced age
Exposure to cold, rain, snow (radiation
       and conduction)
Exposure to wind (convection)
Illness, disease, injuries, e.g., insulin shock,
       myxedema, or burns

Immersion in cold water (conduction)
Inactivity
Malnutrition

Psychosociobehavioral: Accidental

Alcohol consumption
Inactivity
Inadequate clothing (conduction)
Inadequate housing

Lack of permanent housing
Malnutrition
Poverty

Pathophysiological: Inadvertent

Anesthetic gases and medications producing vasodilatation (conduction)
Cold air blowing across client (convection)
Cold anesthetic gases (evaporation)
Cold intravenous solutions or blood transfusions (conduction)
Cold prep solutions (conduction)
Exposed viscera (evaporation)
Exposure to cold operating rooms (radiation)
Inadequate clothing (conduction)
Lying on wet surfaces (conduction)
Surgical procedure

Psychosociobehavioral: Inadvertent

None

Pathophysiological: Intentional

Cooling for surgical procedures (conduction)
Cooling head-injured client

Psychosociobehavioral: Intentional

None

EXPECTED OUTCOMES

Client will become normothermic (36.7° C–37.1° C) ± .2° C (97.3° F–98.8° F).
   Knowledge regarding contributing factors is verbalized.
   Cooling resources are available to intentional cooling of client.
   Warming resources are available to inadvertent and accidentally exposed client.
   Methods to protect from accidental causes are articulated.

INTERVENTIONS	RATIONALE
ACCIDENTAL HYPOTHERMIA **Universal** Monitor core temperature	Core temperatures are the most accurate method of determining hypothermia and can be measured by tympanic, oral, or high rectal methods. Axillary temperatures measure surface or shell temperatures and are not the best method to validate hypothermia.

INTERVENTIONS	RATIONALE
Evaluate level of activity.	Inactivity lowers body heat production through decreased muscle activity.
Evaluate age	Elderly are more susceptible to hypothermia related to decrease in insulating tissue and aged temperature regulation system.
Evaluate nutritional status.	Malnutrition can contribute to hypothermia when there are insufficient substrates for energy production and the release of heat.
Evaluate presence of illness or disease.	Hypothermia may be associated with disease states, e.g., diabetes and myxedema.
Teach first aid methods of rewarming.	Rewarming methods implemented early can prevent problems associated with this diagnosis and include: warm clothing, blankets, shelter, and warm oral fluids.
Teach how to prevent and treat cold water immersion injury.	Immersion in cold water can quickly lead to hypothermia.
Teach how to prevent injuries when exposed to cold, wind, snow, and rain.	Exposure to cold, wind, snow, and rain are primary causes of hypothermia.

Inpatient

Monitor for cardiac arrhythmias.	Cardiac arrhythmias, ranging from premature ventricular contractions to ventricular fibrillation, may occur related to myocardial irritability and depression.
Monitor respiratory rate and oxygen intake.	Hypothermia results in a left shift to the oxyhemoglobin dissociation curve and decreased release of oxygen from hemoglobin.
Monitor environmental temperature.	A warmer room temperature may be required with burn injury to prevent heat loss by conduction.
Implement rewarming measures.	An electric convective warming device is effective in rewarming to promote comfort and reverse physiological changes.

Interventions	Rationale
Community Health/ Home Care	
Evaluate adequacy of housing.	Adequate housing to protect from wind, rain, snow, and cold is a primary preventive measure.
Evaluate financial resources.	Poverty and insufficient food, clothing, and housing are primary contributors to hypothermia.
Evaluate social habits.	Excess alcohol consumption precipitates vasoconstriction followed by vasodilation and heat loss.
INADVERTENT HYPOTHERMIA **Universal** None	
Inpatient Monitor core temperature during surgery.	Symptoms usually begin during surgery and warming measures can be implemented.
Monitor thermal comfort.	Rewarming in the postanesthesia care unit will contribute to thermal comfort.
Recommend head covers.	Approximately 50% of heat loss can occur from the head by conduction and radiation.
Warm prep, irrigating, and intravenous solutions.	Heat loss can be potentiated when solutions that are lower than body temperature are used.
Keep dry.	Lying on wet surgical drapes can potentiate heat loss.
Rewarm and monitor core temperatures in postanesthesia care unit.	Core temperatures should increase as rewarming is initiated. Electric convective warming is more effective than warmed cotton blankets. Anesthetics and other perioperative medications may prevent shivering or piloerection that facilitate rewarming.

Iɴᴛᴇʀᴠᴇɴᴛɪᴏɴs	Rᴀᴛɪᴏɴᴀʟᴇ
Community Health/ Home Care None	
INTENTIONAL HYPOTHERMIA **Universal** None	
Inpatient Monitor bypass pump blood temperature.	Blood is cooled as it circulates through the bypass pump to maintain temperature at desired level. Special surgical procedures, such as coronary artery bypass graft, require cooling to hypothermic levels to induce ventricular fibrillation and decrease metabolic rate.
Monitor cooling blanket.	Cooling blankets for use with head injuries reduce cerebral edema and decrease tissue damage.
Initiate rewarming procedure.	Wrapping in warmed blankets promotes physiological stability and promotes comfort.
Community Health/ Home Care None	

REFERENCES/BIBLIOGRAPHY

Augustine, S.D. (1990). Hypothermia therapy in the postanesthesia care unit: A review. **Journal of Post Anesthesia Nursing, 5**(4), 254–263.

Carpenito, L.J. (1989). **Nursing diagnosis application to clinical practice**. Philadelphia: Lippincott.

Ganong, W.F. (1989). **Review of medical physiology**. Norwalk, CT: Appleton & Lange.

Lilly, R.B. (1987). Inadvertent hypothermia: A real problem. **ASA Refresher Courses in Anesthesiology, 15**(8), 93–107.

Matz, R. (1986). Hypothermia: Mechanisms and countermeasures. **Hospital Practice, 21**(1A), 45–48, 54–58, 65–68.

McFarland, G.K., & McFarlane, E.A. (1989). **Nursing diagnosis & intervention**. St. Louis: Mosby.

Morrison, R.C. (1988). Hypothermia in the elderly. **International Anesthesia Clinics, 26**(2), 124–133.

North American Nursing Diagnosis Association. (1990). **Taxonomy I** (Rev. 1990). St. Louis: NANDA.

Reed, G., & Anderson, R.J. (1988). Management of acute hypothermia. **Hospital Medicine, 24**(1), 155–172.

*Summers, S., Dudgeon, N., Byram, K., & Zingsheim, K. (1990). The effects of two warming methods on core and surface temperature, hemoglobin oxygen saturations, blood pressure and perceived comfort of hypothermic postanesthesia patients. **Journal of Post Anesthesia Nursing, 5**(5), 354–364.

*Summers, S. (in press). Concept analysis of hypothermia. **Nursing Diagnosis**.

Incontinence: Functional

A state in which an individual
experiences involuntary passage of
urine despite a normal urinary tract.

Anne Marie Voith Sherman, R.N., M.S.N.

DEFINING CHARACTERISTICS

Cognitive deficit, memory deficit,
       disorientation
Mobility deficits
Sensory deficits

Voids normal to large amounts
Voluntarily postpones voiding for long
       periods

CONTRIBUTING FACTORS

Pathophysiological

Communication deficits
Deep sleep
Hypnotics, analgesics

Impaired mobility
Increased urine production (as with diuresis)
Stroke or other cerebral injury

Psychosociobehavioral

Inability to locate bathroom
Inattentiveness to the urge to void
Reluctance to use call light or bedpan

Voluntarily postpones voiding for long
       periods

EXPECTED OUTCOMES

Client will experience no incontinent episodes.
       Urge to void is recognized.
       Time between urge and voiding is increased.
       Time to get to toilet is decreased.

INTERVENTIONS	**RATIONALE**
Universal	
Assess need for physical therapy consultation.	Improving mobility will help decrease time between the urge and reaching the toilet.
Consult with physician regarding use of anticholinergics.	Anticholinergics increase warning time by blocking impulses within the sacral reflex arc.
Evaluate medication type and timing and consult with physician for modifications if necessary.	Schedule medications so that incontinence-producing effect is at a time when ability to reach the toilet on time is most likely.
Assess for glycosuria, bacteriuria.	Medical conditions that contribute to incontinence must be ruled out and treated.
Develop scheduled voiding times during waking hours.	Voiding at regular intervals helps prevent overdistention.
Develop a cue that can be used to indicate a need to urinate.	When unable to communicate well verbally, a cue may expedite communication of needs.
Keep bathroom light on and door open at all times.	Confused clients, or those with vision problems may have difficulty locating the bathroom.
Limit diuretics late in the day (e.g., medications, coffee, tea, and alcohol).	Sudden increases in urine output related to the effects of diuretics cause an increased need to void at night when mobility is most impaired.
Modify clothing for easy removal (e.g., Velcro fasteners, loose clothing, and crotchless stockings).	This reduces time and dexterity necessary to remove clothes.
Provide commode at bedside.	If ambulation is difficult, or there is little warning time prior to urinating, a bedside commode is helpful. An upright position allows better emptying of the bladder.
Provide safety bars, raised toilet seat.	Use of the toilet is easier and safer.
Set alarm to void during the night.	Sedatives and hypnotics may "dampen" the urge to void, so that awakening to the urge will not allow the time to get to the toilet.

INTERVENTIONS	**R**ATIONALE
Use an oil-based lubricant on skin after washing.	Oil-based lubricants keep urine away from skin, preventing skin excoriation.
Use sanitary napkins or protective pants during the day.	These products help keep urine away from the skin.
Instruct in therapeutic regimen, its reasons, and complications of incontinence.	Understanding facilitates compliance.
Instruct to seek toilet facility as soon as urge is felt.	Immediate response to the urge to void prevents overdistention.
Instruct to wash perineum after each incontinent episode.	Cleanliness prevents odor, skin irritation, and infection.
Instruct to wipe perineum from front to back.	Wiping from front to back minimizes the introduction of bacteria to the urethral area, preventing infection.
Refer care giver to support group: The Simon Foundation, Box 815, Wilmette, Il 60091; OR Help for Incontinent People, PO Box 544, Union, SC 29373.	Caring for an incontinent person can be stressful.

Inpatient

Assess usual voiding times at home.	Compliance with established schedules promotes continence.
Draw line on floor to bathroom and/or show where the bathroom is.	Confused clients or those with vision problems may have difficulty locating the bathroom.
Leave bedpan within reach.	These items must be readily accessible or incontinence may occur.
Notify staff to respond to call light immediately.	Assistance may be required. If unable to delay urination, incontinence may occur.
Place client in bed closest to the bathroom.	Client will be able to get to the bathroom more quickly.

INTERVENTIONS

RATIONALE

Community Health/ Home Care None	

REFERENCES/BIBLIOGRAPHY

* Heller, B., Whitehead, W.E., & Johnson, L.D. (1989). Incontinence. **Journal of Gerontological Nursing, 15**(5), 16–23.

* Lincoln, R., & Roberts, R. (1989). Continence issues in acute care. **Nursing Clinics of North America, 24**(3), 741–54.

* Long, M.L. (1985). Incontinence. **Journal of Gerontological Nursing, 11**(1), 30–35.

Pannill, F.C., Williams, T.F., & Davis, R. (1988). Evaluation and treatment of urinary incontinence in long-term care. **Journal of the American Geriatrics Society, 36**(10), 902–10.

Voith, A.M. (1988). Alterations in urinary elimination: Concepts, research, and practice. **Rehabilitation Nursing, 13**(3), 122–131.

Incontinence: Reflex

A state in which an individual's micturition is controlled by spinal cord reflex in the absence of higher neural control.

Anne Marie Voith Sherman, R.N., M.S.N.

DEFINING CHARACTERISTICS

No awareness of bladder filling

No urge to void nor feelings of bladder fullness

Uninhibited bladder contraction/spasm at regular intervals

Voids in large amounts

CONTRIBUTING FACTORS

Pathophysiological

Interruption of spinal nerve impulse above the level of S-3.

Psychosociobehavioral

None

EXPECTED OUTCOMES

Client will be continent.
> Regimen for fluid intake is followed.
> A pattern to voiding times is identified.
> Way to trigger voiding reflex is identified OR proper technique for intermittent catheterization is exhibited.

INTERVENTIONS	RATIONALE
Universal	
Assess for urinary retention (see care planning guide, "Urinary Retention, Chronic").	Retention of urine in the form of high post-void residuals frequently occurs with reflex incontinence.
Assess when voiding occurs.	Uninhibited micturition reflex will occur approximately every 250 cc in a normal bladder.
Monitor color, odor, and turbidity of urine.	Characteristics of urine can indicate urinary tract infection or dehydration, both of which contribute to bladder irritability. Bladder irritability will decrease predictability of reflex micturition.
Encourage intake of 1500-2000 cc of fluid per day, unless contraindicated.	Adequate fluid intake aids in the prevention of bladder infections and increases the bladder capacity. Scheduling of fluid intake helps maintain better bladder filling predictability. It may be contraindicated if fluid restrictions are medically necessary.
Attempt to void one-half hour before the expected reflexive voiding by stimulating the reflex arc (e.g., stroke lower abdomen or inner thigh, tap over symphysis pubis), or through intermittent catheterization.	The goal is to successfully void or empty the bladder before the reflex occurs.
Catheterize until residual is below 75 cc if triggering mechanism successful.	High residuals of urine increase the risk of infection.
Encourage reduction/elimination of caffeine and alcohol intake.	These drinks have a diuretic effect and may affect the predictability of reflex voiding.
Offer support and encouragement regarding bladder training.	Incontinence can be very degrading to an individual, and the development of a regimen may take time. Encouragement helps preserve a healthy self-image and promotes compliance.
Set alarm to void during the night.	Scheduled voiding, even during the night, may be necessary to maintain continence.

INTERVENTIONS	RATIONALE
Use an oil-based lubricant on skin after washing.	Oil-based lubricants keep urine away from skin, preventing skin excoriation.
Use external catheter at night.	External catheters allow uninterrupted sleep without incontinence.
Use sanitary napkins or protective pants during the day.	These products help keep urine away from the skin.
Instruct in various triggering methods to initiate voiding, (e.g., stroking inner thigh, pulling lightly on pubic hair, digital stimulation of rectum, stroking glans penis or vulva, and flexing toes.	Different triggering mechanisms work for each individual.
Teach intermittent self-catheterization if the triggering mechanism is ineffective or post-void residuals remain high.	High residual of urine increases the risk of infection.
Instruct in recognition of infection.	Early recognition is important in obtaining early intervention and preventing complications of infection.
Instruct in regimen, its reasons, and complications of incontinence.	Understanding facilitates compliance.
Instruct to wash after each incontinent episode.	Cleanliness prevents odor, skin irritation, and infection.
Instruct to wipe perineum from front to back.	Wiping from front to back minimizes the introduction of bacteria to the urethral area, preventing infection.
Refer care giver to support group: The Simon Foundation, Box 815, Wilmette, IL 60091; OR Help for Incontinent People, PO Box 544, Union, SC 29373.	Caring for an incontinent person can be stressful.

Interventions

Rationale

Interventions	Rationale
Inpatient None	
Community Health/ Home Care None	

REFERENCES/BIBLIOGRAPHY

*Cardenas, D.D., & Mayo, M.E. (1985). Manual stimulation of reflex voiding after spinal cord injury. **Archives of Physical Medicine and Rehabilitation, 66**, 459–462.

*de la Hunt, M.N., Deegan, S., & Scott, J.E. (1989). Intermittent catheterization for neuropathic urinary incontinence. **Archives of Disease in Childhood, 64**(6), 821–824.

Hartman, M. (1978). Intermittent self-catheterization. **Nursing '78, 8**(11), 72–75.

Incontinence: Stress

A state in which an individual expresses the urge to void simultaneously with the loss of small amounts of urine.

Anne Marie Voith Sherman, R.N., M.S.N.

DEFINING CHARACTERISTICS

Dribbling with increased abdominal pressure (e.g., sneezing, coughing, standing) without
  detrusor contraction
Loss of small amounts of urine (less than 50 cc)
Positive Q-tip Test (Q-tip inserted in vagina rises more than 30° at straining)
Unable to start and stop stream while urinating (requires further testing to establish diagnostic
  validity)

CONTRIBUTING FACTORS

Pathophysiological

Degenerative changes in pelvic muscles and structural support
High intraabdominal pressure (e.g., obesity, gravid uterus)
Incompetent bladder outlet
Weak pelvic muscles and structural supports associated with general poor physical condition

Psychosociobehavioral

None

EXPECTED OUTCOMES

Client will remain continent with increased intraabdominal pressure (results can be expected
  in four to six weeks).
  Pelvic floor muscles are correctly identified when performing exercises.
Urinary stream can be started and stopped on command.

INTERVENTIONS

RATIONALE

Interventions	Rationale
Universal	
Assess the presence of urge incontinence (see care planning guide, "Incontinence: Urge").	Stress and urge incontinence frequently occur together.
Consider medical consultation.	If client does not improve within six weeks, has a history of genitourinary surgery, or has a complicated history, medical intervention may be appropriate.
Encourage to decrease or discontinue bouncing exercises.	Bouncing may weaken supporting ligaments. Recommend alternative aerobic exercise like swimming or biking.
Encourage loss of excessive weight.	Weight loss decreases abdominal pressure.
Encourage sit-ups with bent knees.	This exercise improves abdominal muscle tone.
Perform pelvic floor muscle-strengthening exercises (four repetitions, four times daily for three months). (Have client sit with knees apart, feet on floor, and contract perineal muscles as though stopping the expulsion of urine).	This improves muscle tone which is essential to the control and termination of urination.
Initiate biofeedback consultation.	Biofeedback can be useful in helping to learn pelvic floor-strengthening exercises.
Start and stop stream during urination.	The starting and stopping of stream provides immediate feedback that the proper muscles are being used to control micturition and strengthen pelvic floor and sphincter muscles used in resisting release of urine.
Use sanitary napkins or protective pants during the day.	These products help keep urine away from the skin.
Instruct to change protective pads frequently and wash perineum.	Cleanliness prevents odor, skin irritation, and infection.
Instruct in regimen, its reasons, and complications of incontinence.	Understanding facilitates compliance.

Interventions	Rationale
Instruct to wipe perineum from front to back.	Wiping from front to back minimizes the introduction of bacteria to the urethral area, preventing infection.
Instruct to respond immediately to urge to void.	Overdistention of the bladder related to deliberate postponement of voiding further increases supraurethral pressure, increasing likelihood of stress incontinence.
Instruct to sit with firm towel or other object pressing on perineum when incontinence threatens (e.g., cross legs, sit on leg...).	This elevates the perineum, closing the bladder outlet, and stopping the flow of urine.
Instruct to void at precise time intervals.	Scheduled voiding restores confidence in ability to control urine, prevents overdistention, and strengthens pelvic muscles.
Refer care giver to support group: The Simon Foundation, Box 815, Willmette, IL 60091; OR Help for Incontinent People, PO Box 544, Union, SC 29373.	Caring for an incontinent person can be stressful.
Inpatient None	
Community Health/ Home Care None	

REFERENCES/BIBLIOGRAPHY

* Brink, C.A., et al. (1989). A digital test for pelvic muscle strength in older women with urinary incontinence. **Nursing Research, 38**, 196–199.
* Burgio, K.L., Whitehead, W.E., & Engel, B.T. (1985). Urinary incontinence in the elderly: Bladder sphincter biofeedback and toileting skills training. **Annals of Internal Medicine, 104,** 507–515.
Kegel, A.H. (1951). Physiologic therapy for urinary stress incontinence. **JAMA, 146**(10), 915–917.
* Walters, M.D., & Shields, L.E. (1988). The diagnostic value of history, physical examination, and the Q-tip cotton swab test in females with urinary incontinence. **American Journal of Obstetrics and Gynecology, 159**(1), 145–9.

Incontinence: Total

A state in which an individual experiences a continuous and unpredictable loss of urine (NANDA, 1990, p. 29).

Anne Marie Voith Sherman, R.N., M.S.N.

DEFINING CHARACTERISTICS

Constant flow of urine without distention
Unaware of incontinence, despite intact sensory innervation
Unsuccessful treatment of incontinence

CONTRIBUTING FACTORS

Pathophysiological

Cerebral neurological dysfunction
Complete loss of bladder control [atonic (flaccid) bladder]
Fistula
Uninhibited detrusor contraction

Psychosociobehavioral

Inattention to urge to void associated with severe disorientation, memory problems, psychoses

EXPECTED OUTCOMES

Client will experience no complications of incontinence.
    Skin remains intact and free of irritation.
    Urine is clear and free of pathogens.
Client or care giver will understand and maintain therapeutic regimen.
    Therapeutic plan is verbalized.
    Appropriate behaviors are modeled.

323

INTERVENTIONS	**R**ATIONALE
Universal	
Monitor color, odor, and turbidity of urine.	Characteristics of urine can indicate urinary tract infection or dehydration.
Monitor skin integrity.	Skin breakdown is a complication of urinary incontinence.
Offer support and encouragement regarding bladder training.	This helps preserve a healthy self-image and promotes compliance.
Use an oil-based lubricant on skin after washing.	Oil-based lubricants keep urine away from skin, preventing skin excoriation.
Two plans of care for total incontinence may be appropriate. *PLAN A: PROMPTED VOIDING*—Instruct/assist in bladder training as follows: Encourage intake of 1500–2000 cc of fluid per day.	Either method will provide for adequate bladder filling and prevention of infection.
Encourage voiding every two hours by reminding and (as necessary) assisting as needed. If voiding occurs earlier without incontinence, attempt urination two hours after the voiding.	Uninhibited micturition reflex will occur every 250 cc in a normal bladder. The goal is to successfully void before the reflex voiding occurs.
Stimulate primitive reflexes to encourage voiding when scheduled (e.g., drink water, stroke lower abdomen or inner thigh, pour water over perineum, run water in sink, tap over symphysis pubis).	Voiding at regular intervals helps prevent overdistention and may facilitate conditioning of micturition to occur at regular intervals.
Use external catheter intermittently when necessary.	Constant use results in increased risk of infection, irritation, edema, fissures, or necrosis. Intermittent use allows the skin a chance to dry when prompted voiding is not sufficiently successful.

INTERVENTIONS	RATIONALE
Use sanitary napkins or protective pants during the day when out of bed and use waterproof pads or special protective bed sheets when in bed.	These products help keep urine away from the skin.
Instruct to wash perineum after each incontinent episode.	Cleanliness prevents odor, skin irritation, and infection.
Instruct to check external catheter frequently for twisting and leakage and the skin for indications of constriction.	Constant use results in increased risk of infection, irritation, edema, fissures or necrosis.
*PLAN B: CATHETERIZATION—*An indwelling catheter is appropriate when there is high risk for or loss of skin integrity, or a terminal illness is accompanied by great pain. Monitor catheter patency. Keep the drainage bag below the level of the bladder and coil the catheter tubing so there are no dependent loops.	Patency improves drainage and reduces the risk of reflux or retention of urine, reducing risk of infection.
Adapt catheter care techniques to the environment.	The frequency of catheter changes and method of catheter cleaning may be modified in the home environment where the prevalence of harmful organisms is less than in an inpatient setting.
Use a silicone catheter if it is to be left in longer than one week.	A silicone catheter resists crusting and has a larger lumen providing better drainage.
Use a catheter with a lumen that fits the urethra.	If the catheter is too big, it can damage the urethra; if too small, bacteria enter the bladder more easily.
Inpatient None	

INTERVENTIONS

RATIONALE

Community Health/ Home Care	
Refer care giver to support group: The Simon Foundation, Box 815, Wilmette, IL 60091; OR Help for Incontinent People, PO Box 544, Union, SC 29373.	Caring for an incontinent person can be stressful.
Instruct in care of catheter, proper hand washing, and prevention of contamination.	Proper care of the catheter prevents infection.
Instruct in therapeutic regimen, its reasons, and complications of incontinence.	Understanding facilitates compliance.

REFERENCES/BIBLIOGRAPHY

Gross, C. (1990). Bladder dysfunction after stroke: It's not always inevitable. **Journal of Gerontological Nursing, 16**(4), 20–25.

* Hu, T-W., Kaltreider, D.L, & Igou, J. (1989). Incontinence products: Which is best? **Geriatric Nursing, 5**(8), 184–186.

* Kaltreider, L., Hu, T-W., Igou, J.F., Yu, L.C., & Craighead, W.E. (1990). Can reminders curb incontinence? **Geriatric Nursing, 11**(1), 17–19.

* Long, M.L. (1985). Incontinence. **Journal of Gerontological Nursing, 11**(1), 30–35.

North American Nursing Diagnosis Association. (1990). **Taxonomy I** (Rev. 1990). St. Louis: NANDA.

* Schnelle, J.F., et al. (1983). Management of geriatric incontinence in nursing homes. **Journal of Applied Behavioral Analysis, 13** (Summer), 235–241.

* Yu, L.C. (1987). Incontinence stress index: Measuring psychological impact. **Journal of Gerontological Nursing, 13**(7), 18–25.

Incontinence: Urge

A state in which an individual experiences involuntary passage of urine occurring soon after a strong sense of urgency to void (NANDA, 1990, p. 27).

Anne Marie Voith Sherman, R.N., M.S.N.

DEFINING CHARACTERISTICS

Bladder contracture/spasm
Burning on urination
Frequency
Nocturia (greater than two voids during
      hours of sleep)

Urgency
Voiding in small amounts (less than
      100 cc)

CONTRIBUTING FACTORS

Pathophysiological

Decreased bladder capacity (e.g., history of pelvic inflammatory disease (PID), abdominal
      surgeries, indwelling urinary catheter)
Irritation of bladder stretch receptors causing spasm (e.g., bladder infection, alcohol, caffeine,
      increased urine concentration)

Psychosociobehavioral

None

EXPECTED OUTCOMES

Client will be able to postpone voiding 10 minutes past the urge.
      Bladder irritability decreases.
      Bladder capacity increases.
      Appropriate regimen is verbalized.

327

INTERVENTIONS	RATIONALE
Universal	
Assess for the presence of stress and functional incontinence. (Refer to nursing care plan guides for these diagnoses.)	Both of these types of incontinence frequently occur with urge incontinence.
Consult physician regarding possible administration of anticholinergics or smooth muscle relaxants.	Anticholinergics increase warning time by blocking impulses within the sacral reflex arc.
Consult with physician regarding use of imipramine.	Imipramine has anticholinergic and direct relaxant effects on the detrusor and a contraction-enhancing effect on the bladder outlet.
Consult with physician to rule out urinary tract infection (UTI).	UTI can, in and of itself, result in urge incontinence.
Encourage reduction/elimination of caffeine and alcohol intake.	These drinks have a diuretic effect and may affect the predictability of urge to void.
Initiate biofeedback consultation.	Biofeedback can be useful in assisting to learn pelvic floor strengthening exercises and reduce detrusor irritability.
Provide at least 8 oz of fluid with and between meals and in the early evening.	Adequate fluid intake helps prevent bladder infection and reduces bladder irritability. Scheduling of the fluids helps establish a habit which will assure adequate fluid intake.
Use an oil-based lubricant on skin after washing.	Oil-based lubricants keep urine away from skin, preventing skin excoriation.
Use sanitary napkins or protective pants during the day.	These products help keep urine away from the skin.
Instruct in bladder retraining: wait to empty bladder for progressively longer intervals until voiding every three to four hours.	If the bladder is kept completely empty, the result could be a low threshold for the urinary reflex and/or a contracted detrusor with reduced bladder capacity. Progressively longer intervals between voiding helps increase bladder capacity.

INTERVENTIONS	RATIONALE
Instruct in regimen, its reasons, and complications of incontinence.	Understanding facilitates compliance.
Instruct to sit with firm towel or other object pressing on perineum when incontinence threatens (e.g., cross legs, sit on leg...).	This elevates the perineum, closing the bladder outlet, and stopping the flow of urine. This will help delay voiding as attempts are made to progressively lengthen intervals between voiding.
Instruct to wash after each incontinent episode.	Cleanliness prevents odor, skin irritation, and infection.
Instruct to wipe perineum from front to back.	Wiping from front to back minimizes the introduction of bacteria to the urethral area, preventing infection.
Refer care giver to support group: The Simon Foundation, Box 815, Wilmette, Il 60091; OR Help for Incontinent People, PO Box 544, Union, SC 29373.	Caring for an incontinent person can be stressful.
Inpatient None	
Community Health/ Home Care None	

REFERENCES/BIBLIOGRAPHY

* Burgio, K.L., Whitehead, W.I., & Engel, B.T. (1985). Bladder-sphincter biofeedback and toiletting skills training. **Annals of Internal Medicine, 104**, 507–515.

North American Nursing Diagnosis Association. (1990). **Taxonomy I** (Rev. 1990). St. Louis: NANDA.

Greengold, B.A., & Ouslander, J.G. (1986). Bladder retraining. **Journal of Gerontological Nursing, 12**(6), 31–35.

Gross, C. (1990). Bladder dysfunction after stroke: It's not always inevitable. **Journal of Gerontological Nursing, 16**(4), 20–25.

* Lincoln, R., & Roberts, R. (1989). Continence issues in acute care. **Nursing Clinics of North America, 24**(3), 741–54.

Ramphal, M. (1987). Urinary incontinence among nursing home patients: Issues in research. **Geriatric Nursing, 8**(5), 249–254.

Voith, A.M. (1988). Alterations in urinary elimination: Concepts, research, and practice. **Rehabilitation Nursing, 13**(3), 122–131.

Infection: Risk

A state in which an individual is at increased risk for being invaded by pathogenic organisms (NANDA, 1990, p. 13).

Linda S. Baas, R.N., M.S.N., C.C.R.N.

. . . .

RISK FACTORS

Pathophysiological

Advanced age
Decreased normal flora
Decreased tissue perfusion
Hematological disorder
Immature immune system
Immobility
Impaired airway clearance
Impaired nasal warming and filtering of air
Impaired skin or mucous membrane integrity
Inadequate immunization
Ingestion of food containing bacteria or toxins
Injury (e.g., chemical, mechanical, or thermal)
Invasive drainage catheter
Invasive infusion cannula
Invasive monitoring device

Invasive treatment or diagnostic procedure
Metabolic disorder (e.g., anorexia, impaired glucose tolerance, liver dysfunction, malnutrition, or obesity)
Postpartum period
Prematurity
Radiation treatment
Respiratory disorder (e.g., altered breathing patterns, impaired airway clearance, or impaired gas exchange)
Surgical incision
Therapeutic medication regimen (e.g., antimicrobial, antipyretics, immunosuppressants, or steroids)
Transfusion of blood products
Warm moist skin

Psychosociobehavioral

Contaminated work or living environment
Depression
Exchange of body fluids with an infected person
Exposure to a person infected with an airborne pathogen

Exposure to large crowds
Fear
Inadequate personal hygiene
Substance abuse
Stressful life events

331

EXPECTED OUTCOMES

Client will exhibit no signs of infectious process.
>   There is no evidence of fever.
>   There is no evidence of foul odor from wound, draining fluids, or invasive catheter.
>   There is no evidence of adventitious lung sounds.

Client will exhibit no metabolic changes associated with infection.
>   No elimination abnormalities are seen.
>   There is no increase in the basal metabolic rate.
>   No increase in the resting cardiac output is experienced.
>   There is no increase in the resting heart rate or blood pressure.

Client will maintain adequate defense mechanisms to prevent infection.
>   There are no breaks in the skin or mucous membranes.
>   No decrease in leukocytes is seen.
>   There is no lapse in immunizations against communicable diseases.
>   No increase in the pH of body fluids is seen.

Client will reduce exposure to known infectious agents or contaminants.
>   Dress is appropriate for the environment.
>   Food is properly stored, prepared, and eaten in a timely fashion.
>   There is minimal exposure to large groups.
>   There is minimal or no exposure to persons with a known infection.
>   There is no engagement in unprotected sexual intercourse.

INTERVENTIONS / RATIONALE

INTERVENTIONS	RATIONALE
Assess for the presence of risk factors for infection.	Identification of risk factors for infection is the initial step that individualizes the interventions.
Assess for signs or symptoms of an actual infection.	Early identification of an actual infection provides for early initiation of therapy, lessens the impact of the infection, and promotes earlier recovery.
Avoid contact with a known infected person.	By eliminating contact with the pathogen, there is no opportunity for infection.
Maintain integrity of the skin and mucous membranes.	Clean, dry skin provides a barrier to pathogens. Good oral hygiene prevents tooth decay and gum disorders caused by colonization.
Maintain a well-balanced diet.	Adequate nutritional status provides for the integrity of body tissue and the ability to maintain a normal immune response.
Provide for personal hygiene.	Clean clothes and linen maintain integrity of the skin, reducing the possibility of colonization.

INTERVENTIONS	RATIONALE
Wash hands after contact with another person.	Hand washing is the primary intervention to reduce the risk of infection.
Teach guidelines for avoiding infection.	The spread of an infection from an airborne pathogen is reduced by using a handkerchief and hand washing. The spread of a sexually transmitted infection is reduced by using a condom.

Inpatient

INTERVENTIONS	RATIONALE
Assess for signs of infection.	Monitor the vital signs, leukocytes, and cultures to identify the infection early. Early treatment reduces the severity or duration of the infection and lessens the pathophysiologic effects.
Monitor incisions, wounds, and sites of any indwelling catheter or cannula for signs of infection.	Identification of drainage, foul odor, redness, or tenderness can lead to an early determination of infection and treatment.
Provide aseptic care when handling any invasive device or performing wound care.	Reducing the potential for introduction of a pathogen is a primary intervention to reduce the risk of infection. Follow current Centers for Disease Control guidelines for frequency of wound care, change of invasive cannula, and change of administration or monitoring tubing.
Provide measures to ensure adequate oral hygiene.	Provide mouth care at least two to four times per day to reduce the risk of introduction of a pathogen.
Provide measures to ensure adequate skin care.	Daily bathing maintains the integrity of the skin. Frequent turning promotes circulation to dependent areas. Moisturizing the skin reduces dryness and cracking which provide a portal of entry for pathogens.
Turn, cough, and deep breathe every one to four hours.	Pulmonary toilet provides for better aeration of the lungs and reducing the stasis of secretions in the alveoli or airways.
Use universal precautions with all client contact.	Wearing gloves when handling any body fluid reduces the risk of transmitting pathogens.

INTERVENTIONS	RATIONALE
Community Health/ Home Care	
Assess home and work environments for adequate levels of hygiene.	Reduction of contaminants in the environment will reduce the potential for infection.
Assess the adequacy of storage and handling of food products.	Inadequate refrigeration or cooking can result in pathogens or toxins in the ingested food.
Assess adequacy of the removal of waste from the home and work environments.	Disposal of waste through the sewage system or a properly functioning septic tank reduces the spread of infection through a family or community.
Assess ingested water for purity.	Use of tap, bottled, or collected cistern water that is free of pathogens will reduce the risk of infection.
Monitor community for outbreaks of specific infections.	Early identification of epidemiological problems will lead to early treatment intervention, thus reducing the spread of infection in the community.

REFERENCES/BIBLIOGRAPHY

*Baas, L.S., Allen, G.A., Sommers, M.S., & Beiting, A.M. (1987). Predictability of clinical indicators of infection. In A.M. McLane (Ed.). **Classification of nursing diagnoses: Proceedings of the seventh conference,** (pp. 234–238). St. Louis: Mosby.

Garner, J.S. (1985). Centers for Disease Control: Guidelines for prevention of surgical wound infections. In **Guidelines for the prevention and control of nosocomial infection**. Atlanta: Centers for Disease Control.

Gettrust, K.V., Ryan, S.C., & Engelman, D.S. (Eds.). (1985). **Applied nursing diagnosis: Guides for comprehensive care planning**. New York: Wiley.

Kim, M.J., McFarland, G.K., & McLane, A.M. (1989). **Pocket guide to nursing diagnosis** (3rd ed.). St. Louis: Mosby.

North American Nursing Diagnosis Association. (1990). **Taxonomy I** (Rev. 1990). St. Louis: NANDA.

Patrick, M.L., Woods, S.L., Craven, R.F., Rokosky, J.S., & Bruno, P.M. (1991). **Medical surgical nursing: Pathophysiological concepts** (2nd ed.). Philadelphia: Lippincott.

*Sommers, M.S., Baas, L.S., & Beiting, A.M. (1987). Nosocomial infection with four methods of hemodynamic monitoring. **Heart and Lung, 16**, 13–19.

Raffensperger, E.B., Zusy, M.L., & Marchesseault, L.C. (1986). **Clinical nursing handbook**. Philadelphia: Lippincott.

Yannelli, B., & Tu, R.P. (1988). Infection control in critical care. **Heart and Lung, 17**, 596–601.

Injury: Risk

A state in which an individual is at risk of injury as a result of internal and external environmental conditions interacting with the individual's adaptive and defensive resources. (NANDA, 1990, p. 39).

Colleen Lucas, R.N., M.N., C.S.

RISK FACTORS

Internal

Abnormal blood index
Cognitive or emotional impairment
Developmental age
Immune response impairment
Integrative dysfunction

Medication reaction or toxicity
Motor deficits
Nutritional alterations
Sensory-perceptual alterations
Tissue hypoxia

External

Chemical—Drug, poisons, pollutants which are improperly dispensed, contained, marked, stored, or disposed of; use of preservatives
Energy—Incompletely contained or inadequately controlled energy source
Physical—Unsafe design, structure, arrangement, or transport

EXPECTED OUTCOMES

Client will identify factors that increase the potential for injury.
Internal and external factors that can place an individual or groups at risk for injury are listed.
Internal and external factors placing self or others at risk for injury are assessed.
Level of risk is related to available adaptive and defensive resources.
Safety precautions are applied to self, others, and environment in reducing risk for injury.
Measures which will increase safety are identified and implemented.

The modified environment is evaluated and adjusted in accordance with changes in resources.

Client will remain free of bodily injury.

A safe environment is maintained.

INTERVENTIONS	**R**ATIONALE
Universal	
Determine the presence of risk factors for injury and whether the risk factors are internal or external.	The focus of the interventions is directed at lowering the risk for injury by modifying the risk factors. Internal risk factors are more frequently characteristics of the individual and therefore less modifiable than external environmental factors.
Monitor changes.	Changes in risk factors correspond with changes in the level of risk. Knowledge of changes assists in selecting the most effective interventions.
Monitor for malnutrition, vascular disease, impaired mobility, renal and hepatic disease for skin breakdown.	Factors which decrease tissue oxygenation place the client at risk for skin breakdown.
Monitor for alterations in coagulation studies, bleeding times, and platelets.	Increased coagulation and clotting times as well as decreased platelet counts increase the likelihood of bleeding into the tissues and thus increasing tissue damage.
Monitor for changes in white blood cell count and differential.	Alterations in the white blood cell count impair the host response to microorganisms and infection.
Modify and maintain a safe environment.	Modifying the environment reduces the likelihood of injury occurring as a result of external risk factors.
Teach internal and external factors that can place the individual or groups at risk for injury.	Knowledge of risk factors is necessary in order to effect behavior change.
Teach methods for improving the safety of the environment.	Once the environment is evaluated, many options exist for further reducing risks. When these alternatives are understood, informed decisions can be made.

INTERVENTIONS	RATIONALE
Teach safety measures for maintaining a healthy life-style: 1. maintain a well-balanced, healthful diet; obtain annual flu vaccinations 2. visit the doctor regularly for developmental age	A healthy life-style creates an environment in which opportunistic infection is less likely to thrive and when it does occur, can be detected and treated early.
Teach measures to be taken in reducing the risk for injury.	Knowledge of measures which can reduce risk provides empowerment to modify risk profile.
Teach safe medication usage: 1. properly label and store all drugs 2. keep medications out of the reach of children 3. take medications as directed	Clear understanding of how medications are used aids adherence to the regimen. Storing and taking medications as directed helps to achieve the intended therapeutic effect.
Inpatient None	
Community Health/ Home Care None	

REFERENCES/BIBLIOGRAPHY

Fay, M.F., Beck, W.C., Fay, J.M., & Kessinger, M.K. (1990). Medical waste: The growing issues of management and disposal. **ADRN Journal, 51**(6), 1493–1508.

Gettrust, K.V., Ryan, S.C., & Engelmon, D.S. (1985). **Applied nursing diagnosis: Guides for comprehensive planning** (pp. 105–108). New York: Delmar.

*Kent, P., Greenspan, J.R., Herndon, J.L., Mofenson, L.M., et al. (1988). Epidemic giardiasis caused by a contaminated public water supply. **American Journal of Public Health, 78**(2), 139–143.

Kim, M.J., McFarland, G.K., & McLane, A.M. (1989). **Pocket guide to nursing diagnoses**, St. Louis: Mosby.

McFarland, G.K., & McFarlane, E.A. (1989). **Nursing diagnosis and intervention: Planning for patient care**. St. Louis: Mosby.

North American Nursing Diagnosis Association. (1990). **Taxonomy I** (Rev. 1990). St. Louis: NANDA.

Parsons, M.T., & Levy, J. (1987). Nursing process in injury prevention. **Journal of Gerontological Nursing, 13**(7), 36–40.

Rea, J., & Ross, H. Food and chemicals as environmental incitants. **Nurse Practitioner, 14**(9), 17–37.

Vork, K.L., & Olson, D.K. (1990). Asbestos review and update. **AAOHN Journal, 38**(4), 160–164.

Waller, A.E. (1989). Atmospheric pollution. **Chest, 96**(3), 363S–372S.

Knowledge Deficit (Specify)

A state in which an individual experiences an inability to state or explain information or demonstrate a required skill related to health care measures necessary to maintain or improve wellness.

Joan Randall, R.N., M.S.

DEFINING CHARACTERISTICS

Inaccurate follow-through of instruction
Inadequate performance of demonstration of a skill
Inappropriate or exaggerated behaviors, e.g., hysterical, hostile, agitated, apathetic
Lack of recall
Verbalizations indicating inadequate understanding, misinterpretation, or misconception
of desired health behavior

CONTRIBUTING FACTORS

Pathophysiological

Any existing or new medical condition
Severity of illness

Psychosociobehavioral

Cognitive limitations (intellectual)
Complexity of treatment plan
Ineffective coping patterns, e.g., anxiety,
depression, denial of situation,
avoidance of coping
Lack of education or readiness

Lack of interest or motivation to learn
Lack of previous exposure to the experience
Language differences
Uncompensated memory loss
Unfamiliarity with information resources

EXPECTED OUTCOMES

Client will verbalize understanding of desired health behaviors.

Accurate demonstration of desired skill is observed.

Disease process, causes, and factors contributing to disease state are described.

Procedures or health-related practices to control disease or symptoms are verbalized.

Ability to follow prescribed regimen is demonstrated.

Need for additional information regarding desired health behavior is identified.

Less anxiety is experienced related to fear of the unknown, misconceptions, and/or misinformation.

INTERVENTIONS   RATIONALE

INTERVENTIONS	RATIONALE
Universal Assess understanding of prescribed treatment.	Assessment of knowledge base prior to teaching will facilitate a more efficient and successful learning process individualized to specific needs by identifying what content should be presented and how it should be presented.
Assess readiness to learn.	To facilitate successful learning, it is important to assess readiness to learn. The client needs to be free of pain and extreme anxiety to learn. Motivation is an important factor that affects learning. Health beliefs and past experiences related to illness may affect desire to learn.
Assess ability to perform desired health-related care.	Physical limitations or cognitive limitations must be identified and considered when establishing treatment plan. Modification of treatment plan and/or identification of support person may be indicated to facilitate ability to follow prescribed treatment plan.
Assess ability to learn cultural practices, and educational levels.	It is important to assess the educational level and cultural background to facilitate effective teaching-learning process. Individuals learn in their own way. Information must be presented in understandable terms. Cultural practices may influence the learning process.

INTERVENTIONS	RATIONALE
Assess misconceptions of health-related state.	Misinterpretation or misinformation needs to be assessed to facilitate accurate and thorough clarification of information. Anxiety, which affects ability to learn, may be related to misconceptions or misunderstanding of the disease process, possible complications, or seriousness of the disease.
Establish comfortable learning environment.	Environment should be free of distractions and noise. Interactions with individual should be nonjudgmental. Tendency to talk down to client will result in resistance to learning.
Involve client and family in teaching process and planning learning goals.	Encouraging active participation in identifying and planning learning needs will facilitate improved learning by motivation and establishment of realistic goals that client and family support. Encouragement of questions and involvement will enhance learning.
Check for accurate feedback.	Feedback will allow evaluation of learning and understanding, effectiveness of teaching, need for clarification of information presented, or modification of teaching process. Providing feedback enhances awareness of progress and strengthens the learning process and motivation.
Reinforce teaching.	Repeating information, as well as using both verbal and written information, will enhance the learning process. Presenting too much information may inhibit learning. Provide concise pertinent information to strengthen learning process.
Allow practice and demonstrations.	To insure accurate learning and accurate evaluation of ability to perform desired skills, repeat demonstrations need to be observed. Demonstrations of skills will enhance learning and retention. Observations of practicing desired skills allow modifications of treatment plan based on ability to perform the task.
Provide written literature specific to needs.	Written information will reinforce learning by providing a reference resource to clarify information. Written information enhances and clarifies verbal information received.

INTERVENTIONS	RATIONALE
Provide information on community resources.	Information resources in the community will provide additional support which may reduce anxiety, enhance motivation, and enhance compliance to prescribed treatment plan.
Inpatient None	
Community Health/ Home Care None	

REFERENCES/BIBLIOGRAPHY

Carpenito, L.J. (1987). **Nursing diagnosis application to clinical practice** (2nd ed.). Philadelphia: Lippincott.

Gettrust, K.V., Ryan, S.C., & Engelman, D.S. (1985). **Applied nursing diagnosis: Guides for comprehensive care planning**. Albany, NY: Delmar.

Lederer, J.R., Marculescu, G.L., Gallagher, J., & Mills, P. (1986). **Care planning pocket guide: A nursing diagnosis approach**. Menlo Park, CA: Addison-Wesley.

North American Nursing Diagnosis Association. (1990). **Taxonomy I** (Rev. 1990). St. Louis: NANDA.

* Pokorny, B.E. (1985). Validating a diagnostic label: knowledge deficits. **Nursing Clinics of North America, 20**(4), 641–654.

Noncompliance: Dietary

A state in which an individual fails to follow a professionally recommended diet despite knowledge, consent, and demonstrated efficacy of the diet.

Polly Ryan, R.N., M.S.N.

DEFINING CHARACTERISTICS

Denies experiencing problem in following dietary specifications—ever
Failure to achieve desired outcomes (e.g., weight loss, decreased lipid level, lower blood sugar
       Note: These outcomes are only partially determined by dietary compliance)
Lack of familiarity with specifics of diet despite statement that diet is followed
Observation
Reports of significant other that diet has not been followed
Self-reports of noncompliance with diet

CONTRIBUTING FACTORS

Pathophysiological

Diagnosis (e.g., diabetes, hyperlipidemia, obesity)
Physical limitations such as limited mobility, extreme fatigue, pain

Psychosociobehavioral

Failure to believe in need for the diet or
      efficacy of prescribed diet
History of repeated failure to alter dietary
      habits
Inadequate social support

Lack of effective coping mechanisms
Little or no control over diet
Multiple personal, social, or financial
      stressors
No intent to change dietary habits

EXPECTED OUTCOMES

Client will follow professionally recommended diet.

Intention to follow diet is reported.

Specific plans or behaviors are reported which specify how diet is being followed.

Times or situations are reported when diet is difficult to follow.

Management of diet is reported for occasions and changes in routine.

INTERVENTIONS	RATIONALE
Universal Monitor daily intake.	One of the most effective ways of changing dietary patterns is to keep a daily record of food consumed. Self-monitoring changes behavior.
Inform about the benefit(s) of the particular diet and the consequences of not following the diet.	Knowledge and understanding generally require more than a singular explanation. Better understanding of the reasons for specific dietary requirements and the consequences of choosing not to follow the prescribed diet will occur with multiple explanations. Additionally, as more knowledge is gained by the professionals, the specifics of prescribed diets also change. Change in the diet can also occur because of physiological changes.
Utilize resources of a dietitian.	Initial explanation of a dietary prescription is commonly given by a dietitian. Individuals need to know how to access a dietitian with questions and problems.
Help to identify the personal, social, and environmental factors which cue eating behaviors.	Identification of the personal, social, and environmental cues or triggers for eating enables recognition of those factors which cue individual eating habits. Once these are known, pre-planning for how to deal with the cues can occur. Effective methods of managing cues are avoidance (e.g., not buying desserts), distraction (e.g., short walks), substitution (e.g. carrot and celery sticks), relaxation (e.g., deep breathing), or social support (e.g., enlisting the assistance of a buddy).

INTERVENTIONS	RATIONALE
Help to verbalize intentions, a commitment, and describe a specific plan to alter the dietary pattern.	Verbalization of intentions and commitment are known to facilitate behavior change. This can be accomplished by listing the reasons a change in dietary pattern is desired, setting a target date, and having pre-made plans to deal with difficult situations. The pre-made plans need to be tailored to the clients' reasons for their eating habits.
Help to use problem-solving skills when social and environmental factors interfere with usual dietary routine.	Assist in managing social and environmental changes by identifying problems before they occur, pre-planning alternative behavior, role-playing ways to order or decline food, and knowing and/or preparing substitute foods.
Teach how to read labels.	It is important to know specific ingredients which should be included or avoided. Computerized labels listing ingredients can be attached to grocery lists until there is familiarity with various brands. Teaching needs to be done about misleading marketing techniques: e.g., a product can be labeled low in cholesterol but still be high in saturated fats.
Teach that changing behavior requires additional time.	Reading labels when shopping, finding alternative brands, finding and using new recipes, and planning different menus is time consuming. Advise that it will be necessary to spend more than the usual amount of time for several weeks.
Teach that relapse will occur and assist in developing skills necessary to deal with it.	All persons have difficulty maintaining a diet all the time. Therefore, teach to deal with those situations which are risky for persons with specific dietary requirements and how to cope with relapse when it occurs. Instead of being viewed as a failure, a relapse can be framed as an opportunity to better understand feelings and situations in which specific plans and coping skills need to be developed.
Inpatient None	

INTERVENTIONS	**R**ATIONALE
Community Health/ Home Care None	

REFERENCES/BIBLIOGRAPHY

Cameron, R., & Best, J.A. (1987). Promoting adherence to health behavior change interventions: Recent findings from behavioral research. **Patient Education and Counseling, 10**, 139–154.

DiMatteo, M.R., & DiNicola, D.D. (1982). **Achieving patient compliance: The psychology of the medical practitioner's role**. New York: Pergamon.

Falvo, D.R. (1985). **Effective patient education: A guide to increased compliance**. Baltimore: Aspen.

Glanz, K. (1988). Patient and public education for cholesterol reduction: A review of strategies and issues. **Patient Education and Counseling, 12**, 235–257.

Glanz, K., & Mullins, R.M. (1988). Environmental interventions to promote healthy eating: A review of models, programs, and evidence. **Health Education Quarterly, 15**, 395–414.

Green, L.W., Kreuter, M., Deeds, S.G., & Partridge, K.B. (Eds.). (1980). **Health education planning: A diagnostic approach**. Palo Alto, CA: Mayfield.

Guare, J.C., Wing, R.R., Marcus, M.D., Epstein, L.H., Burton, L.R., & Gooding, W.E. (1989). Analysis of changes in eating behavior and weight loss in Type II diabetic patients: Which behaviors to change. **Diabetes Care, 12**, 500–503.

Haynes, R.B., Taylor, D.W., & Sackett, D.L. (Eds.). (1979). **Compliance in Health Care**. Baltimore: Johns Hopkins University Press.

Marlatt, G.A., & Gordon, J.R. (Eds.). (1985). **Relapse prevention: Maintenance strategies in addictive behavior change**. New York: Guilford.

Melnyk, M.A.M. (1988). Barriers: A critical review of recent literature. **Nursing Research, 37**, 196–201.

* Pender, N. (1987). **Health promotion in nursing practice** (2nd ed.). Norwalk, CT: Appleton-Century-Crofts.

* Ryan, P. (1987). Strategies for motivating life-style change. **Journal of Cardiovascular Nursing, 1**, 54–66.

* Smith, A. (1987). Physiology, diagnosis, and life-style modifications for hyperlipidemia. **Journal of Cardiovascular Nursing, 1**, 15–27.

Noncompliance: Prescribed Medication

A state in which an individual fails
to take a therapeutic level of prescribed
medication despite information,
consent, and demonstrated efficacy
of the medication.

Polly Ryan, R.N., M.S.N.

DEFINING CHARACTERISTICS

Failure to achieve desired effects or intended outcomes
Failure to have the prescription filled or reordered
Frequent readmissions or recurrences of problem
Inaccurate reports of the prescribed dose, frequency, or method of administration
Inadequate level of medication as determined by biochemical levels
Inappropriate problem solving (e.g., doubling the dose of a prescribed medication because of
increased symptoms, despite contrary advice)
Self-reports of noncompliance with prescribed medication

CONTRIBUTING FACTORS

Pathophysiological

Allergic response
Confusion and/or memory deficits
Physical limitations such as limited mobility or limited strength
Secondary illness
Side effects

Psychosociobehavioral

Change of routine
Conflicts with other prescribed therapies
Failure to believe in the accuracy of the diagnosis or the efficacy of the treatment
Forgetting
Inadequate support

347

Inconsistent with religious, cultural or social beliefs
Limited resources including, but not limited to: financial, transportation, child care, telephone
Medication taken more than three times per day
More than three prescribed medications
Physician/client relationship
Stigma of chronic illness

Expected Outcomes

Client will take medication as ordered, or discusses discontinuation with a physician.
> Appropriate questions regarding the name, dose, frequency, intended effects, and side effects of the medications are asked.
> A system for taking medication as well as management of change in routines is reported.
> Issues related to forgotten doses and changes in symptoms are problem-solved accurately.
> Knowledge of correct person to contact with questions regarding medications is verbalized.

Interventions	Rationale
Universal	
Assess reason(s) for disregard for medication compliance.	Understanding the factors causing the noncompliance will provide direction for appropriate interventions.
Simplify the drug regimen.	Persons who take more than three medications per day or take a medication more than three times a day are more likely to have problems regularly taking medications. It is important that physicians, nurses, and pharmacists know all the medications currently being taken. Longer acting drugs can be substituted for shorter acting drugs. If noncompliance is a documented problem, reevaluation needs to occur, and only those medications which are essential should be prescribed.
Tailor the medication prescription to the current life-style when possible.	The peak action of a medication, as well as schedule for taking medication, needs to fit with a desired life-style when possible. For example, a grade school teacher might prefer to take a diuretic after school hours, or a night shift worker might prefer to take a three-times-daily medication through the night, not the day.

INTERVENTIONS	RATIONALE
Increase social support.	Any behavior change and maintenance of long-term behaviors is more likely to occur if the individual has social support. Therefore, involve the significant other(s) in the initial instructions and provide with opportunities to identify behaviors which could be most helpful.
Provide verbal and written instructions including the name, dose, frequency, intended effects, and side effects of medication(s).	Instructions should be specific, brief, categorized, prioritized, and spoken or written at an appropriate comprehension and reading level. A pill can be affixed to a written sheet (or with a physician's order, it can be done by a pharmacist) in order to decrease confusion when multiple medications are prescribed. Note: If the prescription is filled with a generic medication, it is the actual medication taken which needs to be affixed to the instructions.
Prepare for expected effects and side effects.	If persons are prepared for the intended or unintended effects of a medication they will be better able to cope with them and make appropriate decisions about them.
Teach about over-the-counter (OTC) medications and foods which may interfere with medication.	OTC medications and foods can potentiate or reduce the effects of some medications. Clients need information specific to their medication. If desired outcomes are not met, this needs to be explored as an alternative reason.
Teach to take medication in association with behaviors regularly performed.	Using regularly performed behaviors as a cue to the performance of a new behavior is a very effective way to establish a new habit, e.g., taking the medication with meals, or when brushing teeth, or before bed.
Advise protection of young children by storing medication appropriately.	Remind about safety precautions which need to be taken for children. Medication should not be stored within the view or reach of young children or kept in easily opened containers in pockets or purses.

INTERVENTIONS	RATIONALE
Teach to request assistance of pharmacist if difficulty arises with child-proof locks.	Compliance with medication prescription has decreased as the result of child-proof containers. Clients who have difficulty opening bottles because of child-proof locks can have their prescription medications bottled differently upon request. Additionally, pharmacists will remove locks on nonprescription medication if requested.
Teach regarding the importance of regularly scheduled checkups.	Any individual who is regularly taking medications should be routinely reevaluated for continued need for the medication and the correct dosage. Additionally, medication-taking behavior is not self-sustaining; rather long-term supervision is necessary.
Teach to reorder medication in a timely fashion.	Teach to reorder medications several days before actually needing it. Additionally, planning and packing for vacations needs to include adequate amounts of medication.
Teach that reminders, pill containers, or calendars can be used when taking multiple medications or when remembering to take medications is a problem.	Medications can be poured for the day, week, or month. Special pill-dispensing containers, fishing tackle boxes, calendars, or other items can be used to arrange medication by the hour or the week. This system visually displays the medication(s), allowing knowledge at a glance what medication should be taken.
Inpatient Involve in a self-medication program.	Several days of in-hospital supervision with new and complex medication prescriptions has been associated with a decrease in noncompliance and errors.
Community Health/ Home Care Recall nonattenders.	Clients, particularly those taking medication(s), who fail to show up for appointments or fail to schedule follow-up appointments should be recalled. Telephone calls and reminder notes have been demonstrated to be effective.

REFERENCES/BIBLIOGRAPHY

Buckalew, L.W., & Sallis, R.E. (1986). Patient compliance and medication perception. **Journal of Clinical Psychology, 42**, 49–53.

Cameron, R., & Best, J.A. (1987). Promoting adherence to health behavior change interventions: Recent findings from behavioral research. **Patient Education and Counseling, 10**, 139–154.

DiMatteo, M.R., & DiNicola, D.D. (1982). **Achieving patient compliance: The psychology of the medical practitioner's role**. New York: Pergamon Press.

Falvo, D.R. (1985). **Effective patient education: A guide to increased compliance**. Rockville, MD: Aspen.

Green, L.W., Kreuter, M., Deeds, S.G., & Partridge, K.B. (Eds.). (1980). **Health education planning: A diagnostic approach**. Palo Alto, CA: Mayfield.

Haynes, R.B., Taylor, D.W., & Sackett, D.L. (Eds.). (1979). **Compliance in health care**. Baltimore: Johns Hopkins University Press.

Haynes, R.B., Wang, E., & Gomes, M.D.M. (1987). A critical review of interventions to improve compliance with prescribed medication. **Patient Education and Counseling, 10**, 155–166.

* Melnyk, M.A.M. (1988). Barriers: A critical review of recent literature. **Nursing Research, 37**, 196–201.

* Pender, N. (1987). **Health Promotion in Nursing Practice** (2nd ed.). Norwalk, CT: Appleton-Century-Crofts.

* Ryan, P. (1987). Strategies for motivating life-style change. **Journal of Cardiovascular Nursing, 1**, 54–66.

Noncompliance: Smoking

A state in which an individual continues smoking despite professional advice to quit and expressed desire for health promotion or improved health status.

Polly Ryan, R.N., M.S.N.

DEFINING CHARACTERISTICS

Observed smoking
Report of significant other
Self-reports of smoking

CONTRIBUTING FACTORS

Pathophysiological

Experiences severe withdrawal symptoms
Multiple addictive behaviors (i.e., drugs and/or alcohol)

Psychosociobehavioral

Continues to "sneak cigarettes" after quitting, denying to themselves that they are still smoking
Denies need to quit smoking either because of feelings of invulnerability or a belief that the current professional information is inaccurate
Denies personal advantage to quitting
Experiences multiple life stresses
Experiences severe withdrawal symptoms
Gains weight after quitting and perceives the weight gain to be intolerable
History of heavy cigarette smoking (i.e., greater than one pack per day)
Intends to continue smoking
Lives, works, and/or socializes with other smokers
Multiple, unsuccessful attempts to quit smoking
Perceives self as unable to quit

EXPECTED OUTCOMES

Client will report complete smoking cessation for one year.
>An intention and commitment to quit smoking is reported.
>Personal reasons for smoking are stated and concrete plans to deal with cues to smoking are made.
>A target date to quit smoking is set.
>Smoking stops.
>The use of effective coping behaviors to deal with withdrawal symptoms, highly tempting situations, and stressful social situations is reported.

INTERVENTIONS	RATIONALE
Universal	
Teach the personal, family, and social consequences of smoking.	Smoking is linked with cancer of the lung, bladder, and pancreas. It is also linked with the development of bronchitis, emphysema, peripheral vascular disease, aortic aneurysm, and coronary heart disease. Spouses of heavy smokers have a higher morbidity rate, and their children have a higher mortality rate. Persons who smoke have a higher rate of absenteeism, and are involved in a greater number of work-related accidents.
Help to identify the reasons for smoking.	Reasons for smoking include stimulation, handling of the smoking material, pleasurable relaxation, tension reduction, craving, and habit. Identification of the reason(s) for smoking enables the development of techniques specifically designed to manage the particular reason(s) for smoking. For example, if smoking is used to manage tension, deep breathing is an alternative method to achieve tension reduction.
Help to identity personal, social, and environmental factors which cue their smoking habit.	Identification of the personal, social, and environmental cues or triggers for smoking enables the recognition of those factors which cue the smoking habit. Once these are known, preplanning can be used to deal with the cues. Effective methods of managing cues are avoidance (e.g., temporarily refraining from coffee), distraction (e.g., short walks), substitution (e.g., gum or hard candy), relaxation (e.g., deep breathing), or social support (e.g., enlisting a friend's assistance).

INTERVENTIONS	**R**ATIONALE
Help to verbalize intentions and a commitment, and describe a specific plan to quit smoking.	Verbalization of intentions and commitment are known to facilitate behavior change. This can be accomplished by clients listing the reason they would like to stop smoking, setting a target date, and having premade plans to deal with difficult situations. The plans need to be tailored to the individual's reasons for smoking and cues or triggers to the smoking behavior.
Prepare for withdrawal symptoms.	Most people who quit smoking experience myriad physical and psychological withdrawal symptoms. The most common withdrawal symptoms include irritability, impatience, hunger, restlessness, frustration, annoyance, anxiety, tenseness, nervousness, increased food consumption, urges for a cigarette, changes in mood, feeling at loose ends, and difficulty concentrating. Clients should know that it is normal to experience these symptoms, that they generally peak between 24 and 48 hours, and gradually disappear within a week or two following cessation.
Teach methods to cope with withdrawal symptoms and use cognitive and behavioral strategies to manage cues and triggers.	Short-term behavioral coping responses include such things as gum chewing, deep breathing, relaxation, doodling, short walks, frequent oral hygiene, and /or distraction. Examples of behavioral responses useful over a long term are regular exercise, stress management, development of a hobby, assertiveness training, and group support. In addition to the behavioral strategies, cognitive coping strategies can be used, for example, assertiveness training, thought stopping, increased self efficacy, and cognitive restructuring.
Prepare for and provide the skills to deal with a potential relapse.	Approximately 70% of persons who quit smoking relapse or return to smoking. Therefore, teach to avoid or manage risky situations and to cope with relapse if it does occur. Instead of a failure, relapse can be framed as an opportunity to learn. Through reflection, greater insight can be gained into those times and situations which are particularly difficult and reassess which cognitive and behavioral strategies were most effective.

INTERVENTIONS	RATIONALE
Inform about available resources including written information and community programs.	Smoking cessation, like any behavior change, is a multi-staged process. In general, phases of behavior change are contemplation, commitment and change, maintenance, or relapse. Different interventions are appropriate for each stage. Information is helpful during contemplation, and specific cognitive and behavioral strategies are effective during early and late phases of quitting.
Inpatient Teach, remind, and support post-operative deep breathing and coughing.	When smoking cessation coincides with a general anesthetic there is a higher risk for post-operative respiratory problems. Secretions tend to be more copious and ciliary action reduced, leading to the risk of ineffective airway clearance and infection. Additionally, increased coughing can lead to increased pain from the surgical wound, and sleep deprivation.
Community Health/ Home Care Participate in the establishment and operationalization of no-smoking policies for schools, health agencies, and public buildings.	Social influences are one of the major determinants of behavior change.
Participate in the use of mass media to communicate information about smoking cessation.	As persons prepare for smoking cessation they think, read, and listen to opinions of others. Information needs to be readily available to the public about the hazards of smoking, the benefits of quitting, and the various methods of quitting.

REFERENCES/BIBLIOGRAPHY

Cameron, R., & Best, J.A. (1987). Promoting adherence to health behavior change interventions: Recent findings from behavioral research. **Patient Education and Counseling, 10**, 139–154.

DiMatteo, M.R., & DiNicola, D.D. (1982). **Achieving patient compliance: The psychology of the medical practitioner's role**. New York: Pergamon.

Falvo, D.R. (1985). **Effective patient education: A guide to increased compliance**. Rockville, MD: Aspen.

Green, L.W., Kreuter, M., Deeds, S.G., & Partridge, K.B. (Eds.). (1980). **Health Education planning: A diagnostic approach**. Palo Alto, CA: Mayfield.

Haynes, R.B., Taylor, D.W., & Sackett, D.L. (Eds.). (1979). **Compliance in Health Care**. Baltimore: Johns Hopkins University Press.

Marlatt, G.A., & Gordon, J.R. (Eds.). (1985). **Relapse prevention: Maintenence strategies in addictive behavior change**. New York: Guilford.

McKool, K. (1987). Facilitating smoking cessation. **Journal of Cardiovascular Nursing, 1**, 28–41.

Melnyk, M.A.M. (1988). Barriers: A critical review of recent literature. **Nursing Research, 37**, 196–201.

Pender, N. (1987). **Health Promotion in Nursing Practice** (2nd ed.). Norwalk, CT: Appleton-Century-Crofts.

Prochaska, J.O., & DiClemente, C.C. (1983). Stages and processes of self-change in smoking: Towards an integrative model of change. **Journal of Consulting and Clinical Psychology, 51**, 390–395.

*Ryan, P. (1990). **Smoking cessation: Subjective reports of withdrawal symptoms**. Unpublished manuscript, Milwaukee: University of Wisconsin—Milwaukee.

Ryan, P. (1987). Strategies for motivating life-style change. **Journal of Cardiovascular Nursing, 1**, 54–66.

Nutrition, Less Than Body Requirement

A state in which an individual experiences an inability to ingest, digest, and/or absorb nutrients in quantities sufficient to fulfill nutritional requirements.

Sharon Willadsen, R.N., B.S.N.
Marilyn Frenn, R.N., Ph.D.

DEFINING CHARACTERISTICS

Body weight 20% or more under ideal for height and frame
Caloric intake (observed or reported) less than minimum daily requirement for current metabolic need
Decreased serum albumin
Decreased serum transferrin or iron-binding capacity
Decreased total protein
Decreased triceps skinfold or midarm circumference, less than 90% of the reference standard
Electrolyte imbalance
Lack of interest in food
Loss of weight with adequate food intake
Poor skin turgor
Recent, unintentional weight loss of 20% or more of usual adult weight
Satiety immediately after ingesting food
Weakness with loss of mobility

CONTRIBUTING FACTORS

Pathophysiological

Alteration in smell
Alteration in taste
Chronic production of sputum
Decreased appetite

Decreased mental status
Decreased salivation
Diarrhea
Dysphagia

357

Dyspnea
Fatigue
Inability to use the muscles needed
      for mastication
Increased metabolic rate
Malabsorption of nutrients
Mechanical obstruction

Muscle weakness and/or paralysis
Nausea and/or vomiting
Pain
Self-care deficit
Stomatitis, glossitis
Surgical interventions

Psychosociobehavioral

Aversion to food
Cultural food preferences
Depressed state
Inability to prepare foods
Inability to procure foods (related to
      physical or financial reasons)

Lack of knowledge regarding nutritional
      needs
Loneliness
Perceived inability to ingest food
Self-induced malnutrition
Stress

EXPECTED OUTCOMES

Client will gain 0.5–1.0 lb/wk until ideal weight is achieved.
    Total caloric intake is increased, preferably by the oral route; second choice, enteral; and
        third choice, parenteral.
    Serum albumin levels are maintained within normal limits.
    Decreased or eradicated nausea, vomiting, diarrhea, and/or stomatitis are experienced.
Client and/or significant other(s) will verbalize a knowledge of nutritional needs.
    An achievable and realistic personal nutritional improvement plan is designed and
        implemented.

INTERVENTIONS

RATIONALE

Universal	
Perform a comprehensive nutritional assessment. This assessment needs to include such things as eating habits and personal preferences.	Formulating a plan that meets the nutritional requirements and is acceptable to the client is based on an accurate collection of information.
Monitor skin turgor and mucous membranes.	Inadequate food/fluid intake causes dehydration. Adequate food/fluid intake increases moistness of oral mucosa, enhances taste, and facilitates swallowing. Fluids also increase excretion of chemotherapeutic agents, thereby decreasing the cause of nausea and vomiting.

INTERVENTIONS	RATIONALE
Help to maintain a food record (food diary).	Objective data can be obtained regarding the types and amounts of food consumed.
Monitor weight daily.	A careful assessment of weight is provided and the effectiveness of interventions used to meet nutritional requirements can be determined.
Monitor bowel function.	Constipation can cause feeling of abdominal fullness, thus decreasing appetite.
Monitor for stomatitis.	Mouth sores decrease the ability and desire to eat.
Specify foods to be eliminated from diet (e.g., very hot or icy cold foods; spicy, acidic, or coarsely textured foods).	Refraining from ingesting these foods minimizes irritation to the oral mucosa. Medications and irradiation can also alter taste sensations.
Use Xylocaine 2% Viscous Solution to anesthetize oral mucosa.	Oral anesthetizing agents decrease pain of mouth sores and improve tolerance of foods.
Provide sufficient fluids with meals.	Decreased salivation makes ingestion of certain foods difficult.
Provide comfort measures such as positioning, analgesics, and/or oxygen.	Pain and/or shortness of breath decrease appetite and ability to eat.
Change consistency of diet to meet needs.	Soft or pureed foods can aid in swallowing and ingesting of food.
Provide alcoholic beverage with meals.	Alcohol can stimulate gastric juices and increase appetite.
Provide small, frequent meals and limit fluids at mealtime.	Large meals three times a day increase a sense of fullness. Smaller meals and less fluid volume at meals facilitate gastric emptying and improve appetite. The small meals are also less overwhelming psychologically.

Interventions	Rationale
Offer high-calorie, low-volume supplements between meals.	Additional caloric intake allows for ingestion of foods in small volumes with high nutrient density.
Encourage periods of exercise, as tolerated.	Exercise acts as an appetite stimulant and aids in digestion.
Compliment for eating well.	Positive feedback reinforces good eating habits.
Elevate head of bed or have client sitting during meals and for one hour after completion of meals.	Proper positioning prevents epigastric discomfort and minimizes potential for aspiration of food.
Offer antiemetics one hour before meals.	Antiemetics suppress the vomiting center in the medulla.
Suggest alternate measures to reduce nausea.	Chewing gum, hard candy, and dry, salty foods such as popcorn or crackers, may aid in controlling nausea and prevent development of an aversion to food.
Provide for rest periods before meals and during meals maintain a quiet, unhurried environment.	Energy is conserved to minimize fatigue at meals.
Assist with eating as needed.	Assistance with eating when physically unable to feed self assures adequate nutritional intake.
Utilize relaxation techniques.	Stress that is reduced or relieved can result in an improved appetite.
Provide adaptive or assistive devices.	Necessary equipment such as plate guards, special utensils, or splints provide independence with meals.
Instruct client and/or significant other(s) in specific nutritional needs, including restrictions.	Education is essential for understanding of specific needs and for follow-through with the nutritional program.

INTERVENTIONS

RATIONALE

Initiate enteral tube feedings as ordered. Include the following:

1. Check for hypoalbuminemia

Hypoalbuminemia is associated with a decrease in colloid osmotic pressure and results in significant intestinal mucosal edema, which impairs intestinal absorption of the enteral feeding and diminishes its effectiveness. Replace-ment of albumin is recommended before enteral feeding is initiated.

2. Insert enteral feeding tube as ordered

The insertion of a patent tube into the stomach provides an alternate route for nutritional support.

3. Administer feedings at room temperature

Abdominal cramping that is associated with tube feeding administration is reduced by careful attention to the temperature of the feeding.

4. Elevate head of bed at least 35°– 40° during tube feeding and for one hour after completion of intermittent tube feedings

Aspiration of the tube feeding is minimized by correct positioning.

5. Check osmolality of medications with dietitian before administration via feeding tube

Medications with osmolalities greater than 700 m0sm/kg can cause diarrhea when given concomitantly with the tube feeding solution. Some examples are: Cimetidine, 4035 m0sm/kg; Sulfamethoxazole-Trimethoprim (Bactrim) Suspension, 4560 m0sm/kg; and Potassium Chloride (KCl) Elixir, 3000 m0sm/kg.

6. Change enteral feeding bag and tubing every 24 hours and rinse with tap water every six hours or following each intermittent feeding

These procedures prevent bacterial contamination of the tube feeding solutions.

7. Monitor intake and output, skin turgor, and stool consistency

Sufficient fluid intake is insured for hydration and fluid overload is prevented.

Interventions

Rationale

Interventions	Rationale
8. Check for tube placement and monitor for gastric residuals every four hours with continuous feeding and before initiation of intermittent feedings. If gastric return is greater than 100 cc, hold feeding for one hour and repeat aspiration before continuing feeding	These precautions prevent aspiration of the tube feeding.
9. Monitor complete blood counts, electrolytes, albumin levels, blood glucose levels, and urea nitrogen	These laboratory studies help determine the effectiveness of the tube feeding regime and also monitor for complications that can occur as a result of this regime.
10. Monitor tube insertion site	Frequent inspection of the site and daily care can assist in the prevention of redness and skin breakdown to the pressure areas.

Initiate total parenteral nutrition as ordered.
Include the following:

Interventions	Rationale
1. Administer all parenteral solutions via IV pump	IV pumps offer the advantage of closely monitoring parenteral solution rate. If parenteral nutrition is given too rapidly, hypermolar diuresis occurs and excess sugar is excreted leading to intractable seizures. If the solution is run too slowly, inadequate nutritional intake is the result.
2. Change dressings every 48 hours using aseptic technique	This allows for close inspection of the insertion site and assists in the prevention of bacterial growth at the site.
3. Change administration tubing and filter daily	This procedure prevents the risk of bacterial contamination to the parenteral solution.
4. Monitor vital signs every four hours	Vital sign changes can signify complications of parenteral administration. Especially note temperature rise, which could signify possible septicemia.
5. Monitor intake and output	Sufficient fluid intake is insured and fluid overload is prevented.

INTERVENTIONS	**RATIONALE**
Inpatient	
Institute a calorie count.	Objective data are obtained on actual caloric intake.
Monitor intake and output.	Adequate fluid intake is insured without the complications of fluid overload.
Monitor results of laboratory studies (serum albumin, total protein, serum transferrin, total lymph, urinary protein, glucose, acetone, 24-hour urinary creatinine, nitrogen, and electrolytes).	Metabolic activity and immune function are carefully assessed through these laboratory studies.
Provide oral care 30 min before meals and frequently between meals.	These activities eliminate foul taste, moisten mucous membranes, and increase taste for food. They also prevent or promote healing of mouth sores.
Open all food containers from food tray and release odors outside the room.	Noxious stimuli caused by the immediate release of combination of odors at the bedside are reduced.
Encourage family to bring foods from home.	Familiar foods may be more appealing to the client.
Provide an optimal mealtime environment (such as a sunroom, lounge, or communal dining area).	A pleasant atmosphere has a positive influence on appetite.
Encourage family and/or friends to visit during meals.	The socialization of being with others while eating is important to many people.
Supervise or assist with menu selection.	Feedback is obtained on awareness of nutritional requirements and specific likes and dislikes and provides opportunity for reinforcement of good eating habits.

INTERVENTIONS	RATIONALE
Initiate referrals as needed (e.g., dietary, occupational and speech therapy, social services, home care).	Appropriate referrals can assist with specific needs and concerns.
Community Health/ Home Care Evaluate the availability of space for food preparation, availability of refrigerator and other kitchen equipment for food preparation, and the presence of a significant other to assist with food preparation.	Assessment of living conditions is obtained and needs determined.
Assess diet of client and/or significant other(s) to determine if basic nutritional needs are met.	Some diet regimens, such as vegetarian diets, lack the proper nutrients to maintain normal body weight. If client fatigues easily, have significant other(s) prepare foods. If client lives alone and is ill, foods should be prepared in advance on days when client is feeling better.
Eat in a positive atmosphere—a favorite table or with family and friends when possible.	A pleasant atmosphere has a positive influence on appetite.
Minimize noxious odors by using foods that need minimal cooking time and have client away from cooking area during preparation.	Noxious odors can give rise to feelings of nausea or aversion to foods.
Make use of kitchen appliances such as blenders, microwaves, and food processors.	Convenience appliances aid in food preparation by decreasing the amount of energy and time spent to prepare foods.
Initiate appropriate referrals for assistive resources as needed (e.g., Meals on Wheels, Food Stamp Program, nutritionist, dentist, occupational therapist, and/or support groups).	Appropriate referrals for assistive resources can assist with specific home care needs and concerns.

REFERENCES/BIBLIOGRAPHY

Bloch, A.S. (1990). **Nutrition management of the cancer patient.** Rockville, MD: Aspen.

* Brinson, R.R., & Kolts, B.E. (1987). Hypoalbuminemia of diarrheal incidence in critically ill patients. **Critical Care Medicine, 15**(5), 506–509.

* Flynn, K.T., Norton, L.C., & Fisher, R.L. (1987). Enteral tube feeding: Indications, practices, and outcomes. **Image: Journal of Nursing Scholarship, 19**(1), 16–19.

Gettrust, K.V., Ryan, S.C., & Schmidt-Engelman, D.S. (1985). **Applied nursing diagnosis: Guides for comprehensive care planning.** Albany, NY: Delmar.

Hermann-Zaidins, M., & Touger-Decker, R. (1989). **Nutrition support in home health.** Rockville, MD: Aspen.

* Niemiec, P., Vanderveen, T., Morrison, J., & Hohenwarter, M. (1983). Gastrointestinal disorders caused by medication and electrolyte solution osmolality during enteral nutrition. **Journal of Parenteral and Enteral Nutrition, 7**(4), 387–389.

The authors wish to acknowledge the consultation of:

Joan Harkulich, R.N., M.S.N.
Director of Research and Professional Services

Barbara Troy, M.S., R.D.
Adjunct Assistant Professor, Marquette University
Milwaukee, WI

Nutrition, Less Than Body Requirement: Risk

A state in which conditions exist that predispose an individual to less intake of nutrients than is required for health.

Marilyn Frenn, R.N., Ph.D.
Sharon Willadsen, R.N., B.S.N.

RISK FACTORS

Pathophysiological

Acute illness

1. Moderate risk (e.g., infection, bleeding, renal impairment)
2. Severe risk (e.g., head injury, major burns, multiple trauma, severe sepsis)

Chronic health problems (e.g., absorptive disorders, anorexia, chemical dependency, confusion, dental caries or periodontal disease, depression)

Dysphagia

Hypermetabolic/catabolic states

Inability to eat for several days prior to admission for acute illness or surgery

Medications that interfere with appetite or eating

Nausea and vomiting

Nothing by mouth (NPO) status supplemented only with low caloric intravenous solutions (e.g., 5% Dextrose in water) for more than three to four days

Responses to illness or disability (e.g., diarrhea, drowsiness, incontinence, pain, reduced ability to smell or taste, requires assistance to eat)

Serum albumin

1. 3.0%–3.4%/g indicates mild visceral protein depletion
2. 2.1%–2.9%/g indicates moderate depletion
3. 2.0% g or less indicates severe depletion

Total lymphocyte count

1. Less than 1500 cells/cu mm indicates risk
2. Less than 900 cells/cu mm indicates severe depletion

Weight loss

1. 10%, no major problems if at ideal weight (Problematic if greater than 5% lost in last month or 10% lost in last six months)
2. 10%–20%, moderate risk
3. Greater than 20%, severe risk
4. Greater than 30%, death due to cardiac malnutrition

Psychosociobehavioral

Food fadism
Inability to procure appropriate foods (e.g., emotional distress, home bound, inadequate income)
Lack of knowledge regarding nutritional needs
Lack of time to prepare nutritious foods
Social isolation
Starvation
Stress

(Additional risks for less vitamins or minerals than Recommended Dietary Allowance [RDA])
Does not eat raw fruits and vegetables (folacin, vitamins A and C)
Low carbohydrate diet (B vitamins, carbohydrates)
Poverty (vitamins)
Over age 65 (protein, calcium, iron, Vitamins A, C, B_1, B_6, and B_{12})
Overuse of alcohol (B vitamins, protein)

EXPECTED OUTCOMES

Client's nutritional intake will be appropriate to body requirements.
Risks for nutritional depletion are identified.
Preventive measures are taken before actual nutritional depletion or other sequelae develop (e.g., impaired healing, impaired weaning from ventilator).

INTERVENTIONS

RATIONALE

INTERVENTIONS	RATIONALE
Universal	
Complete nutritional assessment including:	Early identification of risk can result in more effective treatment, prevention of other health problems, enhanced performance, and enhanced recovery from illness.
1. Anthropometric measurements (skinfold thickness, arm circumference, weight)	
2. Consumption of: calories sufficient to maintain weight	

necessary nutrients relatively more complex carbohydrates, such as whole grain, fruits and vegetables, rather than simple sugars relatively more fish, poultry, and legumes and less red meats relatively more nutrient-rich foods as compared with empty calories. 3. Finances available/used for food 4. Food likes/dislikes 5. General knowledge of nutrition and what constitutes a balanced diet 6. One- to two-day diet history including foods from all four food groups 7. Patterns of eating including three meals per day 8. Persons eating with client 9. Presence of other risk factors for nutritional depletion (e.g., illness) 10. Present and usual weight, patterns of weight loss	
Provide, in collaboration with other disciplines, individual and group health education, prepare and distribute information regarding nutrients necessary for health, risk factors for nutritional depletion, and community resources for subsidized or delivered meal programs.	Maintenance of nutrition can prevent other health problems.
Dietary consult for those at high risk.	Collaboration is essential for quality health care.

INTERVENTIONS	**RATIONALE**
Inpatient	
Include thorough nutritional assessment with each admission (also see "Nutrition, Less Than Body Requirement").	The combination of prior risk factors and stress of illness increases likelihood of nutritional depletion.
Institute calorie count in collaboration with dietitian for those at high risk.	Calorie counts are helpful in identifying problems in consumption.
Review serum albumin, transferrion, and thyroxine-binding proalbumin levels at regular intervals for those at high risk.	Serum albumin levels decline slowly (half-life of 20 days), so levels need to be reviewed frequently. Transferrion and proalbumin are more sensitive indicators of malnutrition.
Community/ Home Health	
Initiate screening and referral for those at high risk.	Screening enables services to be targeted to those in greatest need.

REFERENCES/BIBLIOGRAPHY

Bistran, B. (1988). Nutritional support of the long-term care patient, part II: Nutritional assessment of the elderly. **Nutritional support services, 8**(10), 17–21.

Champagne, M.T., & Ashley, M.L. (1989). Nutritional support in the critically ill elderly patient. **Critical Care Nursing Quarterly, 12**(1), 15–25.

Gettrust K.V., Ryan, S.C., & Engelman, D.S. (Eds.). (1985). **Applied nursing diagnosis**. Albany, NY: Delmar.

Green, M.L., & Harry, J. (1987). **Nutrition in contemporary nursing practice**. New York: Wiley.

* Murphy, L.C. (1989). Establishing and clarifying the etiologies and characteristics of the nursing diagnosis alteration in nutrition: Less than body requirements. In M. Carroll-Johnson (Ed.). **Classification of nursing diagnoses: Proceedings of the eighth conference** (pp. 341–344). Philadelphia: Lippincott.

* Stotts, N.A, & Whitney, J.D. (1990). Nutritional intake and status of clients in the home with open surgical wounds. **Journal of Community Health Nursing, 7**(2), 77–86.

Tramposch, T.S., & Blue, L.S. (1987). A nutrition screening and assessment system for use with the elderly in extended care. **Journal of the American Dietetic Association, 87**, 1207–1210.

The authors wish to thank Barbara Troy, M.S., R.D., Adjunct Assistant Professor, Marquette University College of Nursing, for her consultation regarding this care planning guide.

Nutrition, More Than Body Requirement

A state in which an individual is
experiencing an intake of nutrients
which exceeds metabolic needs
(NANDA, 1990, p. 10).

Marilyn Frenn, R.N., Ph.D.

DEFINING CHARACTERISTICS

Diet history (one to two day)
Expressed concerns regarding nutrition or body weight
Regular intake of nutrients in excess of body needs, (e.g., alcohol, caffeine, calories, cholesterol,
        fat, salt)
Triceps skinfold greater than 15 mm in men, 25 mm in women
Weight 10% over ideal for height and frame = overweight
Weight 20% over ideal for height and frame = obese
Body mass index (BMI = wt in kg/ht. in m^2)
        BMI 25–29.9 = Grade 1 obesity
        BMI 30–40 = Grade 2 obesity
        BMI >40 = Grade 3 obesity

CONTRIBUTING FACTORS

Pathophysiological

Diseases that predispose to weight gain (e.g., Type II diabetes mellitus, Cushing's syndrome,
        thyroid deficiency)
Obesity in one (40% risk) or both (80% risk) parents

Psychosociobehavioral

Behavioral control deficiency
Dependence on prepared or fast foods
Depression

Dysfunctional eating patterns (contextual awareness deficiency)

1. Eating in response to external cues such as time of day, social situation
2. Eating in response to internal cues other than hunger, such as anxiety
3. Use of food as reward or comfort measure

Information deficiency
Less education for women, more education for men
Low income for women, high income for men
Sedentary life-style

Expected Outcomes

Client will maintain weight at satisfactory level for height, frame, and genetic predisposition.
    Nutritional requirements are accurately identified.
    Nutritional intake is appropriate to body energy requirements and expenditures.
    One to two pounds per week are lost until a level appropriate to height and frame is achieved.
Client will demonstrate behaviors to balance intake with energy expenditure.
    Behaviors that contribute to excess intake of nutrients are monitored.
    Responsibility for eating and exercise patterns is acknowledged.
    Contract for behavioral changes is realistic, measurable, and includes rewards for accomplishments.

Interventions

Rationale

Universal

Interventions	Rationale
Assess overall health history, physical examination laboratory data (thyroid function, electrolytes, hematocrit, electrocardiogram if positive cardiac history), weight history since birth, weight of family members and those in household, previous attempts at diet maintenance, one-to two-day current diet history (including likes, dislikes, timing and frequency of meals and snacks, pattern of eating out), feelings about being overweight, pattern of exercise, goals, and mood state.	Comprehensive assessment is necessary to enable accurate planning.

INTERVENTIONS	**RATIONALE**
Assess congruence of actual with perceived body weight to height adequacy.	Perceptions of ideal weight may differ from weight to height ratios recommended for health.
Assess attitudes and motivation for change, as well as level of social support.	Effective life-style changes require integration of personal, behavioral, and social factors (also see "Health Seeking Behaviors—[Specify]").
Evaluate need for and interest in information regarding basic nutrition (e.g., four food groups, balanced meals, food preparation, heart-healthy eating, risk factors for obesity).	Education provided at a time of readiness may prevent reliance on fad diets and allow incorporation of accurate, up-to-date information in establishing a healthy diet.
Assist in choosing a weight control program that provides balanced nutrition and a plan for maintenance.	People lose weight safely and most effectively in programs that specialize in weight loss while providing adequate nutrition.
Provide information about community resources for safe, effective weight loss and dietary referrals as needed.	Those who view themselves as overweight are at risk for weight loss scams and unhealthy degrees of weight loss.
Provide information about ways to avoid empty calorie foods, healthy convenience foods, and restaurants serving heart-healthy menus.	Major barriers to effective weight loss are found in societal patterns of eating and ready availability of less nutritious foods.
Develop group health advocacy programs fostering healthy eating patterns as well as respect for genetic predispositions that may prevent some individuals from achieving societally valued degrees of slimness.	An informed group of clients may support each other and foster improvement in societal patterns of eating.
Teach proper administration and side effects of anorectic drugs (prescription and over-the-counter).	Certain drugs have been effective in promoting weight loss but have important side effects.

INTERVENTIONS	**R**ATIONALE
Inpatient	
Follow specific protocols associated with clinical trials for gastric balloon placement.	Gastric balloons are recommended for use only in clinical trials.
Assist clients who have elected gastroplasty as a treatment for morbid obesity (more than 100 lb. excess weight or refractory to other methods) with pre- and post-operative recovery according to American Society for Clinical Nutrition (1985) guidelines.	Although gastroplasty has not been shown to reduce mortality associated with obesity, it results in longer term weight loss than other methods.
Assist in maintaining exercise program while hospitalized and in monitoring potential side effects of very low calorie diet.	Very low calorie diets may be effective, but require supervision due to possible severe physical and psychological sequelae. Exercise helps to prevent muscle wasting by preserving basal metabolic rate.
Community Health/ Home Care	
Conduct behavioral assessment including motivational analysis, problem identification and clarification, assets and limitations of a behavioral program, environmental supports and restrictions, and presence of psychopathology related to the obesity that may require referral.	In addition to a nutritional assessment, an information base is needed regarding use of behavioral strategies.
Assist with behavioral strategies for weight loss including self-monitoring, stimulus control, contracting, shaping, and positive reinforcement.	Behavioral strategies are most effective when combined with a calorie-reduction diet and exercise.

INTERVENTIONS	RATIONALE
Collaborate with dietitian in calculating optimal weight, assessing calorie needs, and planning balanced reduction diet (500c/da less than prior intake usually results in 1-2 lb per week loss).	Reasonable goals promote weight loss that is physically and psychologically feasible.
Assist to gradually begin exercise program (20 min 3-4 times/wk) unless medically contraindicated.	Regular exercise alone may lead to weight loss in mild obesity. Exercise also promotes maintenance of weight loss by helping to sustain basal metabolic rate.
Maintain patient, flexible, non-judgmental, positive approach.	Losing weight often is frustrating and rapport is important to success.
Develop maintenance program including exercise, support groups, financial contracts, increased number of sessions, and interpersonal problem solving.	Obesity is a chronic health problem. Maintenance programs with these characteristics have been most effective in keeping off excess weight.

REFERENCES/BIBLIOGRAPHY

American Society for Clinical Nutrition Task Force (1985). Guidelines for surgery for morbid obesity. **American Journal of Clinical Nutrition, 42**, 904–905.

Chalmers, K. (1985). Lifestyle counseling: The need for diagnostic clarity. **Journal of Advanced Nursing, 10**, 311–313.

Corrigan, S.A., Raczynski, J.M., Swencionis, C., & Jennings, S.G. (1991). Weight reduction in the prevention and treatment of hypertension: A review of representative clinical trials. **American Journal of Health Promotion, 5**(3), 208–214.

Fine, G. (1987). International conference on obesity. **Nursing** (Oxford), **3**, 616–618.

Frankl, R.T., & Yang, M-U. (Eds.). (1988). **Obesity and weight control**. Rockville, MD: Aspen.

North American Nursing Diagnosis Association. (1990). **Taxonomy I** (Rev. 1990). St. Louis: NANDA.

* Phaosawaske, K., Rice, P., & Wheeler, J. (1988). Obesity: A comparison between the Garren-Edwards gastric bubble and a diet/medication program. **Society of Gastrointestinal Assistants' Journal** (Summer), 14–17.

Rosenblatt, E. (1989). Weight loss counseling in primary care. **Journal of the American Academy of Nurse Practitioners, 1**(4), 112–118.

White, J.H. (1986). Behavioral intervention for the obese client. **Nurse Practitioner, 11**, 27–31.

Nutrition, More Than Body Requirement: Risk

A state in which an individual is at risk of experiencing an intake of nutrients which exceeds metabolic needs (NANDA, 1990, p. 12).

Marilyn Frenn, R.N., Ph.D.

. . . .

RISK FACTORS

Pathophysiological

Diseases that predispose to weight gain (e.g., Type II diabetes mellitus, Cushing's syndrome, thyroid deficiency)
Obesity in one (40% risk) or both (80% risk) parents

Psychosociobehavioral

Dependence on prepared or fast foods
Depression
Dysfunctional eating patterns

1. Eating in response to external cues such as time of day, social situation
2. Eating in response to internal cues other than hunger, such as anxiety
3. Use of food as reward or comfort measure

Less education for women, more education for men
Low income for women, high income for men
Regular intake of nutrients in excess of body needs, e.g.,
    alcohol
    caffeine
    fat and cholesterol
    salt
    relatively more simple sugars than complex carbohydrates, such as whole grain, fruits
        and vegetables
    relatively more red meats and less fish, poultry, and legumes
    relatively more foods with empty calories as compared with nutrient rich foods
Sedentary life-style

EXPECTED OUTCOMES

Client will maintain weight at satisfactory level for height, frame, and genetic predisposition.
    Nutritional requirements are accurately identified.
    Nutritional intake is appropriate to body energy requirements and expenditures.
Client will demonstrate behaviors to reduce risk factors.
    Own risk factors for obesity and excess intake of nutrients are identified.
    Responsibility for eating patterns is acknowledged.
    Plan is identified for balancing intake with exercise to maintain optimal weight for height.

INTERVENTIONS	RATIONALE
Universal	
Assess risk factors and congruence of actual with perceived body weight to height adequacy.	Perceptions of ideal weight may differ from weight to height ratios recommended for health.
Assess attitudes and motivation for change, as well as level of social support.	Effective life-style changes require integration of personal, behavioral, and social factors (also see "Health seeking Behaviors—[Specify]").
Evaluate need for and interest in information regarding basic nutrition (e.g. four food groups, balanced meals, food preparation, heart-healthy eating, risk factors for obesity).	Education provided at a time of readiness may prevent reliance on fad diets and allow incorporation of accurate, up-to-date information in establishing a healthy diet.
Assist in choosing a weight control program that provides balanced nutrition and a plan for maintenance.	People lose weight safely and most effectively in programs that specialize in weight loss while providing adequate nutrition.
Provide information about community resources for safe, effective weight loss and dietary referrals as needed.	Those who view themselves as overweight are at risk for weight loss scams and unhealthy degrees of weight loss.
Provide information about ways to avoid empty calorie foods, healthy convenience foods, and restaurants serving heart-healthy menus.	Major barriers to effective weight loss are found in societal patterns of eating and ready availability of less nutritious foods.

INTERVENTIONS	**R**ATIONALE
Develop group health advocacy programs fostering healthy eating patterns as well as respect for genetic predispositions that may prevent some individuals from achieving societally valued degrees of slimness.	An informed group of clients may support each other and foster improvement in societal patterns of eating.
Inpatient None	
Community Health/ Home Care None	

REFERENCES/BIBLIOGRAPHY

Frankl, R.T., & Yang, M-U. (Eds.). (1988). **Obesity and weight control**. Rockville, MD: Aspen.

Gettrust, K.V., Ryan, S.C., & Engelman, D.S. (1985). **Applied nursing diagnosis: Guides for comprehensive care planning**. Albany, NY: Delmar.

Hytten, F. (1990). Is it important or even useful to measure weight gain in pregnancy? **Midwifery, 6**, 28–32.

* Laffery, S.C. (1986). Normal and overweight adults: Perceived weight and health behavior characteristics. **Nursing Research, 35**(3), 173–175.

North American Nursing Diagnosis Association. (1990). **Taxonomy I** (Rev. 1990). St. Louis: NANDA.

Rosenblatt, E. (1989). Weight loss counseling in primary care. **Journal of the American Academy of Nurse Practitioners, 1**(4), 112–118.

* Stunkard, A.J., Sorenson T.I.A., & Harris, C. (1986). An adoption study of human obesity. **New England Journal of Medicine, 314**, 193–198.

Wright, E.J., & Whitehead, T.L. (1987). Perceptions of body size and obesity: A selected review of the literature. **Journal of Community Health, 12**, 117–129.

Wylie-Rosett, J., Wassertheil-Smoller, S., & Elmer, P. (1990). Assessing dietary intake for patient education planning and evaluation. **Patient Education and Counseling, 15**, 217–227.

Oral Mucous Membrane, Impaired

A state in which an individual experiences a change in the structure and function of the oral mucosa.

Joan Randall, R.N., M.S.

DEFINING CHARACTERISTICS

Atrophy of gums
Coated tongue
Debris desquamation
Dry lips
Dry mouth (xerostomia)
Dry tongue
Edematous mucosa
Halitosis
Hemorrhagic gingivitis
Hyperemia
Leukoplakia
Oral lesions or ulcers
Oral pain/discomfort

Oral plaque
Pain with talking
Reddened mucosa
Reddened tongue
Shiny mucosa
Stomatitis
Swollen buccal glands
Swollen parotid glands
Swollen sublingual glands
Swollen submaxillary glands
Swollen tongue
Thick oral secretions

CONTRIBUTING FACTORS

Pathophysiological

Allergies
Decreased or lack of salivation
Dehydration
Dental caries
Immunosuppression
Infection
Malnutrition

Medication
Mouth Breathing
Trauma—   chemical—   acidic foods
                        alcohol
                        chemotherapy
                        drug therapy
                        noxious agents, e.g., mouthwashes
                        tobacco
            mechanical— braces
                        ill-fitting dentures
                        nasal oxygen
                        radiation therapy (head/neck area)
                        surgical reconstruction or correction
                        tubes (endotracheal/nasogastric)
Vitamin Deficiency

Psychosociobehavioral

Poor oral hygiene

EXPECTED OUTCOMES

Client will have intact oral mucosa.
    Risk factors are described that contribute to altered oral mucosa.
    Measures are participated in which reduce risk factors.
    Importance of oral care is verbalized.
    Oral mucosa is examined daily.
    Dental evaluation is sought at least every six months.
    Oral hygiene regimen is followed daily.
    Oral comfort is verbalized.

INTERVENTIONS	RATIONALE
Universal Assess oral cavity.	Oral assessment of lips, tongue, mucous membranes, gingiva, teeth, dentures, saliva, swallow, odor, voice, taste, and symptoms reported will allow close monitoring of alterations and determine effectiveness of oral care protocols.
Assess current oral care practices.	Use of abrasive toothpastes and hard bristle brushes traumatize the mucosa. Commercial mouthwashes may cause irritation and hypersensitivity stomatitis related to contents, e.g., alcohol, astringents, saccharine for sweetening, dyes.

INTERVENTIONS	RATIONALE
Assess dietary intake pattern.	Lack of nutrients can be a precipitating factor or contribute to delayed healing. Inadequate fluid intake will result in dry mucosa. Foods high in acid content will irritate the mucosa.
Identify substances that irritate oral mucosa.	Use of substances such as tobacco or alcohol will irritate mucosa. Medications such as chemotherapeutic agents may induce stomatitis.
Assess fit of dentures.	Improperly fitted dentures will contribute to irritation of oral mucosa.
Assess for oral lesions.	Cultures of lesions are helpful in indicating if antibiotic mouthwashes are needed.
Initiate oral care.	Frequency of mouth care must be determined individually. Factors such as mouth breathing, intermittent oral suctioning, continuous oxygen inhalation, no oral intake, presence of oral mucosa irritation or lesions require more frequent oral care protocol administration.
Brush teeth with soft bristled toothbrush.	Brushing action helps to loosen debris and plaque.
Floss teeth with unwaxed dental floss.	Flossing helps remove food particles and debris.
Clean dentures and bridge(s).	Removing dentures and cleaning them helps to remove food particles and debris that can be trapped under them.
Rinse mouth with mouthwash.	Use of mouthwash acts to wash away loose debris as well as moisten and soften oral mucosa.
Apply lubricating emollients to lips.	Application of emollient helps to keep lips soft, moist, and intact.
Instruct in proper daily oral care.	Routine oral care will prevent complications and reduce development of dental caries.

INTERVENTIONS	RATIONALE
Instruct in adequate nutrition and hydration.	Oral fluid intake keeps mucous membranes moist. A well-balanced diet helps keep mucosa healthy and intact.
Teach mouth care protocols to be used when oral lesions are present. 1. Remove dentures or other appliances if present Brush teeth gently using soft bristled toothbrush and toothpaste. Brush in a horizontal (back and forth) motion reaching all surface areas of teeth. Rinse mouth with one-half cup of hydrogen peroxide and one-half cup of lukewarm tap water. Swish the mixture around mouth for at least one minute or as long as can be tolerated. 2. Remove dentures or other appliances if present Brush teeth gently using soft bristled toothbrush and toothpaste. Brush in a horizontal (back and forth) motion reaching all surface areas of teeth. Rinse mouth with one-half teaspoon of sodium bicarbonate to one pint of lukewarm tap water. Swish the mixture around mouth for at least one minute or as long as can be tolerated.	Hydrogen peroxide is a foaming agent that removes debris and mucus from the teeth through enzymatic action that destroys bacteria; it has a deodorant effect as it oxidizes odorous gases. Sodium bicarbonate has buffering capacity, provides soothing comfort and symptomatic relief, as well as dissolving mucin, loosening debris and cleaning the mouth.
Provide ice chips or sips of water.	Water or ice chips help prevent drying and promote comfort.

INTERVENTIONS	RATIONALE
Teach daily inspection of oral mucosa.	Close monitoring of oral mucosa will alert client to changes of mucosa or allow evaluation of effectiveness of treatment and provide direction to other appropriate treatment options.
Instruct in cause of alteration of oral mucous membrane.	Better cooperation and compliance will be achieved with adequate knowledge base of cause and effect of alterations. The practice of preventative care and promotion of self-care may be better achieved.
Inpatient Initiate oral care.	Mouth complications can be avoided by scheduling oral hygiene around the clock for the acutely ill.
Obtain order for topical oral antibiotics.	Mycostatin, Nystatin, and Mycelex Troche (clotrimazole) are antifungal antibiotics used for candida and mouth ulcers, often providing symptomatic relief.
Obtain order and administer local anesthetic before meals and as needed (e.g., Xylocaine Viscous Solution).	Local anesthetics swished, swallowed, or expectorated create a numbness in the mouth that will minimize discomfort when eating or swallowing. Food should not be served too hot; avoid acidic, spicy foods.
Obtain order for pain-relieving mouthwash (e.g., Diphenhydramine Elixir plus Maalox or Kaopectate).	Maalox or Kaopectate coat the oral mucosa and Diphenhydramine acts as a local anesthetic. Local application soothes the painful oral mucosa.
Provide with artificial saliva.	Artificial saliva is used with persons with xerostomia and is helpful in keeping oral mucosa moist.
Move endotracheal tube or other mechanical obstruction every day.	Moving tubes/obstructions will minimize trauma and ensure proper cleaning.
Teach to avoid commercial mouthwashes and lemon glycerin swabs.	Lemon-glycerin swabs and commercial mouth washes contain alcohol, which has a drying effect on the mucous membranes.

INTERVENTIONS

RATIONALE

Community Health/ Home Care	
Assess preventative dental practices.	Regular dental consults help identify potential problems and promote comfort.
Instruct in use of assisting devices in performing oral care (e.g., toothettes, irrigating devices).	When brushing is not possible, removal of debris and plaque must be accomplished by other means. Instruction in use of assisting devices helps maintain self-care and promotes independence and compliance.

REFERENCES/BIBLIOGRAPHY

* Dudjack, L.A. (1987). Mouth care for mucositis due to radiation therapy. **Cancer Nursing, 10**(3), 131–140.
* Eilers, J., Berger, A.M., & Petersen, M.C. (1988). Development, testing, and application of the oral assessment guide. **Oncology Nursing Forum, 15**(3), 325–330.
  Gettrust, K.V., Ryan, S.C., & Engelman, D.S. (1985). **Applied nursing diagnosis: Guides for comprehensive care planning**. Albany, NY: Delmar.
  Ziegfeld, C.R. (1987). **Core curriculum for oncology nursing**. Philadelphia: Saunders.

Pain, Acute

A state in which an individual experiences and reports the presence of acute and severe discomfort or an uncomfortable sensation (NANDA, 1990, p. 98).

Judith K. Sands, R.N., Ed.D.

DEFINING CHARACTERISTICS

Agitation and restlessness
Alteration in muscle tone anywhere from listlessness to rigidity
Autonomic responses not seen in chronic, stable pain (diaphoreses, blood pressure and pulse
          rate changes, pupillary dilation, increased or decreased respiratory rate)
Coded or verbal communication of pain descriptors
Distraction behavior (moaning, crying, pacing, seeking out other people/activities, restlessness)
Evidence of inflammation
Facial mask of pain (lackluster eyes, "beaten look," fixed or scattered movement, grimace)
Guarding behavior and splinting of pain site
Inability to concentrate
Irritability
Narrowed focus (altered time perception, withdrawal from social contact, impaired thought
          process)
Self-focusing

CONTRIBUTING FACTORS

Pathophysiological

Invasive diagnostic tests or procedures;
          surgery
Medications or chemicals
Muscle tension or spasm

Tissue hypoxia or inflammation
Tissue injury or trauma
Tissue or organ disease or dysfunction

Psychosociobehavioral

Anxiety and stress
Fatigue
Immobility or poor positioning
Lack of knowledge concerning pain
    control techniques

Personal and cultural responses to the
    phenomenon of pain
Prior experience with acute pain

EXPECTED OUTCOMES

Client will verbalize that pain is relieved or adequately controlled.
    The location and nature of the pain are successfully described.
    Factors that worsen or relieve the pain experience are identified.
    The appropriate use of medications and other pain relief measures are described.
    A feeling of control over the pain experience is related.

INTERVENTIONS	RATIONALE
Universal	
Conduct an accurate and complete ongoing assessment to include the location, duration and severity, and nature of the pain until it is successfully relieved.	Pain is essentially a subjective and changing experience. Intervention strategies are based on information acquired in the assessment.
Utilize established pain assessment tools and rating scales to facilitate accurate ongoing assessment.	Research attempts to define the pain experience have produced excellent tools for use at the bedside, e.g., numerical rating scales, visual analogs, lists of common pain descriptors. These tools profile the pain experience over time and are an excellent adjunct to assessment.
Assess for common nonverbal cues of pain including mood, activity, autonomic nervous system responses, cognitive and behavioral changes.	Visible cues of pain are strongly influenced by the pain tolerance and duration. These cues provide supportive evidence of the presence of pain, but they do **not have** to be present to validate the verbal report of pain. The appropriate planning of intervention in pain relief is dependent upon verbal as well as nonverbal cues, i.e., relaxation or distraction.
Assess for prior experience with acute pain: Usual reaction to pain Past alleviating comfort measures	The pain experience is unique to each client. Response to pain control intervention is influenced by prior experience with acute pain.

INTERVENTIONS	RATIONALE
Personal, religious, or cultural beliefs that influence pain experience Anxiety concerning the use of narcotics and fear of addiction	
Assess the effect of pain on life-style: ADL's, work, leisure, nutrition, sleep, and rest.	Acute pain may occur from a few seconds to as long as six months. The longer the duration of the pain experience the more likely it is that the pain will have a profound impact on all aspects of the life-style.
Assess for factors that decrease pain tolerance.	Pain tolerance is strongly influenced by a wide variety of personal and situational variables, e.g., fatigue, fear, lack of knowledge, and the need to convince care providers of the reality of pain.
Establish a trusting relationship which conveys acceptance of the reported pain experience.	An attitude of acceptance decreases anxiety, enhances the therapeutic relationship, and increases feelings of control, which ultimately affect the response to intervention.
Collaborate with the physician to develop the overall approach to pain management and to evaluate effectiveness.	Collaborative intervention provides the best plan of pain management. The nurse is in the best position to acquire the data necessary to plan pain management strategy and evaluate overall effectiveness with the client.
Collaborate with the client to determine pain management.	Collaboration increases compliance and decreases feelings of powerlessness.
Establish a comprehensive approach to pain which includes not only pharmacologic but also nonpharmacologic management strategies. Nonpharmacologic strategies include: 1. Encourage adequate sleep and rest	Pain is a complex sensory experience which is best managed by an integrated approach to include behavioral, cutaneous stimulation, and cognitive strategies as well as traditional analgesics. Fatigue decreases the ability to tolerate and positively cope with pain, because it leads to anxiety and increased muscle tension.

INTERVENTIONS	**R**ATIONALE
2. Utilize passive and active exercises as appropriate	Exercise increases circulation which promotes healing, prevents the development of joint and muscle deformities, and reduces the chance of constipation, which is a frequent side effect of analgesic use.
3. Maintain proper body alignment and encourage frequent position changes. Support dependent or injured body parts with pillows, slings, or splinting	General comfort measures increase the sense of well-being. The maintenance of good body alignment with support to dependent body parts and frequent position changes promotes circulation, provides comfort, enhances healing, prevents contractures, and decreases fatigue.
4. Utilize massage except where contraindicated	The use of massage causes vascular dilation, inhibits the transmission of pain impulses, and promotes relaxation. Massage is contraindicated when vascular problems such as phlebitis are suspected.
5. Apply dry or moist, warm or cold packs to the painful area	The application of heat or cold causes vascular dilation or constriction, which decreases swelling, promotes healing, and inhibits the transmission of pain impulses. The addition of moisture increases the skin contact, thereby adding to the therapeutic effect.
6. Apply contralateral stimulation	Contralateral stimulation is useful for phantom pain or cast discomfort and causes circulation and sensation to be diverted away from the pain.
7. Teach relaxation and distraction techniques, i.e., slow rhythmic breathing, visual concentration, listening to music, conversation, imagery	Relaxation and diversion promotes anxiety and muscle tension reduction, increases comfort, and diverts attention from pain by providing the central nervous system with competing sensory stimuli and blocking the pain perception. Ongoing evaluation of these techniques is essential, since response varies and can change.
Teach a preventative or early response approach to pain.	Preventative administration eliminates the roller coaster effect, provides a constant blood level, reduces anxiety, and ultimately reduces the total 24-hour dose.
Teach about the nature, effect, side effects of any pain medications used.	Knowledge increases compliance, provides a sense of self-control, and insures the safe administration of drugs.

INTERVENTIONS

RATIONALE

Interventions	Rationale
Inpatient Monitor the continuing need for and response to pain medication.	Ongoing assessment at the bedside determines whether the medication orders are appropriate in type, amount, route, and frequency of administration.
Monitor vital signs frequently when narcotics are administered.	Physiologic response to narcotic analgesics varies significantly, particularly with IV administration. Respiratory depression, hypotension, decreased consciousness, and nausea and vomiting are important side effects to note.
Use pain flow sheets to monitor the occurrence of pain, use of medications, and the effectiveness of the protocol.	The use of bedside flow sheets establishes a concrete and objective record of the pain experience, and provides for evaluation by the primary nurse and physician, especially when there are multiple care givers.
Administer analgesics, using the dose and route that provide for optimal relief.	The oral route of administration is the preferred route, and a wide variety of analgesics are available in oral form. If the oral route is inappropriate, i.e., immediately after surgery or when nothing by mouth (NPO) is necessary, the intravenous (IV) route is preferable to provide freedom from pain and guaranteed absorption. Patient-controlled analgesia (PCA) has been shown to provide the most satisfactory mode of administration, and frequently the total doses are lower.
Administer analgesics on a routine rather than as needed (p.r.n.) for severe ongoing pain.	Routine and around-the-clock medication administration prevents the pain from becoming severe and uncontrollable due to the addition of anxiety and muscle tension.
Offer to administer analgesics prior to activity and scheduled treatment.	Based on the plan of care, periods of increased pain are predictable. The administration of preventative analgesia allows for the comfortable participation in strategies aimed at healing. Being pain free enough to ambulate, cough, and deep breathe assists in preventing lung congestion, constipation, and other side effects of narcotics.

INTERVENTIONS	**R**ATIONALE
Utilize appropriate equianalgesic doses and drugs when switching from parenteral to oral non-narcotic medications.	Morphine is used as a standard against which the effectiveness of analgesia is typically measured. Knowledge of equianalgesics is essential to ensure that sustained pain relief is achieved. Oral administration usually requires higher doses but can be given less frequently.
Teach to report the incidence of pain promptly.	The preventative approach emphasizes intervening before the pain becomes severe; but fear of addiction may interfere with asking for analgesia. Preventative administration eliminates the roller coaster effect, provides for a constant blood level, reduces anxiety, and lowers the total 24-hour dose.
Reassure concerning the facts of narcotic tolerance, dependency, and addiction.	There is frequent confusion about drug terminology and needless worry about addiction. Drug tolerance is an inevitable and relatively rapid physiologic response to repeated narcotic administration, and over time a prescribed dose begins to lose effectiveness. Drug dependence is also an inevitable physiologic outcome of repeated narcotic use, and withdrawal symptoms are experienced if there is rapid discontinuation. Addiction is a behavioral pattern characterized by overwhelming preoccupation with the acquisition and use of the drug and is not the outcome of properly managed acute pain.
Community Health/ Home Care Assess knowledge concerning the nature and expected duration of the pain and the various components of the pain management regimen.	Pain management is a complex and multifaceted process, which involves learning new skills and safely administering potentially dangerous drugs in the home environment.
Encourage to include adequate rest and sleep in the daily life-style.	Fatigue decreases the ability to tolerate and positively cope with pain. Energy is depleted by efforts to deal with pain, and this necessitates planning for additional sleep and rest each day.
Provide accurate information about the physiologic basis of pain and the expected course, if known.	Surgical incisions, fractures, and most uncomplicated injuries follow fairly predictable pain patterns. Knowing what to expect decreases fear of the unknown, increases feeling of control, and adds comfort.

INTERVENTIONS	**R**ATIONALE
Teach the importance of staying active and involved in normal activities, particularly outside the home.	Daily activities provide for significant natural distraction from the pain experience. Being active reduces the severity of constipation, which frequently accompanies analgesic use.
Incorporate the family into the pain relief regimen if possible.	Dissemination of responsibility increases cohesiveness and feelings of control, provides mutual support of positive coping behaviors, decreases anxiety, and enhances the safety necessary in the use of medications.

REFERENCES/BIBLIOGRAPHY

American Pain Society. (1988). Relieving pain: An analgesic guide. **American Journal of Nursing, 88**(5), 816–825.

Cogan, R.D., Waltz, W., & McCue, M. (1987). Effects of laughter and relaxation on discomfort thresholds. **Journal of Behavioral Medicine, 10**, 139–144.

Coyle, N. (1987). Analgesics and Pain. **Nursing Clinics of North America, 22**(3), 727–741.

Harrison, M., & Cotanch, P.H. (1987). Pain: Advances and issues in critical care, **Nursing Clinics of North America, 22**(3), 691–697.

Jones, L. (1987). Patient controlled analgesia. **Orthopedic Nursing, 6**, 38–41.

* Kleiman, R.L., Lipman, A.G., & Hare, B.D. (1988). A comparison of morphine administered by patient controlled analgesia and regularly scheduled intramuscular injection in severe post operative pain. **Journal of Pain Symptom Management, 3**, 15–22.

Kleiman, R.L., Lipman, A.G., Hare, B.D., & MacDonald, S.D. (1987). PAC vs. regular injections for severe post op pain. **American Journal of Nursing, 87**(11), 1491–1492.

Lisson, E.L. (1987). Ethical issues related to pain control. **Nursing Clinics of North America, 22**(3), 649–659.

McCaffery, M. (1987). A practical "portable" chart of equianalgesic doses. **Nursing 87, 17**(8), 56–57.

McCaffery, M. (1987). Giving meperidine for pain: Should it be so mechanical? **Nursing 87, 17**(4), 60–64.

McCaffery, M., & Beebe, A. (1989). **Pain: Clinical manual for nursing practice**. St. Louis: Mosby.

Melzak, R. (1987). The short form McGill pain questionnaire. **Pain, 30**, 191–197.

North American Nursing Diagnosis Association. (1990). **Taxonomy I** (Rev. 1990). St. Louis: NANDA.

Olsson, G., & Parler, G. (1987). A model approach to pain assessment. **Nursing 87, 17**(5), 52–57.

* Swinford, P. (1987). Relaxation and positive imagery for the surgical client: A research study. **Perioperative Nursing Quarterly, 3**, 9–16.

Vandenbosch, T.M. (1988). How to use a pain flow sheet effectively. **Nursing 88, 18**(8), 50–51.

Watt-Watson, J.H. (1987). What do we need to know about pain? Assessing pain and giving narcotics. **American Journal of Nursing, 87**(9), 1217–1218.

* Whipple, B. (1987). Methods of pain control: Review of research and literature. **Image, 19**(3), 142–146.

Pain, Chronic

A state in which an individual experiences pain that continues for more than six months in duration. (NANDA, 1990, p. 99).

Judith K. Sands, R.N., Ed.D.

DEFINING CHARACTERISTICS

Altered ability to continue previous activities
Anger or frustration
Anorexia
Changes in sleep patterns, insomnia
Color changes in the affected area
Depression
Difficulty concentrating
Disruption of personal, sexual, family, and social relationships

Facial mask, flat affect
Fatigue and loss of energy
Feelings of worthlessness and powerlessness
Guarded movement
Muscle spasm, reflex abnormalities
Physical and social withdrawal
Verbal report of pain experienced for more than six months
Weight changes

CONTRIBUTING FACTORS

Pathophysiological

Musculoskeletal injury, inflammation, or degeneration
Neoplastic tissue invasion or destruction
Organ inflammation or dysfunction

Peripheral nerve dysfunction, inflammation, or injury
Vascular spasm

Psychosociobehavioral

Lack of knowledge concerning pain management strategies
Personal and cultural responses to the phenomenon of pain
Personal or social adjustment problems

391

EXPECTED OUTCOMES

(Note: Due to the nature of chronic pain, the goals are all long-term.)
Client will verbalize that pain is reduced to a controllable level.
Client will verbalize an increasing ability to adequately cope with the pain experience.
Client will acquire knowledge about appropriate analgesics and nonpharmacologic pain control strategies.
Client will express satisfaction with the overall quality of life.

INTERVENTIONS	RATIONALE
Universal (See also care planning guide, "Pain, Acute.") Accurately assess the pain experience.	All management and strategies begin with a detailed assessment of the physical experience of pain. In addition to standard pain assessment tools, pain diaries provide insight into the location, intensity, and duration of the pain over time.
Assess factors which affect the incidence and severity of the pain or influence pain tolerance.	The presence and severity of chronic pain are influenced by a variety of personal and environmental factors, which can be used to evaluate the potential effectiveness of different approaches to pain management.
Assess the impact of the pain on ADLs, energy, sleep patterns, occupational and recreational pursuits, and intrapersonal relationships.	Chronic pain is a devastating problem, precisely because it can negatively impact on virtually any aspect of daily life. The importance of each factor is unique to the individual. Understanding the nature and importance of the factors allows the plan of care to be appropriately targeted to the priority areas.
Assess identified coping style for dealing with the chronic pain and evaluate its overall effectiveness.	The stressor of chronic pain triggers highly individual responses which reflect unique coping styles and strengths. Pain management strategies which build on coping strengths are most effec-tive. New strategies attempt to broaden the coping resources and reinforce existing positive approaches.
Assess the current chronic pain management protocol, including the use of analgesics or other drugs.	A variety of approaches may be utilized to manage the chronic pain. Each component of the current plan is carefully evaluated before new strategies are devised. Over-the-counter analgesic products are frequently overlooked in

INTERVENTIONS	**R**ATIONALE
	the discussion of analgesic approaches but play an important role in home management.
Convey a message of acceptance for the reports of pain.	Many health care personnel have negative feelings toward chronic pain and consider the pain to be primarily psychological and therefore somehow "less real." A trusting relationship cannot be established without clear reassurance that the reality of the pain is accepted.
Assist to set realistic goals concerning the pain.	Complete pain relief is not typically a realistic goal, as knowledge concerning pain management is far from complete. A realistic goal considers the nature of the pain pathology, its expected pattern, and the setting and resources available for management.
Assist to reduce or eliminate the factors that increase the frequency or intensity of the pain or decrease pain tolerance.	Stress, fatigue, boredom, overexertion, and environmental conditions are among the factors which commonly influence the perception of pain. Modifying ADLs to minimize the influence of these factors assists in stabilizing the unpredictability of the pain experience.
Provide with accurate information about the causes of the pain, if available.	No pain is imaginary but not all pain can be successfully traced to an identifiable pathophysiologic base. Teaching about the pain reinforces the message of acceptance of its presence and at least partially addresses the crucial question of why. An understanding of cause also supports appropriate decision making concerning diagnostic testing and treatment options.
Teach or reinforce the correct use of cutaneous stimulation therapies such as heat and cold, massage, and transcutaneous electrical nerve stimulator (TENS) units.	Chronic pain is managed holistically, and every attempt is made to avoid excessive reliance on analgesic medications. Cutaneous stimulation strategies apply the gate control theory of pain, blocking or interfering with pain transmission. They also relax muscles and enable the client to maintain or increase activity.
Teach the importance of remaining as active as possible but avoiding fatigue.	Remaining involved in normal activities supports the sense of self-worth and role competence. Activities are also excellent distractors

INTERVENTIONS	RATIONALE
	from the pain experience. The presence of pain, however, requires energy for coping and does increase fatigue. And, in cyclical fashion, fatigue increases the awareness of pain. A balance of activity and rest is most effective.
Inpatient Assess the ability of the pain protocol to deal with the new or increased stresses associated with hospitalization.	Chronic pain fluctuates significantly in intensity and duration over time. The stress of disease exacerbation and hospitalization can significantly disrupt the balance and effectiveness of the total pain management program, necessitating adjustments.
Administer analgesics, orally if possible, at doses that are sufficient to satisfactorily relieve the pain and on a schedule that sustains therapeutic blood levels.	Exacerbations or crises of the pain are treated aggressively. Analgesics are administered in doses that succeed in controlling the pain. Oral administration on a scheduled rather than PRN basis establishes and maintains therapeutic blood levels of the drug and eliminates the experience of peaks and troughs of effectiveness.
Avoid the sudden withdrawal of narcotic or sedative medications.	The abrupt withdrawal of narcotic or sedative medications can precipitate painful withdrawal symptoms in drug-dependent persons. Any change in route, dose, or drug is made with careful attention to equianalgesic properties of the ordered drugs to ensure ongoing effective analgesia.
Teach cognitive and behavioral strategies that can enhance the sense of control over the pain experience. These may include relaxation, distraction, guided imagery, and hypnosis.	Cognitive strategies, relaxation strategies in particular, reduce anxiety and muscle tension which are clearly associated with an increased pain awareness. The ability to maintain or restore a sense of control over the pain experience represents active coping rather than passive victimization by the pain.
Community Health/ Home Care Assess the support systems which are available to implement the pain management regimen.	The management of chronic pain is time-consuming, often expensive, and extremely lonely work. A data base about physical, financial, and personal resources available in the home setting

INTERVENTIONS	**RATIONALE**
	allows for appropriate selection of long-term management strategies.
Assess family members'/ significant others' knowledge and beliefs about the pain and clarify misconceptions.	An environment of suspicion, hostility, or overt pity concerning the chronic pain state results in conflict or alienation. Clarification of misunderstandings or feelings concerning chronic pain best supports an optimal home care environment.
Offer management strategies which are congruent with natural coping styles.	Cognitive/behavioral pain control strategies are most effective when they are congruent with the client's innate value and belief systems and support accustomed patterns of coping. The placebo effect plays a role in pain management. Strategies which are not believed in or accepted are rarely evaluated as effective.
Encourage adherence with a regular exercise or conditioning regimen. Initiate referrals to physical therapy, if appropriate.	Improving overall muscle tone and general physical conditioning enhances general health, promotes restful sleep, and increases the overall sense of well-being. Rehabilitation specialists are involved when specific limitations or concerns regarding the cardiovascular or musculoskeletal system exist.
Explore the use of anti-depressants to correct sleep disturbances.	Sleep problems seriously complicate the entire chronic pain cycle. Sleep deprivation worsens fatigue, increases pain awareness, and decreases pain tolerance. Depression ensues, which typically worsens sleep problems. Tricyclic anti-depressants are successfully used at bedtime to interrupt the cycle and support restful sleep.
Provide factual information about the risks of tolerance and dependence associated with chronic narcotic use.	Narcotic analgesics are not the preferred approach for dealing with chronic pain, but their use may be both appropriate and necessary. Accurate information about the associated side effects, risks, and benefits is provided to ensure safe administration and prevent unnecessary anxiety over the attendant risks of dependence and addiction.
Help to adapt diet, fluid, and activity to deal with anticipated drug side effects.	Gastric irritation, sedation, and constipation are associated with the ongoing use of analgesic drugs. Most of these effects can be successfully

INTERVENTIONS	RATIONALE
	dealt with by increasing the intake of fiber and fluids and buffering drugs with food. Sedation is usually mild but safety concerns, particularly those associated with driving or operating machinery, are carefully considered.
Initiate referrals to pain management centers if available.	The appropriate management of chronic pain is a complex process, which is frequently best managed by pain specialists when these resources exist. Information about location, available services, and basic costs are provided, particularly when the pain experience is consuming virtually all of the available energy.
Explore the need for additional assistance in coping with the chronic pain.	Depression is an expected outcome of chronic pain, but exacerbations of pain or the occurrence of incidental life stressors may precipitate a crisis of control and even the risk of suicide. Prompt referral to professional assistance is initiated when evidence exists that coping resources are being exhausted.

REFERENCES/BIBLIOGRAPHY

Graffman, S., & Johnsonn, A. (1987). A comparison of two relaxation strategies for the relief of pain and its distress. **Journal of Pain Symptom Management, 2**(4), 229–231.

Lisson, E.L. (1987). Ethical issues related to pain control. **Nursing Clinics of North America, 22**(3), 649–659.

McCaffery, M., & Beebe, A. (1989). **Pain: Clinical manual for nursing practice**. St. Louis: Mosby.

North American Diagnosis Association. **Taxonomy I** (Rev. 1990). St. Louis: NANDA.

Pearson, B.D. (1987). Pain control: An experiment with imagery. **Geriatric Nursing, 8**, 28–30.

Perlman, S.L. (1988). Modern techniques of pain management. **Western Journal of Medicine, 148**, 54–61.

Roberts, A.H. (1987). Literature update: Biofeedback and chronic pain. **Journal of Pain Symptom Management, 2**, 169–171.

Turk, D.C., Rudy, T.E., & Stieg, R.I. (1988). Chronic pain and depression. **Pain Management, 1**, 17–25.

Wallace, J. (1987). Morphine sulfate administered sublingually to control chronic pain. **Oncology Nursing Forum, 14**, 66–68.

Whipple, B. (1987). Methods of pain control: Review of research and literature. **Image, 19**(3), 142–146.

Wright, S. M. (1987). The use of therapeutic touch in the management of pain. **Nursing Clinics of North America, 22**(3), 705–713.

Parental Role Conflict

A state in which parent(s) or person(s)
performing the parental role(s)
experiences dissonance regarding
performance in response to crisis.

Ann Moore, R.N., M.Ed.

DEFINING CHARACTERISTICS

Demonstrated disruption in caretaking routines

Expresses concerns about changes in parental role, family functioning, family communication, and/or family health

Expresses concerns about perceived loss of control over decisions relating to their child

Expresses concerns/feelings of inadequacy to provide for infant's/child's physical and emotional needs during hospitalization, while in the home, or if placed outside of the home (e.g., foster care)

Lack of expression of a clear idea of what the parental roles are and how to effect these for the benefit of the infant/child

Reluctance to participate in usual caretaking activities even with encouragement and support

Verbalization, demonstration of feelings of guilt, anger, fear, anxiety, and/or frustrations about effect of child's physical and/or psychological dysfunctioning upon the family process

CONTRIBUTING FACTORS

Pathophysiological

Chronological age of parent(s) and siblings

Parental physical or psychological disturbance prior to onset of crisis

Psychosociobehavioral

Change in marital status

Family size

Home care of a child with special needs (e.g., apnea monitoring, postural drainage, hyperalimentation, attention deficit hyperactivity disorder, oppositional defiant disorder)

397

Interruptions of family life due to home care regimen (treatments, health care givers, lack of respite)
Intimidation with invasive or restrictive modalities (e.g., isolation, intubation), specialized
     care centers, policies
Lack of available support systems
Lack of knowledge
Pre-crisis level of coping
Presence of additional stressors (financial, legal, employment)
Separation from child due to chronic illness (either physical or psychological)
Unmet social/emotional needs of parent(s)
Unrealistic expectations of self and/or infant/child
Unrealistic expectations of the outcome of care

Expected Outcomes

Client will perform parental role functions that foster healthful life style for self and
     infant/child/family.
     Dysfunctional nature/aspects of current level of functioning are identified.
     In collaboration with treatment team members, activities are developed that foster
          improved physical and psychological functioning.
     Assistance/support is identified that may be required.
     Role performance improvement is facilitated in cooperation with treatment team members.

Interventions	Rationale
Universal In collaboration with parent(s), develop a plan of care.	Enlisting the parent(s) from the beginning fosters compliance with the plan of care by reestablishing the sense of control.
Determine abilities to perform in-home care necessary for the treatment of the child.	Accurate identification of what can and will be done offers a sense of caring for the parents, as well as the infant/child. Requiring performance of procedures that discomfit could lead to procedures being performed inaccurately, as well as reinforcing feelings of inadequacy.
Teach procedures and coping strategies within the realm of identified abilities.	Educational/coping methods will be better utilized if viewed as within parents' ability.

INTERVENTIONS	RATIONALE
Provide time for questions to be answered and for feedback regarding return performances of any procedures that parent(s) will be implementing.	Feedback facilitates a trusting relationship and provides opportunities for confidence to be bolstered.
Provide information regarding support groups within the local community.	Additional support groups of people who have experienced similar concerns/feelings provide role models and other avenues for expression of feelings.
Inpatient Evaluate for risk of altered parenting following discharge.	This assessment provides additional information that may help with discharge and/or respite care planning.
Determine need for community health/home health care. Provide adequate private time to verbalize feelings.	Inadequate time to verbalize feelings and concerns with hospital staff may result in further feelings of inadequacy and lack of control.
Involve in as many aspects of inpatient care as possible (within legal limits).	Involvement alleviates feelings of loss of control and facilitates compliance after discharge.
Instruct about the need for continued care after hospitalization. Identify the benefits and limitations.	Providing a thorough explanation of all possible options for care upon discharge allows an opportunity for an informed decision. Making an informed decision facilitates alleviation of guilt.
Community Health/ Home Care In collaboration with the parent(s) and inpatient treatment team, develop a plan of care to be implemented within the home.	The parenting/nurturing figures living with the child need to be intimately involved with the plan development, implementation, evaluation, and any necessary alterations to the plan.

INTERVENTIONS	RATIONALE
Determine a schedule of in-home appointments and provide a copy of the schedule for the parent(s).	A schedule for house calls must be set in conjunction with the parent(s) needs and schedule. By setting the time only according to convenience to the health care professional, involvement from the family may be compromised. Also, written reminders serve as recall prompts when making other plans.
Develop goals to be evaluated during each house call/ home visit.	Goal-setting and evaluation provide immediate feedback regarding progress.
Offer verbal encouragement and verbal praise to the parent(s).	Positive reinforcement increases desired behaviors.
Determine the mode of understanding that is most often used, i.e., visual, auditory.	Providing tools, graphs, audio and/or visual tapes that provide role-modeling situations and other information is best incorporated when the information is provided within the best mode of learning.

REFERENCES/BIBLIOGRAPHY

See bibliography for "Parenting, Altered."

Parenting, Altered

A state in which an individual acting as a caretaking person is experiencing dysfunctional responding in the areas of affecting, cognating, and/or behaving during interactions with other person(s), i.e., the focus(es) of the caretaking responsibilities.

Ann Moore, R.N., M.Ed.

· · · · · · · · · · ·

DEFINING CHARACTERISTICS

Abandonment
Child receives care from multiple caretakers without consideration for the needs of the infant/ child
Compulsively seeking role approval from others
Constant expression (verbal and nonverbal) of disappointment in gender, temperament, and/or physical characteristics of the infant/child
Expressions (verbal and nonverbal) of resentment towards the infant/child
Frequent accidents
Frequent illness
Growth and development lag(s) in the infant/child
History of child abuse or abandonment by primary caretaker
Inappropriate caretaking behaviors (toilet training, safety, exercise, sleep/rest, feeding, language development)
Inappropriate or inconsistent discipline practices
Inappropriate visual, tactile, auditory stimulation
Inattention to infant's/child's needs
Incidence of physical and psychological trauma
Lack of parental attachment behaviors
Negative attachment of meanings to infant's/child's characteristics
Negative identification of infant's/child's characteristics
Noncompliance with health appointments for self and/or infant/child
Runaway

Verbal and nonverbal disgust at body functions of infant/child
Verbalizes desire to have child call himself/herself by first name versus traditional cultural
       tendencies
Verbalization of role inadequacy
Verbalization that child cannot be controlled

CONTRIBUTING FACTORS

Pathophysiological

Familial history of mental illness
Limited cognitive functioning
Limited language abilities in both the caretaker and the child
Mental and/or physical illness
Multiple pregnancies
Organicism related to alcohol and/or other substance abuse

Psychosociobehavioral

Alcohol and/or other substance abuse
Ineffective role model
Interruption in bonding process, i.e., maternal, paternal, other
Lack of available role model
Lack of knowledge
Lack of or inappropriate response of infant/child to relationship
Lack of role identity
Lack of support between/from significant other(s)
Meets own needs before the needs of the infant/child
Negative influences upon the child from peers; this influence is beyond the control of the
       parent(s)
Parental guilt
Parental overpermissiveness
Parental overprotection
Perceive threat to own survival—physical and emotional
Physical and psychosocial abuse of nurturing figure
Poor, inconsistent communication within the relationship
Presence of stress (financial, legal, recent crisis, cultural move)
Unmet social/emotional maturation needs of parenting figure(s)
Unrealistic expectation for self, infant/child, partner
Unrealistic parental demands

EXPECTED OUTCOMES

Client (caretaking individual) will initiate and continue practicing infant/child care that fosters
       age-appropriate physiological and psychological development.
       Developmental milestones are attained.

Medical appointments are made and kept.
Normal developmental milestones are verbalized.
Activities that foster physical and psychological development are described and initiated.
Assistance/support that may be required is identified.
Episodes of inflicting either physical or psychological pain onto the infant/child do not occur.

INTERVENTIONS

RATIONALE

Universal

Interventions	Rationale
Assess for history of altered parenting.	Clients with a history of difficulties with parenting have a greater tendency for future difficulties. An awareness of the unique set of circumstances within which the client(s) finds self provides vital information for determining interventions that would be most effective.
Assess for previous health care interventions related to problematic relationships between parent(s) and infant(s)/child(ren).	Historical assessment provides information related to methods which have previously been implemented, what has and has not worked, and how unalterable the current level of functioning may be.
Assess for actual physical and/or psychological abuse.	Severe stress conditions strain a person's ability to cope and may lead to abusive situations. In addition to facilitating development of preventive measures, many state laws require that all nurses report situations of abuse to a designated authority/agency.
Assess the physical and developmental levels of the infant/child.	The infant's/child's physical and developmental levels are, in part, a reflection of the environment within which he or she is being raised. Additionally, baseline data provide critical information when evaluating the nursing process and considering adjustments for the plan of care.
Conduct a family history.	Genetic information is relevant information when determining biopsychosocial interventions.
Teach the extent to which the infant/child can function within a nurturing/caring environment.	Realistic expectations must be described to the parent(s) to foster reasonable limitations.

INTERVENTIONS	**RATIONALE**
Teach interventions which foster the infant's/child's advancement to age-appropriate developmental levels (these interventions may be physiological, cognitive, affective, and/or behavioral in nature).	Parental training is crucial when attempting to impact upon/change the infant's/child's current level of functioning. Increasing parental skills fosters confidence when interacting with the infant/child, thus increasing a sense of well-being. Proper instructions facilitate consistency with discipline practices, and consistency strengthens trust within the relationship. Since health care professionals are not in the home throughout the entire day, parental training enables the child to be exposed to the benefits of teaching around the clock.
Institute necessary referrals. These include inpatient medical or psychiatric facilities.	The nurse must be cognizant of other professional disciplines and agencies which may be of service to the parent(s)/family.
Emphasize importance of scheduling and keeping all medical appointments.	Ongoing physical and developmental assessments and interventions for infants/children are essential. Early identification of problems is facilitated by ongoing assessment. Maintaining necessary medical appointments as the infant/child grows provides opportunities to ensure proper immunizations. Current immunizations aid not only the infant/child but the community at large.
Obtain signed authorization for release of information before providing data to outside agencies (unless an emergent situation develops).	The parent(s) has a legal right to know to whom information about their situation is going. Laws regarding confidentiality require signed release forms unless an emergent situation develops.
Inpatient None	
Community Health/ Home Care In collaboration with the parent(s), develop a plan of care to be implemented within the home.	The parenting/nurturing figures living with the child need to be intimately involved with the plan development, implementation, evaluation, and any necessary alterations to the plan.

INTERVENTIONS	**R**ATIONALE
Determine a schedule of in-home appointments and provide a copy of the schedule for the parent(s).	A schedule for house calls must be set in conjunction with the parent(s) needs and schedule. By setting the time only according to convenience to the health care professional, involvement from the family may be compromised. Also, written reminders serve as recall prompts when making other plans.
Develop goals to be evaluated during each house call/home visit.	Goal-setting and evaluation provide immediate feedback regarding progress.
Offer verbal encouragement and verbal praise.	Positive reinforcement increases desired behaviors.
Determine the mode of understanding most often used, i.e., visual, auditory.	Providing tools, graphs, audio and/or visual tapes that provide role-modeling situations and other information is best incorporated when the information is provided within the best mode of learning.

REFERENCES/BIBLIOGRAPHY

Bartz, W.R., & Rasor, R.A. (1978). **Surviving with kids, A lifeline for overwhelmed parents**. San Luis Obispo, CA: Impact Publishers.

Bee, H. (1989). **The developing child**. New York: Harper & Row.

Dangel, R.F., & Polster, R.A. (Eds.). (1984). **Parent training, Foundations of research and practice**. New York: Guilford.

Ginott, H.G. (1965). **Between parent and child, New solutions to old problems**. New York: Macmillan.

North American Nursing Diagnosis Association. **Taxonomy I** (Rev. 1990). St. Louis: NANDA.

Roberts, S.L. (1978). **Behavioral concepts and nursing throughout the life span**. Englewood Cliffs, NJ: Prentice-Hall.

Travis, G. (1976). **Chronic illness in children, Its impact on child and family**. Stanford, CA: Stanford University Press.

Stuart, G.W., & Sundeen, S.J. (1987). **Principles and practice of psychiatric nursing**. St. Louis: Mosby.

Parenting, Altered: Risk

A state in which an individual acting as a caretaking person is at risk to experience dysfunctional responding in the areas of affecting, cognating, and behaving during interactions with other person(s), i.e., the focus(es) of the caretaking responsibilities.

Ann Moore, R.N., M.Ed.

RISK FACTORS

Pathophysiological

Any physical illness

Psychosociobehavioral

Alcohol and/or other substance abuse
Familial history of mental illness
Ineffective role model
Interruption in bonding process, i.e., maternal, parental, other
Lack of available role model
Lack of knowledge
Lack of or inappropriate response of infant/child to relationship
Lack of role identity
Lack of support between/from significant other(s)
Limited cognitive functioning
Limited language abilities in both the caretaker and the child
Meets own needs before the needs of the infant/child
Mental illness
Multiple pregnancies
Negative influences from child's peers; these may not be under the influence of the parent(s)
Organicism related to alcohol and/or other substance abuse
Overprotection

Parental guilt
Parental overpermissiveness
Perceive threat to own survival—physical and emotional
Physical and psychosocial abuse of nurturing figure
Poor, inconsistent communication
Presence of stress (financial, legal, recent crisis, cultural)
Unmet social/emotional maturation needs of parenting figure(s)
Unrealistic demands
Unrealistic expectation for self, infant/child, partner

EXPECTED OUTCOMES

Client (caretaking individual) will initiate and continue practicing infant/child care that fosters age-appropriate physiological and psychological development.
Developmental milestones are attained.
Medical appointments are made and kept.
Normal developmental milestones are verbalized.
Activities that foster physical and psychological development are described and initiated.
Assistance/support that may be required is identified.
Episodes of inflicting either physical or psychological pain onto the infant/child do not occur.

INTERVENTIONS / RATIONALE

Universal	
Assess for history of altered parenting.	A history of parenting difficulties predisposes a parent(s) to have a greater tendency for future difficulties. An awareness of the unique set of circumstances within which the client(s) finds self provides vital information for determining interventions that would be most effective.
Assess for previous health care interventions related to problematic relationships between parent(s) and infant(s)/child(ren).	Historical assessment provides information related to methods which have previously been implemented, what has and has not worked, and how unalterable the current level of functioning may be.
Assess for potential as well as actual physical abuse.	Severe stress conditions strain the ability to cope and may lead to abusive situations. In addition to facilitating development of preventive measures, many state laws require that all nurses report situations of abuse to a designated authority/agency.

INTERVENTIONS	RATIONALE
Assess the physical and developmental levels of the infant/child.	The infant's/child's physical and developmental levels are, in part, a reflection of the environment within which he or she is being raised. Additionally, baseline data provide critical information when evaluating the nursing process and considering adjustments for the plan of care.
Obtain signed authorization for release of information before providing data to outside agencies (unless an emergent situation develops).	Parents have a legal right to know to whom information about their situation is going. Laws regarding confidentiality require signed release forms unless an emergent situation develops.
Conduct a family history.	Genetic information is relevant information when determining biopsychosocial interventions.
Teach the extent to which the infant/child can function within a nurturing/caring environment.	Realistic expectations must be described to foster reasonable limitations.
Teach interventions which foster the infant's/child's advancement to age-appropriate developmental levels (these interventions may be physiological, cognitive, affective, and/or behavioral in nature).	Parental training is crucial when attempting to impact upon or change the infant/child's current level of functioning. Increasing skills fosters confidence when interacting with the infant/child, thus increasing a sense of well-being. Proper instructions facilitate consistency with discipline practices, and consistency strengthens trust within the relationship. Since health care professionals are not in the home throughout the entire day, parental training enables the child to be exposed to the benefits of teaching around the clock.
Institute necessary referrals.	The nurse must be cognizant of other professional disciplines which may be of service to the parent(s)/family.
Emphasize importance of scheduling and keeping medical appointments.	Ongoing physical and developmental assessments and interventions for infants/children are essential. Early identification of problems is facilitated by ongoing assessment. Maintaining necessary medical appointments as the infant/child grows provides opportunities to ensure proper

INTERVENTIONS	RATIONALE
	immunizations. Current immunizations aid not only the infant/child but the community at large.
Inpatient None	
Community Health/ Home Care In collaboration with the parent(s), develop a plan of care to be implemented within the home.	The parenting/nurturing figures living with the child need to be intimately involved with the plan development, implementation, evaluation, and any necessary alterations to the plan.
Determine a schedule of in-home appointments and provide a copy of the schedule for the parent(s).	A schedule for house calls must be set in conjunction with parental needs and schedule. By setting the time only according to convenience to the health care professional, involvement from the family may be compromised. Also, written reminders serve as recall prompts when making other plans.
Develop goals to be evaluated during each house call/home visit.	Goal-setting and evaluation provide immediate feedback regarding progress.
Offer verbal encouragement and verbal praise.	Positive reinforcement increases desired behaviors.
Determine the mode of understanding that is most often used, i.e., visual, auditory.	Providing tools, graphs, audio and/or visual tapes that provide role-modeling situations and other information is best incorporated when the information is provided within the best mode of learning.

REFERENCES/BIBLIOGRAPHY

See bibliography for "Parenting, Altered."

Personal Identity Disturbance

A state in which an individual experiences an inability to perceive self from nonself (NANDA, 1990, p. 91).

Cynthia C. Valentin, R.N., Ph.D.

DEFINING CHARACTERISTICS

Subjective Reports

A fear of going "crazy"
Being an outside observer of self's mental or bodily processes
Feeling insecure or inferior
Feeling like one's thoughts and actions are being carried on mechanically
Feeling separated, isolated, or unreal
Feelings are frozen and thoughts seem strange
In extreme states one no longer feels like one has a body
No longer feeling like oneself, but not like one is becoming someone else
Not feeling in complete control of one's actions (including speech)
Objects in the external world are perceived as altered in size or shape
Parts of body or mind are strange and do not belong to the person
People and objects are unreal or distant
The outside world is unreal, alien, or strange
Unexperienced feelings appear familiar—as having been perceived before
World appears dream-like and/or frightening

Objective Observations

Acknowledgment of disturbed sense of reality confusion
Appearance of bewilderment
Appearance of "lifelessness"—lacking in spontaneity or animation
Identity confusion
Information-processing difficulties
Intact reality testing
Loss of ego boundaries

Marked distress
Memory disturbances—amnesia, memory distortion
Obsessive rumination
Somatic concerns
Thought/judgment impairment

CONTRIBUTING FACTORS

Pathophysiological

Affective disorders
Anxiety disorders
Brain tumor
Epilepsy
Flashbacks
Medications (e.g., Valium (benzodiazepine); phenothiazines; antidepressants)
Previous head injury
Schizophrenia

Psychosociobehavioral

Amnesic state induced by alcohol
Anxiety
Déjà vu experience
Depersonalization experience and/or disorder
Depression
Derealization experience
Drug-induced states of unreality (e.g., hallucinogens: LSD/Mescaline, marijuana)
Ego boundary distortion
Emotional shock
Flashbacks
Hyperventilation
Inability to cope with anger or aggressive impulses
Multiple-personality disorder
Post-trauma stress response
Psychogenic amnesia
Psychogenic fugue
Separation anxiety/problems
Severe physical and/or sexual abuse

EXPECTED OUTCOMES

Client will verbalize feeling "of being in touch with" or an integration among own thoughts, feelings, and behaviors.
Factors that contribute to own stress response (dissociation) are identified.
The role that anxiety and dissociation play in the process of avoidance is verbalized.

Awareness of own physical, emotional, intellectual, and spiritual boundaries is verbalized.
Adaptive coping strategies as healthy alternatives for anxiety relief are verbalized.
Personal identity is maintained even during times of extreme stress.

INTERVENTIONS	RATIONALE
Universal Ascertain whether the personal identity disturbance is a primary disorder (e g., depersonalization disorder), or a symptom of other psychiatric and/or medical problems. Refer to a physician for medical and/or psychiatric assessment and treatment.	The focus of the interventions will be influenced by the etiologies of the disturbance and therefore are essential for proper treatment planning.
Perform a meticulous physical and psychosocial assessment. 1. Explore for evidence of organic causes for the dissociative reactions 2. Identify possible sources of the anxiety reaction	Many clients exhibit behaviors that resemble organic conditions (including post-concussional amnesia and temporal lobe epilepsy); thus organic bases for responses must be ruled out before proceeding with treatment. It's important that differentiation between possible "fundamental sources" of the anxiety be identified early, as a wide range of psychiatric disorders include dissociation-type responses as part of the clinical symptom pattern. Depending upon the disorder, a variety of interventions might be appropriate.
Utilize a supportive therapeutic approach. 1. Clarify role and expectations thereof in nurse-client relationship 2. Approach in a nondemanding, nonaggressive manner 3. Be aware that the nurse's attitude can serve as an assistance or hindrance for expansion of self-awareness	Supportive therapy enhances ego strengths and existing adaptive coping strategies. Exploring and clarifying role(s) assists in establishment of healthy boundaries. An impersonal attitude or criticism can result in a decrease in the client's self-esteem. The placement of excessive demands (in terms of self-exploration and self-disclosure) can result in a challenge to the self-concept, causing withdrawal and utilization of defenses to protect against the pain.

INTERVENTIONS	RATIONALE
Explore adaptive and maladaptive responses to conflict. 1. Discuss by way of contrast the difference between adaptive and maladaptive responses 2. Explore advantages and disadvantages of maladaptive responses 3. Utilize facilitative communication with supportive confrontation	It is necessary to explore the factors that contribute to the inhibiting of self-growth. Exploring the disadvantages to the maladaptive response assists in gaining insight into any secondary gains obtained from the self-defeating behaviors.
Teach about proper use of anxiolytic agents when prescribed by physician. 1. Inform about the potential dependency (exception, Buspirone) that can develop with long-term use 2. Caution not to change dose without physician consent 3. Alert to the potentiating effect of alcoholic beverages when taken in conjunction with medication 4. Caution not to ingest caffeinated beverages, as they decrease the desired effects of the medication 5. Alert to necessity of informing physician of any over-the-counter and other prescribed medications being consumed	Proper instruction and administration of anxiolytic agents insure reduction of anxiety, allowing development and use of healthy coping skills.

Inpatient

Assess for "bewilderment," or presence of words/phrases indicating a splitting off from the self.	A dissociative state indicates the presence of a high degree of anxiety.

INTERVENTIONS	RATIONALE
Ensure safety by providing a safe, nonthreatening environment. 1. Provide activities that are simple and allow individual to progress at own pace 2. Assess readiness for group participation activities 3. Monitor by frequent observations	Inattention to safety needs may occur. A nonthreatening environment aids in anxiety reduction.
Support reality and ego boundary establishment by confirming client's identity. 1. Let clients know who is approaching them. Use pronouns that convey separation between people, e.g., "It is eight o'clock, time for your breakfast" 2. Orient to time and place 3. Describe your perceptions concretely, so that all feedback is reality based	Supporting reality promotes the establishment of ego integrity.
Assist in decision making; however, encourage whenever possible to engage in own decision making related to here-and-now issues.	The goal is to enhance ego strength and self-esteem building without creating undue stress that could accompany the inability to make "wise decisions."
Assist in gaining understanding about the effects of anxiety and the consequences of dissociation. 1. Discuss how dissociation serves as an unconscious protection against acknowledging the disorganizing effects of anxiety 2. Discuss ways in which dissociation serves as a	The main focus of the conversation is the gentle uncovering of the affect and the reality of the conflicts and pain. As insight is gained into symptoms/disorder, an understanding of their role in the dysfunction occurs. With this increased understanding comes the potential to choose other approaches/behaviors that are more supportive of integrated adaptive functioning.

INTERVENTIONS	RATIONALE
defense against experiencing overwhelming pain 3. Help to see the outcomes of using dissociation as a method of coping with stress	
Teach stress management techniques. 1. Instruct in stress reduction exercises 2. Discuss approaches for problem identification and explore alternative solution options 3. Identify ways to get in touch with feelings and how to express them in a safe manner	Stress reduction approaches provide healthy alternatives for the relieving of anxiety. When anxiety level is decreased, unaccessed feelings will be experienced. It is important to assist in labelling these feelings and how to express them safely so as to decease fear and the potential for becoming overwhelmed with emotions. Problem-solving approaches enhance skill building and self-esteem development.
Community Health/ Home Care Teach awareness of subtle mood changes experienced within self in various settings (e.g., home, work). 1. Suggest use of a journal to record thoughts, feelings, and behaviors from daily experiences	The use of a journal supports the acknowledgment of thoughts, feelings, and behaviors as being separate from those of others (reinforces boundaries). This reinforces continued awareness of own ideas and emotional responses to various experiences. It assists in gaining greater awareness of the various environmental cues that lead to stress reactions.

REFERENCES/BIBLIOGRAPHY

American Psychiatric Association. (1987). **Diagnostic and statistical manual of mental disorders** (3rd ed. rev.). Washington, DC: American Psychiatric Association.

* Anderson, G. (1988). Understanding multiple personality disorder. **Journal of Psychiatric Nursing, 26**(7), 26.

Bellak, L., & Siegel, H. (1983). **Handbook of intensive and emergency psychotherapy.** Larchmont, NY: C.P.S.

Cox, H.C., et al. (1989). **Clinical applications of nursing diagnoses.** Baltimore: Williams & Wilkins.

Doenges, M., Townsend, M., & Moorehouse, M. (1989). **Psychiatric care plans—Guidelines for client care.** Philadelphia: Davis.

Freedman, A.M., Kaplan, H.I., & Sadlock, B.J. (1988). **Comprehensive textbook of psychiatry.** Baltimore: Williams & Wilkins.

Haber, J., Hoskins, P., Leach, A., & Sideleau, B. (1987). **Comprehensive psychiatric nursing.** New York: McGraw-Hill.

Kolb, L.C., & Brodie, H.K. (1982). **Modern clinical psychiatry.** Philadelphia: Saunders.

* Morris, M.M., & Myton, C.L. (1988). Ego function. Enhancement through social interaction. **Journal of Psychosocial Nursing, 24**(12), 17–22.

Perko, J., & Kreigh, H. (1988). **Psychiatric and mental health nursing—A commitment to care and concern.** Norwalk, CT./San Mateo, CA: Appleton & Lange.

Stuart, G., & Sundeen, S. (1987). **Principles and practice of psychiatric nursing.** St.Louis/ Washington/Toronto: Mosby.

Townsend, M.C. (1988). **Nursing diagnoses in psychiatric nursing—A pocket guide for care plan construction.** Philadelphia: Davis.

Varcarolis, E.M. (1990). **Foundations of psychiatric mental-health nursing.** Philadelphia: Saunders.

Yura, H., & Walsh, M.B. (1988). **The nursing process—Assessing, planning, implementing, evaluating.** Norwalk, CT./San Mateo, CA: Appleton & Lange.

Physical Mobility, Impaired

A state in which an individual experiences a limitation of ability for independent physical movement (NANDA, 1990, p. 71). (See also, care planning guide, "Disuse Syndrome: Risk.")

Brenda S. Nichols, R.N., D.N.Sc.

DEFINING CHARACTERISTICS

Decreased muscle strength, control, mass, or endurance
Impaired coordination
Impaired memory or intellectual capacity
Imposed restriction of movement due to a mechanical device or medical order
Inability to move purposefully within the physical environment
Limited range of motion
Reluctance to attempt movement

CONTRIBUTING FACTORS

Pathophysiological

Musculoskeletal impairments—for example:
    Arthritis (all types)
    Atrophy
    Bursitis
    Contractions—spastic or flaccid
    Decreased muscle mass
    Dislocation of joints
    Edema
    Hypercalcemia
    Hypothyroidism
    Myalgias
    Osteomyelitis
    Paget's disease
    Sprains
    Subluxation
    Systemic lupus erythematosus
    Trauma
Neuromuscular impairments—for example:
    Alcoholism
    Burn injuries
    Cerebral palsy
    Cerebrovascular accident
    Decreased level of consciousness

Demyelinating diseases—
amyotrophic lateral sclerosis,
multiple sclerosis, muscular
dystrophy, myasthenia gravis,
poliomyelitis
Drug side effects
Obesity
Parkinson's disease
Peripheral neuritis
Sensory deficits associated with pain
Sensory-perceptual impairment
Spinal cord injury or impairment
(compression of nerve root,
paraplegia, quadriplegia)
Tetanus

Vitamin deficiencies (Vitamin B_{12}
and thiamine)
Pain
Treatment-related conditions
Amputations
Bradytherapy (radiation therapy)
Chemotherapy
Depressant effect of anesthesia
and/or narcotic analgesics
Medical equipment—braces, cast,
dressings, intravenous tubing,
monitoring equipment, splints,
tubes, ventilators, wounds
Nausea
Nutritional deficit

Psychosociobehavioral

Aging
Intolerance to activity
Mental problems—e.g., depression, severe anxiety, bipolar disease (manic-depressive)

EXPECTED OUTCOMES

Client will perform locomotion activities independently or with assistive devices, as appropriate.
Sitting position can be assumed.
Transfer to and from chair is performed.
Ambulation is observed and/or reported.
Client will remain free of musculoskeletal problems.
Contractures are prevented.
All joints are moveable.
Muscle atrophy is minimized.
Proper body alignment is maintained.
Client will experience no complications of immobility.
Circulatory system:
Peripheral pulses (pedal and radial) are normal.
No edema is present in feet and/or legs.
No irregular heart sounds are audible.
No evidence of venous thrombosis is present. No pain in calves, thighs, or in thoracic region.
No falls are experienced due to orthostatic hypotension (no dizziness, etc., upon ambulation).
Gastrointestinal systems:
Normal bowel patterns, sounds, formed semisoft stools at least every third day and no abdominal distention are maintained.

A normal appetite and adequate dietary intake are maintained.
No weight changes are experienced.
Genitourinary system:
  Normal urinary output and elimination patterns are maintained.
  Adequate hydration is maintained.
  No renal calculi develop.
  Bladder distention is prevented.
Integumentary system:
  Intact skin is maintained with no reddened areas.
  Skin turgor is normal.
Neurological system:
  No changes in level of consciousness are experienced.
  No psychosocial problems develop and/or remain.
Respiratory system:
  Lung fields have no rales or rhonchi audible with stethoscope.

INTERVENTIONS	RATIONALE
Universal Assess and document: 1. All factors that impair physical mobility 2. Daily functional ability 3. Functional Mobility Classification score (see appendix A).	Determining factors that impair physical mobility establishes baseline data which allow for goal-setting and identifying milestones.
Monitor for effects of replacement drugs when indicated, as follows: 1. Thyroid hormone: Evaluate client for decrease in symptoms of hypothyroidism: weight loss, increased activity level, appetite and sense of well-being. Monitor for signs of toxicity: insomnia is usually the earliest symptom, irritability, nervousness, heat intolerance, pulse rate increases.	Monitoring for side effects and adverse reactions of treatment allows for prompt intervention if necessary.

INTERVENTIONS

RATIONALE

Interventions	Rationale
2. Vitamin B$_{12}$: Evaluate for no further progression in neurological deterioration: gait stabilization, awareness of surroundings, stabilization of fine motor tremors. Rarely does toxicity occur with vitamin administration. Monitor during the first 48 hours of therapy for signs of hypokalemia (profound muscle weakness or paralysis, irregular heart rate, etc.). 3. ACTH and/or corticosteriods: Evaluate for therapeutic action-increased joint mobility, decreased pain. Observe for adverse reactions: abdominal pain, black tarry stools, hypertension, edema, muscle cramping, bone pain, increased bruising, or altered wound healing.	
Perform range-of-motion exercises to joints, unless contraindicated, progressing from passive to active exercises as tolerated.	Exercises prevent joint contracture, muscle weakness, and atrophy.
Turn and position frequently and establish turning schedule for dependent clients; post schedule at the bedside and monitor frequency of turning.	Movement prevents skin breakdown by relieving pressure.
Give skin care to prominent areas or potential breakdown areas with every other turn.	Skin care to bony prominences encourages circulation to the area and keeps the area intact.

INTERVENTIONS	RATIONALE
Place joints in functional positions on an alternating schedule. (Use of trochanter roll along thigh, abduction of thighs, high top shoes, small pillow under head).	Placement of limbs in anatomical position using these aids prevents musculoskeletal deformities (contractures).
Promote progressive mobilization within the limits of tolerance. Determine distance walked and increase daily.	Activity maintains muscle tone and prevents complication of immobility.
Administer medications prescribed to control pain.	Pain interferes with the ability to ambulate and inhibits muscle movements.
Place items within reach of unaffected arm if one-sided weakness or paralysis is present.	Positioning allows independent access to items and promotes self-help.

Instruct client and family/significant other(s) in the following interventions:
    Mobility regimen
    Range-of-motion exercises
    Quadricep setting exercises
    Transfer techniques
    Skin inspection
	Pertinent information encourages preparation for participation in recovery and prevention of the complications of immobility.

Inpatient

Perform baseline assessments of:
    Circumferences of affected and unaffected body parts
    Joint motion
    Muscle strength (may use dynamometer to determine handgrip strength), resistance, gait, coordination, movement.
	Data obtained serve as a baseline which will be used for comparison.

INTERVENTIONS	RATIONALE
Assess mechanical devices to prevent possible injuries as follows: 1. Ace bandages—ensure even distribution, wrap distal to proximal, observe for skin irritation, improper distribution of bandage, reapply bandage at least twice per day (unless contraindicated—pressure dressing, etc.)	Circulation can be adversely affected by the presence of Ace bandages. Improperly applied bandages enhance the potential for skin breakdown.
2. Cast—assess for complaints of pain, examine skin color for pallor, check for pulse at least every four hours	Pain, pallor, pulselessness are key signs of compartment syndrome.
3. Sling—check for correct application, ensure that sling is loose around neck and not tied at the nape of neck	Improper application forces the extremity into improper alignment. Slings should never be closed along the spinal cord, due to the potential for spinal root damage.
4. Traction devices—assess for correct alignment of bones and position of weights, ensure that weights hang freely; check pulse quality, skin temperature, capillary refill; assess for changes in sensation, mobility, skin irritation	Skin color, temperature, and sensation, as well as pulse quality, are indicators of circulatory and neuromuscular status.
Monitor for presence of hypercalcemia by assessing: Changes in mental status, muscle weakness or flaccidity, nausea, vomiting, anorexia, cachexia, cardiac arrhythmias, daily intakes and outputs (to determine if polyuria is present).	With immobility, calcium is not deposited into bone, thus increasing the circulating calcium. Calcium depresses the nervous system, central nervous system reflexes become sluggish, the QT interval of the heart decreases, and constipation and lack of appetite occur.

INTERVENTIONS	**RATIONALE**

Assist, if spasticity occurs, as follows:
    Avoid stimulating extremities or muscle groups
    Prevent fatigue
    Prevent chills
    Provide or assist with non-pharmacological measures for reducing spasticity (e.g., biofeedback, warm bath, whirlpool, local applications of heat or cold)
    Administer muscle relaxants (e.g. baclofen, dantrolene) to relieve muscle spasticity
	Spasticity interferes with ambulation and mobility. Spasticity follows the initial period of flaccidity.

Utilize full-length mirrors to aid in awareness of body position.	Mirrors help to visualize body positions when the brain is not interpreting stimuli correctly.

Implement measures to prevent falls:
    Keep bed in low position with side rails up
    Keep needed items within easy reach
    Use lap belt
    Have call bell within easy reach
    Avoid unnecessary clutter in room
    Accompany during ambulation utilizing a transfer safety belt if indicated
    Provide ambulatory aids (cane, walker) if weak or unsteady
    Do not rush
    Allow adequate time for trips to the bathroom
	Safety measures limit the potential for falling and decrease the fear of injury.

INTERVENTIONS	RATIONALE
Perform actions (e.g., range of motion exercises, active and passive exercises, increased ambulation) which will improve strength and activity tolerance	
Reward attempts at physical mobility.	Praising rewards effort and provides motivation for further activity.

Promote rest and reduce fatigue as follows:
    Organize care to allow short rest periods prior to initiation of activity and at intervals during the day
    Minimize external environmental stimuli between activities
    Assist with self-care needs with encouragement to increase daily activity.
	Energy is required for movement. If fatigued, the body has less energy for mobility.

If hypercalcemic or at risk, encourage foods high in sodium (unless contraindicated by other preexisting conditions).	Sodium competes with calcium reabsorption in kidney tubules.
Teach how to move body in bed (e.g., hook arm through side rail to assist in turning self, use flexor spasm of knee to help swing legs over side of bed during transfer to and from wheelchair).	Client participation promotes self-esteem.
Teach to perform active and active-resistive exercises.	Exercise enhances muscle strength and decreases the complications of immobility.
Instruct client and significant other(s) in correct use of mobility aids; allow time for client-controlled demonstration.	Proper utilization of aids is essential to mobility.

INTERVENTIONS	RATIONALE
Teach to avoid over-the-counter antacids which contain calcium (e.g., OS-Cal, Tums) if hyper-calcemic.	Some medications contain calcium, which may further increase hypercalcemia.
Community Health/ Home Health Evaluate and modify, as indicated, the living arrangements: 　　Toileting facilities 　　Potential household hazards (e.g., phone cords, extension cords, area rugs, waxed floors) 　　Good lighting in bedrooms, halls, closets, and particularly around the bed 　　Install handrails in bathroom 　　Non-skid flooring 　　Use of straight-backed, firm chairs—avoid use of rockers, deep soft chairs, etc.	A safe environment is a requirement for mobility.
Identify external resources to carry out mobility regimen— (e.g., stroke program, American Heart Association, National Multiple Sclerosis Society).	Client and significant others will need to have resources available.
Keep room temperature below 75°F, and avoid using hot water for bathing.	Increased body temperature will increase the metabolic rate and decrease the amount of energy available for mobility.
Evaluate, modify, and reteach gait, if indicated, including the following: 　　Slow, steady gait with feet apart providing for a wide base of support 　　Use non-skid shoes (rubber soled, firm)	Measures need to be taken which will improve quality of ambulation and prevent falls.

INTERVENTIONS

RATIONALE

Interventions	Rationale
Teach the client and family about nutritional needs to prevent complications of immobility (e.g., high protein, high fiber diet and fluids to 2000-3000 cc/da, as tolerated.	High protein foods are needed to provide for the energy requirements during ambulation. High fiber content is needed to avoid constipation (a frequent complication of immobility). Fluids are required to adequately hydrate the individual, prevent constipation, and avoid renal problems associated with higher calcium levels.
Teach to use energy-saving techniques, e.g., use a chair while showering, sit to brush hair and teeth, use an electric razor.	Energy is required for movement, and activities should be planned to allow for the greatest reserve.

REFERENCES/BIBLIOGRAPHY

Beare, P.G., & Myers, J.L. (1990). **Principles and practices of adult health nursing**. St. Louis: Mosby.

Carpenito, L.J. (1987). **Nursing diagnosis: Application to clinical practice** (2nd ed.). Philadelphia: Lippincott.

Creason, N.S. (1985). Validating the nursing diagnosis of impaired physical mobility. **Nursing Clinics of North America, 20**(4), 669.

Gordon, M. (1987). **Nursing diagnosis: Application and process** (2nd ed.). New York: McGraw-Hill.

Guyton, A.C. (1981). **Textbook of medical physiology** (6th ed.). Philadelphia: Saunders.

Jennings, M.C. (1988). **Nursing care planning guides for home health care.** Baltimore: Williams & Wilkins.

McKenry, L.M., & Salerno, E. (1989). **Mosby's pharmacology in nursing** (17th ed.). St. Louis: Mosby.

North American Nursing Diagnosis Association. **Taxonomy I** (Rev. 1990). St. Louis: NANDA.

Olson, E.V. (1967). The hazards of immobility. **American Journal of Nursing, 67**(4), 780–797.

Sundberg, M.C. (1989). **Fundamentals of nursing with clinical procedures** (2nd ed.) Boston: Jones & Bartlett.

Taylor, C., Lillis, C., & LeMone, P. (1989). **Fundamentals of nursing**. Philadelphia: Lippincott.

APPENDIX A: Suggested Code for Functional Level Classification

0	Completely independent
1	Requires use of equipment or device
2	Requires help from another person for assistance, supervision, or teaching
3	Requires help from another person and equipment or device
4	Is dependent, does not participate in activity

Code adapted by North American Nursing Diagnosis Association. **Taxonomy I.** (Rev. 1990). St. Louis: NANDA. p. 71. From Jones, E., et al. **Patient classification for long-term care: Users' manual**. HEW, Publication No. HRA-74-3107, November 1974.

Poisoning: Risk

A state in which an individual is at accentuated risk of accidental exposure to or ingestion of drugs or dangerous products in doses sufficient to cause poisoning (NANDA, 1990, p. 41).

Colleen Lucas, R.N., M.N., C.S.

RISK FACTORS

Internal

Altered drug metabolism
Cognitive or emotional difficulties
Errors in self-medication
Lack of drug and safety education
Lack of financial resources
Lack of safeguards within work setting
Multiple diseases
Reduced vision

External

Contaminated water supply
Deliberate act of war contaminating air, water, soil
Illicit drugs contaminated with poisonous additives
Inadequately processed or improperly stored food
Ingestion of poisonous vegetation
Large supplies of drugs and multiple drugs available in home
Unlocked medicine cabinets in reach of confused or emotionally unstable persons
Unprotected contact with heavy metals, chemicals, chemotherapeutic drugs
Use of paint, lacquer, etc. in poorly ventilated area

EXPECTED OUTCOMES

Client will list factors that increase the risk for poisoning.
    Internal factors that influence defensive resources are identified.
    External factors that increase poisoning risk are identified.
Client will apply safety precautions in modifying the environment to reduce risk.
    Measures to improve the safety of the environment are identified.
    Measures to improve safety are implemented.
    Effectiveness of modifications and revised actions are evaluated.
Client will remain free of poisoning.
    Hazards within the environment are reduced or nonexistent.
    There is no exposure to poisons.
    Medications are safely administered as prescribed; follow-up on side effects occurs as
        directed.
    Self-exposure is prevented through the use of protective clothing and equipment.

INTERVENTIONS	RATIONALE
Universal	
Continuously monitor the environment of the confused or emotionally disturbed for changes that increase the risk for poisoning.	In the presence of altered judgment, most environments present safety hazards. Continuous monitoring will provide early warning for need of intervention.
Advocate for environmental controls on disposal of toxic wastes and pollutants; advocate for safety standards in laws governing the licensing of institutions housing individuals with impaired judgment.	Nurses are leaders in health care and through a collective voice, shape state and national health policy, as well as setting safety standards.
Establish and enforce monitoring standards for high-risk groups (i.e., workers with chemicals, nurses administering chemotherapy, clients receiving anticoagulants).	Exposure and level of toxicity can be determined through consistent screening programs (i.e., liver function tests, urinalysis, blood work).
Keep medicine cabinets locked and medicines, chemicals, and other poisons out of reach of those with impaired judgment.	Decreasing access reduces the risk of poisoning.

INTERVENTIONS	RATIONALE
Assist in reviewing medications and discarding medications which are outdated, no longer prescribed, or no longer in use.	Discarding old medications avoids polypharmacy, overmedicating, undermedicating, and drug interactions, as well as helping to achieve the intended therapeutic response.
Set up a self-medication regimen using a daily, weekly, or other dispensing device.	A self-medication regime enhances compliance.
Teach precautions and clothing to use in preventing exposure to known poisons in the environment.	Impervious barriers prevent direct contact with poisons causing tissue trauma or absorbed through the skin; masks prevent inhalation of aerosolized or gaseous poisons.
Teach safe food preparation and storage.	Bacteria grow and form toxins in improperly stored or prepared food. County extension services provide free information on home canning and food storage. The right temperature must be reached and maintained for a prescribed amount of time in order to kill bacteria and prevent toxin production. Once correctly prepared, food must also be stored via canning, refrigeration, or freezing.
Teach safe medication use: 1. Dose, time, route, side effects 2. Read label and accurately dispense drugs, using good light 3. Storage 4. What to do if a dose is missed 5. Follow-up with MD	Knowledge of medications assists adherence to achieving safe therapeutic levels. Doubling up on missed doses and overlooking side effects can lead to poisoning.
Teach methods for protecting self and others when exposure to poisons is anticipated: 1. Follow specified instructions for disposal of chemicals, household poisons, and medications 2. Discard tainted food products	Measures for protection, when correctly followed, decrease the risk for poisoning in the presence of chemicals, gases, and other toxic substances.

INTERVENTIONS	**R**ATIONALE
3. Boil water or use special purification tablets when bacterial contamination is suspected 4. Adequately ventilate areas where paints and other chemicals are in use	
Teach how to discriminate between poisonous and non-poisonous plants.	Many outdoor (and some indoor) plants are poisonous and if mistaken for a nonpoisonous variety (e.g., berries or mushrooms), can cause severe toxicity or death.
Inpatient None	
Community Health/ Home Care None	

REFERENCES/BIBLIOGRAPHY

Davis, N.M., & Cohen, M.R. (1989). Today's poisons: How to keep them from killing your patients. **Nursing 89, 19**(1), 49–51.

Garrison, S.J., & Henson, H.K. (1990). Dilantin toxicity and vegetative depression: A report of two cases. **Archives of Physical Medicine and Rehabilitation, 71** (May), 422–23.

Gettrust, K.V., Ryan, S.C., & Engelmon, D.S. (Eds.) (1985). **Applied nursing diagnosis: Guides for comprehensive planning** (pp. 105–108). Albany, NY: Delmar.

Iobst, W.F., Bridges, C.R., & Regan-Smith, M.G. (1989). Antirheumatic agents: CNS toxicity and its avoidance. **Geriatrics, 44**(4), 95–102.

Kim, M.J., McFarland, G.K., & McLane, A.M. (1989). **Pocket guide to nursing diagnoses**. St. Louis: Mosby.

McFarland, G.K., & McFarlane, E.A. (1989). **Nursing diagnosis and intervention: Planning for patient care**. St. Louis: Mosby.

North American Nursing Diagnosis Association. **Taxonomy I** (Rev. 1990). St. Louis: NANDA.

Post-Trauma Response

A state in which an individual experiences an event outside the range of usual human experience. The event has the potential to interfere with the individual's ability to function either at the time of the event or later.

Marcia Williams, R.N., M.S.N.
Alice Kramer, R.N., B.S.N.

DEFINING CHARACTERISTICS

Avoidance

Deliberate efforts to avoid thoughts or feelings associated with the event
Deliberate efforts to shun activities or situations that arouse recollections of the event
Diminished interest in significant activities
Feeling of detachment or estrangement from others
Restricted range of affect, e.g., unable to feel love or spontaneous enjoyment
Sense of a foreshortened future

Repetitive Responses

Increased arousal symptoms, e.g., difficulty falling or staying asleep, irritability or outbursts of anger, difficulty concentrating, hypervigilance, exaggerated startle response
Intense psychological or physiologic distress at exposure to events that symbolize or resemble an aspect of the event, such as anniversary of the event
Recurrent and intrusive distressing recollection of the event
Repetitive, distressing dreams of the event
Sudden acting or feeling as if the event were recurring, which includes a sense of reliving the experience; flashback episodes; illusions; and hallucinations

CONTRIBUTING FACTORS

Pathophysiological

None

Psychosociobehavioral

Serious threat or harm to a significant other
Serious threat to one's life or physical integrity
Sudden destruction of one's home or community
Witnessing injury or death of another person
Note: The above could be a result of either natural traumatic events such as floods, earthquakes, hurricanes, epidemics or man-made traumatic events such as wars, crime, vehicular accidents, fires, industrial disasters

EXPECTED OUTCOMES

Client will integrate the traumatic event into his/her personal history and will have a renewed enthusiasm for the future.
   The traumatic event and its impact on his/her life is acknowledged.
   Willingness to participate in the recovery process is verbalized (e.g., talking or expressing through art, music, emotion, journaling).
   There is evidence of a decrease of the trauma response symptoms (e.g., flashbacks, sleeplessness, isolation, avoidance).
   Support persons and resources are identified and utilized.
   Ability to problem solve and set goals is demonstrated.
   Expressions and actions indicative of hopefulness are evidenced.

INTERVENTIONS	RATIONALE
Universal Assess the magnitude and impact of the traumatic event, including the following: 1. Determine that there has been exposure to a traumatic event 2. Evaluate the magnitude of the event (e.g., number of persons injured, duration of event)	The assumption should not be made that each person will have the same intensity or response to a given traumatic event.

INTERVENTIONS

RATIONALE

3. Assess the personal impact of the event (e.g., personal vulnerability, intolerance to suffering and carnage)

4. Determine the client's traumatic response as witnessed by health care professionals, family, and friends

---

Provide the opportunity to tell the story of the traumatic event and include the following:

1. Provide a safe, quiet, private environment. Retelling of the event may be extremely distressing

2. Evaluate the need for a family/friend to be present for support during the retelling. It is for the client to choose whether or not to involve significant others

3. Utilize active listening skills, i.e., open-ended questions, expressions of empathy, nonhurried approach

4. Allow client to proceed at own pace

5. Acknowledge the impact of the event for the client

6. Acknowledge feelings that surface during this phase, but do not dwell on the feelings

Telling the story recreates the experience and is the first step in the recovery process known as debriefing. It is optimal to provide debriefing within 48 hours to one week post-event. Defenses which are high the first 24–48 hours tend to relax, allowing interventions to be more effective.

INTERVENTIONS

Guide to re-experience the emotions felt before, during, and immediately after the traumatic event. (Note: Although we encourage the exploration of feelings as part of recovery, clients are never forced to reexperience feelings or details against their will. Denial/avoidance, especially earlier in recovery, is often an important protective mechanism.) Include the following:

1. Help to focus on the feelings associated with the event

2. Discuss further the feelings that surfaced with the original telling of the story of the traumatic event

3. Normalize the feelings and give permission for their expression. Expression of homicidal or suicidal thoughts require immediate mental health evaluation

4. Be alert to emotional escalation that may result in feelings of loss of control or panic. By remaining calm and maintaining a quiet environment, the client will be helped to regain control

5. Help to understand the link between the event and current emotional response (e.g., anger, depression, anxiety)

RATIONALE

Many powerful emotions (e.g., rage, fear, guilt, shame) result from a traumatic event. If these emotions do not surface, they could have detrimental effects on the mental and physical health of the client.

INTERVENTIONS

RATIONALE

Evaluate coping strategies, including the following:

1. Identify the coping strategies used during and since the event (e.g., exercise, rest, alcohol, drugs)

2. Help identify past successful strategies

3. Recognize and support religious and cultural values in dealing with the event

4. Identify level of hopefulness toward the future

5. Identify the quality and quantity of support available

6. Identify willingness to access available support systems

7. Identify symptoms associated with the traumatic event

8. Identify the presence and extent of repetition and avoidance responses (see "Defining Characteristics")

9. Evaluate for psychosomatic responses such as headache, GI symptoms, muscular aches. (Note: Psychosomatic responses are legitimate health changes resulting from high-level or long-term stress.)

10. Determine any significant change in mentality, daily activities or relationship interactions

11. Evaluate the presence of ineffective coping strategies as evidenced in the severity of symptoms

The quality and quantity of coping strategies used will determine the speed and extent of recovery.

INTERVENTIONS	RATIONALE
Provide education for client and significant others, including the following: 1. Help to understand the relationship between coping strategies and responses/symptoms 2. Discuss the importance of selecting effective, nonharmful coping strategies over ineffective strategies that may have been used in the past 3. Identify characteristics of hopefulness and steps to be taken in response 4. Normalize the post-trauma response to the significant others 5. Discuss possible future post-trauma responses and effective coping strategies 6. Identify community resources that would be available 7. Convey that time and effort will be needed to integrate the traumatic event into personal history	In crisis, fear of the unknown can create resistance to healing. Education provides the realistic information about the traumatic event, which will reduce alarm and allow the client and significant others to work together toward recovery.
Prepare for reentry phase, including the following: 1. Help identify a companion if client is unable to stay home alone 2. Assist in planning a telephone network strategy for support on difficult days 3. Rehearse response to invasive questioning by the curious 4. Help the client who is willing to be involved with the media	The purpose of the reentry phase is to ready the client to face life without the constant availability of professional support.

INTERVENTIONS	RATIONALE
to better understand the possible outcome of such action. (Note: Clients may be eager to give interviews without being aware of the emotional impact that results from the exposure.) 5. Evaluate willingness to access community resources 6. Identify resource people to contact who have also experienced this or similar traumatic events 7. Identify available community professionals who can assist if problems persist or resurface	

Inpatient

INTERVENTIONS	RATIONALE
Assess for repetitive responses and/or avoidance behaviors.	Nightmares, flashbacks, and hypervigilance may be indicators of continued trauma.
Evaluate ability to interact with staff and others.	Avoidance behavior may be a coping strategy.
Evaluate the need for an advanced nurse practitioner or psychiatric consult.	A consultant may be necessary for assisting in problem solving and intervention; however, the primary nurse must take steps to insure that the care remains holistic and does not become fragmented.
Evaluate the impact of the traumatic event on ability to resume life (e.g., ability to return fully to work, marital harmony, resumption of activities of daily living[ADL]).	The potential exists that the greater the physical injury, the less ability there may be to deal immediately with the emotional aspects of the traumatic event.
Evaluate readiness and ability to learn.	People in crisis or in post-trauma recovery have decreased concentration and learning ability.
Provide a quiet environment.	A calm, unhurried approach will decrease the likelihood of a startle response.

INTERVENTIONS	RATIONALE
Maximize the number of hours of uninterrupted rest and/or sleep and note presence of restlessness or intrusive dreams.	The quantity and quality of sleep may be interrupted by the impact of the traumatic event.
Initiate follow-up referrals as indicated.	Referral to home care agency, support group, or individual/family counseling may be warranted to assist post discharge.
Community Health/ Home Care Assess for repetitive responses and/or avoidance behaviors that can be observed in community setting.	Nightmares; flashbacks; diminished interest in significant activities at home, work, or school may be indicators of continued trauma.
Assess ability to care for self, perform parenting responsibilities, and attend to home/work duties.	Evaluating for evidence of proper diet, cleanliness, and order of environment; care of children, pets, etc. will indicate how effective coping strategies are.
Assess for safety hazards which may result from the following: 1. Sleep deprivation—may result in decreased ability to operate industrial machinery, make critical decisions, drive a car, etc. 2. Flashbacks—may result in interrupted concentration or mood swings that can affect both work and home environment 3. Startle response—loud, unexpected noises may affect job performance	People experiencing stress, especially after a traumatic event, are at increased risk for injury because of their potential for sleep deprivation, loss of concentration, and impaired ability to make decisions.
Assess the significant other's ability and willingness to be involved.	Effective recovery occurs more often when a support system is available.

INTERVENTIONS	**R**ATIONALE
Evaluate for compliance with follow-up care.	Post-trauma response support groups, individual therapy, and keeping physician's appointments will aid in the recovery process.

REFERENCES/BIBLIOGRAPHY

American Psychiatric Association. (1987). **Diagnostic and statistical manual of mental disorders** (Third Edition, revised). Washington, D.C.: American Psychiatric Association.

*Carpenito, L.J. (1989). **Nursing diagnosis: Application to clinical practice** (3rd ed.). (pp. 574–580). Philadelphia: Lippincott.

Doenges, M., & Moorhouse, M. (1988). **Nursing diagnosis with interventions** (2nd ed.). (269–275). Philadelphia: Davis.

Jones, D.R. (1985). Secondary disaster victims: The emotional effects of recovering & identifying human remains. **American Journal of Psychiatry, 142(3)**, 303–307.

Mitchell, J. (1987). Effective stress control at major incidents. **Maryland Fire & Rescue Bulletin, 9**(6).

Mitchell, J. (1988). Stress: Development and functions of a critical incident stress debriefing team. **Journal of Emergency Medicine, 13(12)** 43–46.

North American Nursing Diagnosis Association. **Taxonomy I** (Rev. 1990). St. Louis: NANDA.

*Rubin, J.C. (1990). Critical incident stress debriefing: Helping the helpers. **Journal of Emergency Nursing, 16**(4), 255–258.

Williams, T. (Ed.). (1987). **Post traumatic stress disorders: A handbook for clinicians**. (19–31). Cincinnati: Disabled American Veterans National Headquarters.

Powerlessness

A state in which there is a perception that one's own action will not significantly affect an outcome; a perceived lack of control over a current situation or immediate happening (NANDA, 1990, p. 95).

Lynda Slimmer, Ph.D., R.N.

DEFINING CHARACTERISTICS

Apathy/passivity
Dependence on others that may result in irritability, resentment, anger, guilt, or depressed affect
Expressions of doubt, dissatisfaction, or frustration regarding ability or inability to perform
      expected activities
Nonparticipation in care or decision making
Reluctance to express true feelings, fearing alienation from others
Verbal expression of having no control over situations, outcomes, or self-care

CONTRIBUTING FACTORS

Pathophysiological

Illness-related loss of control over physical or mental integrity

Psychosociobehavioral

Experience or perception of failure
Interpersonal relationships which include consistent negative feedback/no positive feedback
Life-style of helplessness, resulting from difficulty accomplishing developmental tasks and a weak
      identity
Loss of significant other beyond one's control and incomplete grief work
Nongrowth-promoting health care environment which fosters dependency beyond physical and
      mental needs

EXPECTED OUTCOMES

Client will demonstrate increased control over activities and situations.

Situations are identified in which powerlessness is felt.

Controllable and uncontrollable situations and outcomes are discriminated.

Acceptance of situations and outcomes over which one does not have control are verbalized.

Realistic goals are set, and alternative behaviors to increase control are tried.

Independent problem-solving behavior occurs.

Decisions are made related to care, and active involvement in care is evident.

Appropriate role functioning and coping skills are demonstrated.

Mood is appropriate.

Assertive behaviors in interpersonal interactions are used.

Positive feelings regarding ability to perform ADLs is verbalized.

An increased sense of control over present situations and future outcomes is verbalized.

INTERVENTIONS	RATIONALE
Universal	
Assess when feelings of loss of control began.	The identification of contributing factors and stressful events related to powerlessness provides direction for intervention.
Assess what situations cause feelings of powerlessness.	The appropriate planning of interventions is dependent on knowing if the perception of powerlessness is limited and situational or global.
Assess locus of control.	Interventions are more directive when the locus of control is external.
Assess for attempts to regain control.	Present ability to regain control is dependent on the recall of what has been effective and ineffective in the past.
Assess for symptoms of depression and make referrals if needed.	A perception of powerlessness can lead to clinical depression requiring medical intervention.
Establish a therapeutic and facilitative relationship.	A safe environment allows for the expression of feelings, the practicing of new behaviors, the feeling of being understood and accepted.

INTERVENTIONS	RATIONALE
Facilitate expression of feelings through therapeutic communication skills, i.e., active listening, reflection, paraphrasing; and provision of opportunities to express feelings in nonverbal ways, i.e., writing, drawing, physical exercise.	Expression of feelings releases anxiety that contributes to the perception of powerlessness, and initially the nonverbal expression may be less difficult.
Seek input in decisions about care.	Demonstrating that personal choices are available decreases feelings of loss of control.
Modify the environment to facilitate an active role in care.	The perception of powerlessness causes an assumption that an internal, personal limitation is responsible for the inability to perform self-care. Modification of the environment demonstrates that the problem may be external and serves to increase the perception of abilities.
Be directive in involvement in care, gradually adding new activities.	Powerlessness leads to lack of desire to be involved; a directive approach increases participation if there is a belief that action will result in failure. If, however, the nonparticipation is a rational, conscious choice, control is being exhibited and force only serves to increase the perception of loss of control.
Encourage risk-taking situations in which there can be success.	Reaching beyond a minimal level of achievement increases self-confidence and decreases the perception of powerlessness.
Offer feedback on appropriateness of goals set to regain control.	Unrealistic goals set one up for failure and reinforce the perception of powerlessness.
Provide positive feedback for constructive methods to regain control.	Positive feedback reinforces the behavior, increases self-confidence, and decreases the perception of powerlessness.
Discuss causes of difficulty in making needs known, and fears about expressing true feelings.	Feelings of powerlessness increase when one does not assert needs or passively accepts directives. Awareness is the first step toward change.
Use cognitive therapy techniques to modify perceptions of loss/failure.	The aim of cognitive therapy is to monitor the prevalence of negative self-talk and to assist the reality testing of self-deprecatory thoughts.

INTERVENTIONS	RATIONALE
Help to find alternative roles and interests.	Acquiring new roles and interests increases self-esteem and the perception of control if physical or mental impairments have caused actual loss of control over past roles and activities.
Counsel family members to increase sensitivity to client's imposed loss of control.	In an attempt to be caring, families may foster dependence, which serves to increase the perception of powerlessness.
Teach how to discriminate between controllable and uncontrollable situations.	Perceptions of personal weakness decrease with the recognition that some situations are intrinsically and universally outside control.
Teach decision making/problem solving/coping skills.	Adding to the repertoire of behaviors that facilitates control of self and the environment decreases the possibility of the return of the perception of powerlessness.
Use role playing to teach assertive communication skills.	Assertive behavior facilitates control of self and the environment. Behavior reversal is an effective way to learn new behaviors.
Provide information about the illness and treatment plan.	Knowledge decreases fear of the unknown and the perception of powerlessness over the unknown.
Inpatient Be sensitive to and limit incidents and institutional policies that induce powerlessness, i.e., medical jargon, rigid schedules.	Powerlessness is often a response to a non-growth-promoting health care environment that fosters dependency beyond what is necessary.
Avoid a paternalistic approach.	Making decisions for the client fosters the sense of loss of control even when it is done in an attempt to be caring.
Encourage a collaborative relationship when planning and implementing care.	Collaboration increases the belief that control is not being taken away.
Explain treatment procedures.	Knowledge about the purpose and schedule of treatments decreases the perception of unpredictability and the development of the perception of powerlessness.

INTERVENTIONS	RATIONALE
Reinforce the right to ask questions.	Information decreases the fear of the unknown and the perception of powerlessness over the unknown. Nonassertiveness needs reassurance that the environment is a safe place to ask questions.
Community Health/ Home Care	
Encourage family members to allow independent role activities within abilities.	In an attempt to be caring, family members may foster dependence, which serves to increase the perception of powerlessness.
Support involvement in community self-help groups.	Self-help groups provide both the empathy and supportive confrontation that is necessary to counter negative cognitions not reality based.

REFERENCES/BIBLIOGRAPHY

Abramson, L., Seligman, M., & Teasdale, J. (1978). Learned helplessness in humans: Critique and reformulation. **Journal of Abnormal Psychology, 87**(1), 49–74.

Doenges, M., & Moorhouse, M. (1988). **Nursing diagnoses with interventions** (2nd ed.). Philadelphia: Davis.

Doenges, M., Townsend, M., & Moorhouse, M. (1989). **Psychiatric care plans: Guidelines for client care**. Philadelphia: Davis.

Kim, M., McFarland, G., & McLane, A. (1989). **Pocket guide to nursing diagnoses** (3rd ed.). St. Louis: Mosby.

*LeSage, J., Slimmer, L., Lopez, M., & Ellor, J. (1989). Learned helplessness experienced by the elderly in long-term care. **Journal of Gerontological Nursing, 15**(5), 9–15.

McFarland, G., & McFarlane, E. (1989). **Nursing diagnosis and intervention: Planning for patient care**. St. Louis: Mosby.

McFarland, G., & Wasli, E. (1986). **Nursing diagnosis and process in psychiatric mental health nursing**. Philadelphia: Lippincott.

North American Nursing Diagnosis Association. **Taxonomy I** (Rev. 1990). St. Louis: NANDA.

*Slimmer, L., LeSage, J., Lopez, M., & Ellor, J. (1990). Helping those who don't help themselves. **Geriatric Nursing, 11**(1), 20–22.

*Slimmer, L., Lopez, M., LeSage, J., & Ellor, J. (1987). Perceptions of learned helplessness. **Journal of Gerontological Nursing, 13**(5), 33–37.

Stuart, G., & Sundeen, S. (1987). **Principles and practice of psychiatric nursing** (3rd ed.). St. Louis: Mosby.

Townsend, M. (1988). **Nursing diagnoses in psychiatric nursing: Pocket guide for care plan construction**. Philadelphia: Davis.

Protection, Altered

A state in which an individual experiences a decrease in the ability to guard the self from internal or external threats such as illness, infection, or injury (NANDA, 1990, p. 45).

Joan T. Harkulich, R.N., M.S.N.

DEFINING CHARACTERISTICS

Altered clotting
Anorexia
Chilling
Cough
Deficient immunity
Dementia
Disorientation
Dyspnea
Fatigue
Immobility
Impaired healing

Insomnia
Itching
Maladaptive stress response
Neurosensory alterations
Night sweats
Perspiring
Predisposition to infections
Pressure sores
Restlessness
Weakness
Weight loss

CONTRIBUTING FACTORS

Pathophysiological

Abnormal blood profiles (e.g., leukopenia, thrombocytopenia)
Acute phase of an illness or condition (e.g., onset of pneumonia or urinary tract infection 24–48 hours postpartum, 24–48 hours postsurgery, 24–48 hours after hospital admission)
Advanced age
Chronic illness (e.g., multiple sclerosis, diabetes mellitus, anemias, chronic obstructive lung disease)
Critical illness (e.g., renal disease, leukemias, AIDS)
Drug therapy (e.g., antineoplastic drugs, corticosteroids)

Inadequate nutrition
Mental retardation
Presence of foreign bodies in system (e.g., transplant, catheter, tracheostomy)
Treatments (e.g., chemotherapy, radiation)

Psychosociobehavioral

History of alcoholism
History of drug misuse and/or abuse
Homelessness

EXPECTED OUTCOMES

Client will exhibit no signs or symptoms of additional illness, infections, or injuries.
　　Health practices are listed which are to be used to ward off infections, illness, or injury.
　　Hazards in the environment are identified and eliminated.
　　"Safe sex" is practiced.
　　Physician is notified of any unusual symptoms.
　　Medical and nursing appointments are kept.
　　Medication, nutrition, and nursing regimes are understood and adhered to closely.
　　Universal Precautions, when necessary, are understood and practiced.

INTERVENTIONS | RATIONALE

Universal	
Assess for the risk of falling.	Bruised or broken bones, torn ligaments and tendons, as well as other problems, compromise the protective ability.
Assess for deep vein thromboses (cramping, positive Homan's sign, and/or pain in the calf).	Thrombi can occur in clients with anemia or other abnormal blood profiles. Care must be taken to prevent pulmonary emboli.
Assess the prothrombin time (PT) as well as the medication regime during anticoagulation therapy.	Keeping the PT within normal limits poses a problem to nurses. It is important to be aware of potential drug interactions that prolong PT (e.g., glucogon, antibiotics) and shorten PT (e.g., antacids, barbituates.)
Assess clients at risk for decubitis ulcer formation.	Assessing general physical condition, level of consciousness, activity, mobility, incontinence, and nutrition will supply the nurses with risk factors and allow nurses to implement preventative care.

INTERVENTIONS	RATIONALE
Employ Universal Precautions.	These precautions will protect both care givers and other clients from infections.
Manage problems with nausea and vomiting. Make suggestions such as: eat small meals often, avoid greasy foods, eat dry foods like toast or crackers, drink liquids one-half hour to one hour before meals, try cold entrees, rest after meals with upper body elevated, and replace vomited foods and electrolytes with ginger ale, juice, broths, or bouillon.	These practices will decrease weight and electrolyte loss and prevent opportunity for illness.
Incorporate a mild exercise program into the regimen of the chronically ill.	Exercise will encourage physical fitness and positive feelings about self.
Apply creams, lotions, and soaps and shampoos for dry skin.	Dry skin can increase the likelihood of skin breakdown. The application of moisturizing agents will diminish dry skin.
Use artificial tears if problems exist producing liquid from the lacrimal glands.	Use of eye drops provides moisture and prevents irritation and the potential for infection.
Catheterize intermittently rather than placing an indwelling urinary catheter, whenever possible.	Intermittent catheterization decreases the risk of infection because of the limited amount of time in the urethra and bladder.
Educate to the importance of closely adhering to the prescribed medication regimen and avoid the introduction of over-the-counter medications or alcohol without physician approval.	Drug therapy is a frequently used mode of treatment. The introduction of other medications and/or alcohol could cause drug/drug or drug/alcohol interactions.
Educate the homeless to the availability of free clinics and other agencies within the community.	Because of poor eating and health habits, as well as exposure to the elements, the homeless are susceptible to many chronic illnesses and infections.

INTERVENTIONS	RATIONALE
Educate those with neurosensory alterations of potential hazards and safety measures to be taken.	Because of diminished sensation, care must be taken when, e.g., ambulating, performing foot care, and working around stoves and hot oil.

Inpatient

INTERVENTIONS	RATIONALE
Assess for headaches, change in level of consciousness, impaired communication skills, or visual disturbances.	These symptoms could indicate neurological changes, e.g., intracranial bleed or other problem.
Assess clients who have a foreign substance within the body (e.g., tracheostomy, A/V fistula graft) for signs and symptoms of infection or rejection.	Detecting indications of infection or rejection early in the process provides an opportunity for immediate action to treat it.
Monitor clients receiving invasive therapies for weight loss, skin irritation, change in vital signs, or other indications of complications.	Prompt intervention will prevent/limit complications.
Use a safety alert sticker on the chart and care plan, and over the bed.	A notice will draw attention to the staff that client is at risk for falls.
Remove soiled linens and other articles frequently from the client's environment.	Soiled material can be a carrier of contaminants.
Initiate an infection control reporting form.	Tracking infections will alert staff of clients who are at greatest risk or need special care.
Place at risk client in reverse isolation.	Greater protection from infection can be provided when susceptible clients are separated from others.
Encourage coughing and deep breathing exercises.	Respiratory passages will clear and complications will be avoided.
Educate client and family members about Universal Precautions.	The spread of infection can be prevented if safeguards are taken.

INTERVENTIONS	**R**ATIONALE
Community Health/ Home Care	
Assess the general health of the client and family with careful attention to the primary caregiver.	Primary care givers frequently experience fatigue, exhaustion, and sleep deprivation, making them more vulnerable to illness.
Use a home safety assessment tool.	A careful assessment will help point out safety practices to decrease the likelihood of injury.
Educate families of older adults about risk factors which might produce falls (e.g., loose mats, electric cords in walkways, footpath irregularities, steps, change in position, medications which may impair judgment, overuse of restraints, absence of a rubber mat in the bath tub, and absence of grab rails in the bathroom).	Alerted family members may be able to prevent falls in the home.
Educate to the importance of good personal hygiene, drinking adequate amount of fluids, eating a well-balanced diet, exercising, and avoiding contact with people with infectious diseases.	A healthy life-style will lower the chances of succumbing to illness.
Educate the sexually active about safe sexual practices.	Knowledge about the mode of transmission of infection may prevent its spread.
Suggest use of respite care or day care if available in the community.	Respite care can provide relief for a primary care giver and allow time to take care of own physical and emotional needs.

REFERENCES/BIBLIOGRAPHY

Berne, A.S., Dato, C., Mason, D.J., & Rafferty, M. (1990). A nursing model for addressing the health needs of homeless families. **Image**, 22(1), 8–13.

Calkins, M.P., Namazi, K.H., Rosner, T.T., Olson, A., & Brabender, B. (1990). **Home modifications: Responding to dementia**. Chardon, OH: Heather Hill.

* Campbell, A.J., Borrie, M.J., Spears, G.F., Jackson, S.L., Brown, J.S., & Fitzgerald, J.L. (1990). Circumstances and consequences of falls by a community population 70 years and over during a prospective study. **Age and Ageing, 19**, 136–141.

Campbell, E.B., Williams, M.A., & Mlynarczyk, S.M. (1986). After the fall—Confusion. **American Journal of Nursing, 86**(2), 151–154.

Froberg, J.H. (1989). The Anemias: Causes and courses of action. **RN**, May, 42–49.

Gallagher, M.T., & Wyland, N.L. (1986). Leukemia: When white cells run wild. **RN**, November, 33–39.

Herbelin, K., & McElroy, D. (1990). Infection control under OBRA '87. **Contemporary Long-Term Care, 13**(2), 60–62.

Higgins, L.B. (1990). New Medicare/Medicaid requirements. **Contemporary Long-Term Care, 13**(3), 63–64.

* Holman, R.C., et al. (1990). Age and human immunodeficiency virus infection in persons with hemophilia in California. **American Journal of Public Health, 80**(8), 967–969.

Krokosky, N.J., & Vanscoy, G.J. (1989). Running an anticoagulation clinic. **American Journal of Nursing, 89**(10), 1304–1306.

North American Nursing Diagnosis Association. **Taxonomy I** (Rev. 1990). St. Louis: NANDA.

Olson, E.V. (1990). The hazards of immobility. **American Journal of Nursing, 90**(3), 43–49.

Parsons, M.T, & Levy, J. (1987). Nursing process in injury prevention. **Journal of Gerontological Nursing, 13**(7), 36–40.

Plawecki, H.M., Brewer, S., & Plawecki, J.A. (1987). Chronic renal failure. **Journal of Gerontological Nursing, 13**(12), 14–17.

Pritchard, V. (1988). Geriatric infections: The urinary tract. **RN**, May 36–38.

Snyder, T.E. (1989). An exercise program for dialysis patients. **American Journal of Nursing, 89**(3), 362–364.

Spellbring, A.M., Gannon, M.E., Klecker, T, & Conway, K. (1988). Improving safety for hospitalized elderly. **Journal of Gerontological Nursing, 14**(2), 31–37.

Taber, J. (1989). Nutrition in HIV infection. **American Journal of Nursing, 89**(11), 1446–1456.

Teutsch, E., & Hill, M. (1987). Sjogren's syndrome—Adding moisture to your life. **American Journal of Nursing, 87**(3), 326–329.

* Thorne, S.E., & Robinson, C.A. (1989). Guarded alliance: Health care relationships in chronic illness. **Image, 21**(3) 153–157.

Tideiksaar, R. (1989). Home safe home. **Geriatric Nursing, 10**(6), 280–284.

Tynan, C., & Cardea, J.M. (1987). Home health hazard assessments. **Journal of Gerontological Nursing, 13**(10), 25–27.

* Ward, M.C., Gundroo, R.J., Bailey, R.J., Mehta, T.V., & Vallon, A.G. (1990). Effect of investigation on the management of elderly patients with iron deficiency anaemia. A**ge and Ageing, 19**(3), 204–206.

Whedon, M.B., & Shedd, P. (1989). Prediction and prevention of patient falls. **Image, 21**(2), 108–114.

* Wineman, N.M. (1990). Adaption to multiple sclerosis: The role of social support, functional disability, and perceived uncertainty. **Nursing Research, 39**(5), 294–299.

Woods, N.F., Yates, B.C., & Primono, J. (1989). Supporting families during chronic illness. **Image, 21**(1), 46–50.

* Wright, B.A., Aizenstein, S., Vogler, G., Rowe, M., & Miller, C. (1990). Frequent fallers. **Journal of Gerontological Nursing, 16**(4), 15–19.

Rape-Trauma Syndrome

A state in which a survivor responds behaviorally, cognitively, emotionally, and physically to an act of sexual violence. There is an acute phase of disorganization and a longer phase of reorganization. (Note: In most of the current literature on rape and treatment thereof, the term survivor is used in place of the term client. That terminology is used here.)

Carrol A.M. Smith, R.N., M.S.

DEFINING CHARACTERISTICS

Acute Phase

Anger
Anxiety
Calm and subdued affect (occasionally)
Crying
Disruption of sexual functioning
Embarrassment
Fatigue
Fear
Feelings of helplessness
Gastrointestinal irritability
Genitourinary disturbances (including
        pregnancy and/or sexually
        transmitted diseases)

Inability to make decisions
Physical trauma
Restlessness
Self-blame
Shock and disbelief
Skeletal muscle tension
Sleep pattern disturbances
Tension headaches
Thoughts of revenge
Withdrawal from usual social contact

Long-term Reorganization Phase

Change in appearance
Continued anxiety and fear

452

Depression

Increased motor activity, i.e., changing residence, travelling, changing phone number

CONTRIBUTING FACTORS

Pathophysiological

Current physical status, i.e., concurrent acute or chronic illness, handicapping conditions

Psychosociobehavioral

Age

Circumstances of the rape

Cultural beliefs concerning sexuality and
    sexual assault

Current and past stressors

Developmental level

Gender

Personal values and attitudes

Sexual orientation

EXPECTED OUTCOMES

Survivor will integrate role as a survivor of sexual assault and function at appropriate developmental, physical, and psychosociobehavioral levels.

Freedom from medical and physical symptoms and complications of sexual assault is experienced.

Decreased levels of acute-phase emotional responses such as anxiety, guilt, lack of trust are demonstrated.

Situational support from health care professionals, educated volunteers, and family and personal social network is received.

Suicidal ideation and dependence on alcohol or drugs as a coping mechanism is not present.

Behaviors consistent with mastery of feelings of fear and powerlessness is demonstrated.

INTERVENTIONS	RATIONALE
Universal	
Evaluate and document general condition and specific needs immediately.	Individual treatment based on the physical and emotional symptoms during the acute phase are crucial to long-term recovery.
Provide counseling and support by specially prepared personnel.	Needs are best met by caretakers who know the symptoms and phases of rape-trauma syndrome and who will provide the kind of specific short- and long-term intervention necessary for resolution of the trauma. Effective coping is promoted through counseling.

INTERVENTIONS	**R**ATIONALE
Provide health teaching and anticipatory guidance specific to the situation.	Survivors must know the legal, physical, and emotional consequences of sexual assault in order to take an active part in making choices for self-care. Anticipatory guidance provides preparation for unexpected reactions in self, significant others, and friends, as well as for the chain of events if charges are pressed against the perpetrator.
Demonstrate acceptance of any affect displayed.	Survivor affects can range from calm and subdued to crying, anger, and disbelief. These affects are dependent upon survivor coping skills, **not** on the believability of the rape report.
Inpatient (Emergency Room Care) Secure a complete history and provide thorough physical examination.	The history and physical are necessary for evaluation of injury and potential for pregnancy in the female. The physical examination also includes evidence collection, which may be used if charges are pressed.
Assess level of fear and coping abilities prior to discharge.	The survivor, unless seriously battered, will need to face leaving the protection of the emergency care setting. Immediate, overwhelming fears may prevent even simple self-care upon discharge.
Provide tests for sexually transmitted disease.	The sexual assault can result in transmission of any of the sexually transmittable diseases including human immunodeficiency virus.
Offer prophylactic medications and postcoital contraception with appropriate counseling.	An understanding of the sequelae of the prophylaxis and post-coital contraception is essential in order to make an informed choice.
Inform of legal rights and obtain informed consents for all procedures.	Informed persons, even at times of great stress, can be assisted in taking action in behalf of themselves, which enhances compliance, decreases feelings of powerlessness, and ultimately fosters recovery.

INTERVENTIONS	RATIONALE
Provide privacy for all immediate crisis care activities.	Vulnerability is extreme immediately post-trauma. An environment which shields from any further trauma by unfeeling bystanders, and has an ambiance in which fears, anxieties, and concerns may be expressed without fear of rejection or criticism, decreases feelings of vulnerability.
Help to recover a sense of control and empowerment (allow choices to be made regarding care, etc.).	The assailant renders most survivors powerless by the very act of sexual assault. Any means which can help to regain feelings of a sense of control and empowerment fosters resolution of the acute phase.
Listen carefully to the account of the assault.	Nonjudgmental listening to the full description of the event provides a necessary catharsis.
Assist in identifying whom to notify about the assault for assistance and support.	Skilled support personnel help the survivor to be protected as much as possible from having to deal with negative reactions from others in the immediate acute phase.
Assist with necessary referrals and follow-up information.	Anxiety and extreme stress require repeated verbal and written information to facilitate follow-through.
Community Health/ Home Care Provide follow-up telephone calls.	Coping abilities are enhanced when continuity is provided by initial caretaking system.
Provide or refer for long-term counseling.	Eventual integration of the significant life event and reorganization of life patterns depend on the ability to work through the memories and sequelae of the assault with a qualified counselor.
Complete follow-up care for sexually transmitted diseases (STD) or pregnancy.	The physical sequelae of STD/pregnancy require resolution for a return to overall health.

INTERVENTIONS	**R**ATIONALE
Refer for education in self-defense and other deterrent tactics.	Increased feelings of safety and sense of power are experienced when specific tactics are learned that could be used in behalf of the self.
Provide public education regarding sexual assault.	Myths about sexual assault and the criminal justice system must be dispelled in order to increase public awareness and concern for the needs of survivors.

REFERENCES/BIBLIOGRAPHY

Bourque, L.D. (1989). **Defining rape**. Durham, NC & London: Duke University Press.

Brownmiller, S. (1975). **Against our will: Men, women and rape**. New York: Simon & Schuster.

*Burgess, A.W. (Ed.). (1985). **Rape and sexual assault; A research handbook**. New York: Garland.

*Burgess, A.W., & Holmstrom, L.L. (1974). Rape trauma syndrome. **American Journal of Psychiatry, 131**(9), 981–986.

*Burgess, A.W., & Holmstrom, L.L. (1979). Adaptive strategies and recovery from rape. **American Journal of Psychiatry, 136**(10), 1278–1283.

*Burgess, A.W., Jacobsen, B., Thompson, J.E., Baker, T., & Grant, C.A. (1990). HIV testing of sexual assault populations: Ethical and legal issues. **Journal of Emergency Nursing, 16**(5), 331–8.

Dennis, L.I. (1988). Adolescent rape: The role of nursing. **Comprehensive Pediatric Nursing, 11**, 59–70.

*Gise, L.H., & Paddison, P. (1988). Rape, sexual abuse and its victims. **Psychiatric Clinics of North America, 11**(4), 629–648.

Kim, M.J., McFarland, G.K., & McLane, A.M. (1991). **Pocket guide to nursing diagnoses** (4th ed.). St. Louis: Mosby.

Ledray, L.E. (1986). **Recovering from rape**. New York: Henry Holt.

Ledray, L.E. (1990). Counseling rape victims: The nursing challenge. **Perspectives in Psychiatric Care, 26**(2), 21–26.

McFarland, G.K., & McFarlane, E.A. (1989). **Nursing diagnosis and intervention: Planning for patient care**. St. Louis: Mosby.

Minden, P. (1989). The victim care service: A program for victims of sexual assault. **Archives of Pediatric Nursing, 3**(1), 41–46.

Warshaw, R. (1988). **I never called it rape: The Ms. report on recognizing, fighting, and surviving date and acquaintance rape**. New York: Harper & Row.

Rape-Trauma Syndrome: Compound Reaction

A state in which the survivor of a sexual assault has either a past or current history of additional physical, psychiatric, or social difficulties.

Carrol A.M. Smith, R.N., M.S.

DEFINING CHARACTERISTICS

Same as for Rape-Trauma Syndrome with the following additions:
- Psychiatric illness
- Reliance on alcohol or drugs
- Suicidal ideation or self-destructive behavior

CONTRIBUTING FACTORS

Pathophysiological

Current symptoms of a pathophysiological condition of any kind

Psychosociobehavioral

Financial difficulties
History of psychiatric illness
Inability to handle stress
Multiple prior losses (especially in elderly)
Presence of Rape-Trauma Syndrome

EXPECTED OUTCOMES

Same as for Rape-Trauma Syndrome with the additional short-term goals:
- Freedom from harm to self or others is experienced.
- Physical problems are not increased.

457

INTERVENTIONS	RATIONALE
Universal Same as for Rape Trauma Syndrome with the following addition: Assume a secondary position to other health care providers with whom survivor may already be in treatment.	Working closely with other agencies/providers allows for support without interfering with previously designed treatment modalities. Interference could cause disruption or regression.
Inpatient Same as for Rape Trauma Syndrome.	
Community Health/ Home Care Same as for Rape Trauma Syndrome with the following additions: Assess periodically for suicidal or homicidal ideation, as well as other aggressive or self-destructive behavior.	Periodic assessment allows for early intervention.
Assess periodically for physical symptoms.	Physical symptoms may become exacerbated and need to be treated as soon as possible.

REFERENCES/BIBLIOGRAPHY

See "Rape-Trauma Syndrome."

Rape-Trauma Syndrome: Silent Reaction

A state in which a survivor suffers the sequelae of sexual assault without help, because the assault is never reported to anyone. A psychological burden results from the unsettled feelings and reactions which are the same as in "Rape Trauma Syndrome." Any subsequent life event may reactivate the trauma syndrome.

Carrol A.M. Smith, R.N., M.S.

DEFINING CHARACTERISTICS

Same as for Rape-Trauma Syndrome with the following additions:
> Avoidance of relationships with significant sexual other
> Dreams of violence and/or nightmares
> Increasing anxiety during interview, i.e., stuttering, silence, blocking of associations
> Marked change in sexual behavior
> No discussion of the sexual assault
> Sudden onset of phobic reactions

CONTRIBUTING FACTORS

Pathophysiological

Same as for Rape-Trauma Syndrome

Psychosociobehavioral

Same as for Rape-Trauma Syndrome with the following additions:
> Denial
> Fear of ridicule or not being believed
> Intense shame, embarrassment, guilt, self-blame
> Knowing the assailant
> Lack of understanding and confusion about what has occurred

Perceived lack of emotional support
Protection of loved ones or of "male image"

EXPECTED OUTCOMES

Same as for Rape-Trauma Syndrome.

INTERVENTIONS

RATIONALE

Universal Provide counseling and support by specially prepared personnel.	The needs of the survivor are best met by caretakers who know the symptoms and phases of rape trauma syndrome and who will provide the kind of specific short- and long-term intervention necessary for resolution of the trauma. Counseling must be made available to promote effective coping.
Inpatient (None, unless the silent reaction is discovered at the time of a subsequent sexual assault; at that time the inpatient interventions would be the same as for Rape Trauma Syndrome.)	
Community Health/ Home Care Same as in Rape Trauma Syndrome with the following addition: Pay special attention to assisting survivor in determining reasons for initial silence.	In order to achieve resolution of the assault, part of that resolution includes dealing with factors underlying the initial silence.

REFERENCES/BIBLIOGRAPHY

See "Rape-Trauma Syndrome."

Relocation Stress

A state in which an individual experiences physiological and/or psychological disturbances as a result of a transfer from one environment to another.

Christine Brugler, R.N., M.S.N.
Joan T. Harkulich, R.N., M.S.N.

DEFINING CHARACTERISTICS

Anger
Anxiety
Apprehension
Change in behavior (confusion, disorientation, negativism)
Change in eating patterns
Change in sleep patterns
Demonstration and verbalization of dependency
Demonstration and verbalization of insecurity in new living situation
Demonstration and verbalization of lack of trust in staff
Depression
Grief
Increased stress on family relationships
Increased use of drugs and alcohol
Increased verbalization of needs
Loneliness
Loss of bladder control
Physical deterioration
Psychosomatic illnesses
Weight change
Withdrawal

CONTRIBUTING FACTORS

Chronic or debilitating illness
Diminished sensory perception (limited vision, hearing)
Financial or other worries or concerns
History of depression
History of recent multiple losses
History of resistance to change
Loss of control or decision-making skills
Loss of support systems
Negative experiences with previous moves
Presence of confusion/disorientation

EXPECTED OUTCOMES

Client will verbalize positive statements in regard to acceptance of the new environment.
> Rationale for change is identified.
> Participation in decision-making activities is taken.
> Feelings of control and self-confidence are expressed.
> Stress management techniques are demonstrated.
> New bonds with people are established.
> Participation in activities at new location is sought.

INTERVENTIONS

RATIONALE

Universal

Interventions	Rationale
Obtain a complete nursing history including (a) the circumstances which precipitated the relocation and (b) how past relocations have been managed.	The nursing history will give insights into individual idiosyncrasies which will help with developing the care plan. Exploring the past relocations will provide a more complete understanding of the problems.
Assess problems within the family structure which are related to relocation.	All family members exhibit stress when a relocation occurs and may benefit from interventions to resolve that stress.
Encourage meaningful activities.	Older/home-bound client—Arts and crafts will give meaning to many empty hours during the day; parties will provide a fun activity and break the monotony of long dull days; movies, games, trips, and other interesting activities will be a healthy diversion for the relocated older client living in a new area.
Provide a list of organizations (Welcome Wagon, churches, Parents Without Partners, singles' groups, senior citizens' groups).	These types of organizations may help client form new relationships and become acquainted with positives in the new area.
Show concern and empathy and use listening skills.	This will help build a trusting relationship.
Encourage verbalization of feelings, especially release of negative feelings.	Allowing this kind of verbalization will help the adjustment.
Encourage to begin a journal to work through various emotions.	Writing in a journal might be very therapeutic.

INTERVENTIONS	RATIONALE
Assist in choosing problem-solving skills or suggest solutions to problems.	The nurse could be the medium to help the adjustment to the new environment.
Reassure during every interaction.	The client might feel lonely, worried, and fearful and reassurance will allay these feelings.
Share suggestions of sleep inducers such as: warm milk, backrubs, use of white noise, and/or music.	Sleep patterns might be disturbed when environment is changed. Lights, noise, and appearance of the new sleeping room will not be the same as was customary in the old room.
Encourage to participate in a support group composed of other newly relocated persons.	Support groups are a valuable way to promote and hasten relocation adjustment.
Refer to a social worker, psychiatrist, physician, occupational therapist, dietitian, and/or activity therapist.	Many of these experts can help the adjustment to the new location.
Instruct how to participate in a healthy life-style and seek help for any signs or symptoms of illnesses.	Persons under stress have reduced immunity to illnesses and need to be alerted to the proper methods to avoid and report any disease processes.
Instruct the family in regard to community services which are available to relocated members.	This referral is essential to the family that is not familiar with the area.

Inpatient

Assess the need for an intra-institutional move (a move within the same institution) and make sure that it is a team decision.	A team might suggest other alternatives to a move and bypass the relocation.
Assess levels of confusion upon admission and regularly afterwards for clients involved in an intra-institutional or inter-institutional move.	Use of a tool to assess confusion (Ludwick's) immediately after the move and regularly afterward would be helpful in monitoring the medication regimen and other interventions.

INTERVENTIONS	RATIONALE
Assess the ability to adjust to the new room or institution and repeat directions to the bathroom, times of meals, visiting hours, and other information as often as necessary.	When first relocating to another facility or area, stress may be high enough to block the ability to listen or remember directions.
Communicate choices in regard to space, room arrangements, and decorations.	The ability to make choices in "home territory" areas will hasten adjustment and lessen stress.
Offer special food or treats to improve the appetite.	Weight loss might occur following the relocation.
Institute hug/touch therapy in the form of dance therapy, pet therapy, intergenerational visits, and touching by the staff.	These therapies may give a sense of belonging and self-worth.
Ask another inpatient to befriend a relocated client.	This will provide a sense of importance and belonging as well as offer friendship.
Allow to revisit friends and staff on the "old" unit.	This will help avoid a sense of abandonment.
Make certain that eye glasses, dentures, hearing aids, and any other adaptive devices arrive with the client.	It will be easier for adjustment to a new facility if personally needed aids are available.
Choose, when possible, a room that is similar to the existing room if movement within the facility is necessary (same bed location, same view, same area, and environmental outlay).	Carefully choosing a new room will make adjustment easier.
Offer consistency of care (same daily staff, same environment, same daily routine).	Consistency will hasten adjustment.

INTERVENTIONS	RATIONALE
Support the prior roommate to prevent feelings of responsibility for the move, and feelings of guilt or abandonment.	The roommate may feel responsible for the move, and reassurance from the staff needs to be provided.
Encourage the prior roommate to visit.	Because a relationship has already been developed between these clients, a feeling of loss could occur if visitation is not permitted or encouraged.
Reassure, when a move interinstitutionally is necessary, that return to familiar facility and friends is probable.	Many long-term care clients view the facility as their home. Reassurance is needed, if realistic, that return to familiar surroundings will occur.
Encourage to eat in the dining room or day room with others if possible.	Eating is a social affair and appetite and relationships may improve with company.
Use a "Do not disturb" sign on the door, if requested, and always knock before entering.	This will afford a sense of territorial security.
Help maintain relationships (help write letters, post cards, greeting cards, and assist with phone calls).	Maintaining relationships will lessen feelings of abandonment and keep family ties throughout institutionalization.
Communicate with staff from the previous facility or unit regarding specific client information.	Continuity of care will be evident, which will ease the relocation.
Instruct in regard to personal use of public areas.	Most relocated clients feel insecure and will not move chairs, TVs, and other objects unless given permission to do so.
Communicate with family members regarding relocation and adjustment to solicit their help.	Family member support can be beneficial to hasten adjustment.
Instruct staff members never to move objects or personal belongings without permission.	This practice reinforces the autonomy of the client and the need for control over certain space.

INTERVENTIONS	**R**ATIONALE
Community Health/ Home Care Assess family member's health promotion histories (immunizations, dental visits, well-child visits, health care follow-ups, prescription refills).	Moving is often a hectic time and such matters may be overlooked.
Assess the needs of the relocated family and offer the help that is necessary.	Newly relocated family members might need help, but may not know where to seek it.
Assess the adjustment to the move of each family member and single out those members who might need more assistance.	All family members will not adjust the same way to relocation, and some members will need more assistance than others.
Assist the parents in conveying a positive attitude regarding the move to the other family members: (1) Provide reassurance and positives in regard to the move; (2) Provide understanding instead of punishment for adverse reactions to the move, for example, bedwetting; (3) Provide a list of organizations, for example, Boy Scouts, Girl Scouts, Campfire Girls, Catholic Youth Organization, and church groups.	These strategies will lessen the feelings of loss of control and "not belonging" on the part of children in the family. If there are any problems with the children within the family structure, the entire family suffers.
Advise parents to allow children some choices in the new home such as room arrangements, rooms, colors, decorations, and new furniture purchased.	These types of choices will help family members adjust to the move more easily.
Advise parents to communicate with their children's teachers, guidance counselors, and school psychologists.	These professionals will help families cope with apparent problems.

INTERVENTIONS	**R**ATIONALE
Share with parents the importance of their presence during the transition.	Although new routines will be developed, the parents' visibility will provide a sense of stability for the children.
Educate family members in regard to signs of depression, lowered self-esteem, and dependence on drugs and/or alcohol.	A relocation could produce these kinds of problems, and families could learn to help each other and seek help in the community (Alcoholics Anonymous, drug counselor, psychiatrist, psychologist, or marriage counselor).
Encourage family members to discuss with each other the effects of the relocation.	Communication among family members is essential during this time.
Teach family members to write down important phone numbers and have them available by the phone for all family members to use.	Hunting for phone numbers during a family crisis is not ideal. Include on this list: physicians, dentists, podiatrist, poison center, emergency center, relatives' phone numbers, schools, and places of employment—and continue to add to this list as needed.

REFERENCES/BIBLIOGRAPHY

Amenta, M., Weiner, A., & Amenta, D. (1984). Successful relocation of elderly residents. **Geriatric Nursing**, November/December, 356–360.

Ardrey, R. (1966). **The territorial imperative: A personal inquiry into the animal origins of property and nations** (1st ed.). New York: Atheneum.

*Bellin, C. (1990). Relocating adult day care: Its impact on persons with dementia. **Journal of Gerontological Nursing, 16**(3), 11–14.

*Borup, J.H. (1982). The effects of varying degrees of interinstitutional environmental change on long-term care patients. **The Gerontologist, 22**(41), 405–417.

Brooke, V. (1989). How Elders adjust. **Geriatric Nursing**, March/April, 66–68.

Brooks, J.W. (1989). Preparing for relocation. **Contemporary Long-Term Care, 12**(12), 46–48.

Brugler, C. (1986). **The defining characteristics of translocation syndrome—A validation study.** Unpublished paper. Kent, OH: Kent State University Press.

Chenita, W.C. (1983). Entry into a nursing home as a status passage: A theory to guide nursing practice. **Geriatric Nursing**, Mar/Apr, 92–97.

*Dimond, M., McCance, K., & King, K. (1987). Forced residential relocation: Its impact on the well-being of older adults. **Western Journal of Nursing Research, 9**(4), 445–464.

Ebersole, P., & Hess, P. (1990). **Toward healthy aging: Human needs and nursing response**. (pp. 315–328). St. Louis: Mosby.

Engle, J.L. (1985). Temporary relocation: Is it stressful to your patients? **Journal of Gerontological Nursing, 11**(10), 28–31.

Engle, V. (1986). Bridging the research gap between acute and long-term care of older adults. **Image, 18**(4), 148–150.

Foreman, M.D. (1990). Complexities of Acute Confusion. **Geriatric Nursing, 11**(3), 136–139.

Gordon, M. (1985). **Manual of nursing diagnosis** (p. 214). New York: McGraw-Hill.

Hall, E.T. (1966). **The Hidden Dimension**. New York: Doubleday.

* Harkulich, J., & Brugler, C. (1989). Nursing diagnosis/translocation syndrome: Expert validation study. **People to People Journal**.

Harkulich, J., & Brugler, C. (1989). Relocation of institutionalized residents. **Today's Nursing Home, 10**(10), 24–25.

Harkulich, J., & Brugler, C. (1990). **Relocation and the resident: Information for family and friends**. Beachwood, OH: Care Services.

King, K.S., Dimond, M., & McCance, K.L. (1987). **Coping with relocation. Geriatric Nursing, 8**(5), 258–261.

Lange, J.L. (1980). Voluntary relocation among the Elderly: Nursing implications. **Journal of Gerontological Nursing, 6**(3), 405–407.

Ludwick, R. (1981). Assessing confusion: A tool to improve nursing care. **Journal of Gerontological Nursing, 7**(8), 474–477.

Maas, M.L., Hardy, M.A., & Craft, M. (1990). Some methodologic considerations in nursing diagnosis research. **Nursing Diagnosis, 1**(1), 24–30.

Marsico, T., & Puskar, K.R. (1986). Family relocation: Helping children adjust. **Pediatric Nursing, 12**(2), 108–110.

Matter, D.E., & Matter, R.M. (1988). Helping young children cope with the stress of relocation: Action steps for the counselor. **Elementary School Guidance and Counseling, 23**, 23–29.

* Puskar, K.R. (1986). The usefulness of Mahler's phases of the separation-individuation process in providing a theoretical framework for understanding relocation. **Maternal-Child Nursing Journal, 15**(1), 15–22.

Puskar, K.R. (1990). Relocation support groups for corporate wives. **American Association of Occupational Health Nurses, 38**(1), 25–31.

Rantz, M., & Egan, K. (1988). Reducing death from transition syndrome. **Today's Nursing Home, 9**(8), 24.

Rosswurm, M.A. (1983). Relocation and the elderly. **Journal of Gerontological Nursing, 6**(12), 632–637.

* Thomasma, M., Yeaworth, R.C., and McCabe, B.W. (1990). Moving day: Relocation and anxiety in institutionalized elderly. **Journal of Gerontological Nursing, 16**(7), 18–24.

Weiss, M.D. (1989). Relocating families: An overlooked market segment for nursing. **American Association of Occupational Health Nurses, 37**(11), 454–458.

* Yazdanfar, D.J. (1990). Assessing the mental status of the cognitively impaired elderly. **Journal of Gerontological Nursing, 16**(9), 32–36.

Role Performance, Altered

A state in which an individual or others see an actual or perceived disparity in meeting role obligations or expectations.

M. Kathleen Eilers, R.N., M.S.N.

DEFINING CHARACTERISTICS

Change in others' perception of role
Change in physical capacity to resume role
Change in self perception of role
Change in usual patterns of responsibility

Conflict in roles
Denial of role
Lack of knowledge of role

CONTRIBUTING FACTORS

Pathophysiological

Cognitive/perceptual difficulties
Mental retardation

Physical/mental illness

Psychosociobehavioral

Change in occupation
Changed expectations, new role
Conflict situations
Cultural transitions
Developmental crisis
Developmental transitions

Inability to learn new role requirements
Inadequate supports/resources
Lack of role model
Role ambiguity/incongruity
Role incompatibility

EXPECTED OUTCOMES

Client will express satisfaction about functioning in a new or changed role.
    Feelings about role loss are verbalized.
    Appropriate knowledge and skill for role mastery is demonstrated.
    Client will demonstrate reduced or alleviated role distance.

Role perceptions are verbalized.

Awareness of and ability to meet role expectations are expressed.

Client will resolve role conflicts.

Factors contributing to role conflict are verbalized.

Strategies to resolve conflict are developed.

Strategies to resolve conflict are implemented.

Client will demonstrate role competence.

Knowledge necessary for role competence is acquired.

Skills necessary for role performance are demonstrated.

INTERVENTIONS

RATIONALE

Universal	
ROLE LOSS: Inability to perform in previously prescribed role.	
Evaluate level of role loss. Assist in identifying role loss or change.	Specific identification of how role has changed and what components of previous roles can continue needs to occur.
Facilitate grieving response to experienced role loss.	Role loss can precipitate a threat to the individual's self-concept.
Educate about altered functional capacity and how it affects role performance.	Specific knowledge about limitations assists with adjustment.
Explore available option for role change or adjustments. Provide anticipatory guidance for life-stage role transitions.	Planning for role transitions can reduce anxiety.
ROLE DISTANCE: Role behavior differs from socially prescribed expectations.	
Explore and clarify perceptions of role performance in a psycho/social/cultural context.	Cultural and social values influence role performance.
Show respect for existing belief systems and values that support role expectations.	Showing respect can improve a sense of self-worth and foster an atmosphere conducive to change.
Model role behaviors that must be learned.	Observation of appropriate behaviors strengthens learning.

INTERVENTIONS	RATIONALE
Refer to appropriate community groups for support.	Peer support strengthens role behaviors.
ROLE CONFLICT: Incompatible or incongruent expectations within a certain role. Evaluate level of role conflict. Assist in exploring issues surrounding role conflict and identifying sources of stress.	Role conflict is experienced as frustration, since there may be feelings of being torn in opposite directions or feelings of inadequacy or unsuitability for performing certain roles.
Offer clarification and rectify misunderstandings. Explore compromise options. Offer supportive guidance for determining priorities. Offer family or group meetings to clarify conflicting role expectations.	Often there are cultural/social expectations that certain attributes go with certain roles. Role conflict can be caused by the incongruity between the individual's and others' expectations.
Foster effective communication and problem-solving skills.	Open dialogue can provide an opportunity for clarification and validation of feelings and concerns. Utilizing effective problem-solving strategies promotes confidence and a sense of ownership of choices made.
ROLE FAILURE: Inability to meet expectations of a prescribed role or derive satisfaction from role. Evaluate level of role failure. Assist in identifying reasons for role failure. Assess readiness to learn required role functions.	Psychological and physical readiness must be in place in order for learning to occur.
Facilitate expressions of fear and disappointment about encountered failure. Assist in recognizing strengths and abilities. Involve others as appropriate in clarifying expectations and giving feedback.	Support and direction from significant others is necessary.

INTERVENTIONS	RATIONALE
Use role modeling and role rehearsal to teach knowledge and skills.	Modeling and rehearsal strengthen learning.
Offer praise for accomplishments.	Positive reinforcement enhances learning.
Inpatient None	
Community Health/ Home Care None	

REFERENCES/BIBLIOGRAPHY

Kanter, F. H., & Goldstein, A. (Eds.). (1975). **Helping people change**. Elmsford, NY: Pergamon.

Kolb, L.C., Keith, H., & Brodie, H. (1982). **Modern clinical psychiatry** (10th ed.). Philadelphia: Saunders.

McFarland, G.K., & McFarlane, E. A. (1989). **Nursing diagnosis and intervention**. Philadelphia: Mosby.

Millon, T. (1969). **Modern psychopathology: A biosocial approach to maladaptive learning and functioning**. Philadelphia: Saunders.

North American Nursing Diagnosis Association. **Taxonomy I** (Rev. 1990). St. Louis: NANDA.

Stuart, G., & Sundeen, S. (1983). **Principles and practice of psychiatric nursing** (2nd ed.). St. Louis: Mosby .

Self-Esteem Disturbance: Chronic Low

A state in which an individual has long-standing negative self-evaluation/feelings about self or self capabilities (NANDA, 1990, p. 89).

Joan Norris, R.N., Ph.D.

DEFINING CHARACTERISTICS

Evaluates self as unable to deal with events
Exaggerates negative feedback about self
Excessively seeks reassurance
Expression of shame and/or guilt
Frequent lack of success in work or other life events
Hesitant to try new things/situations
Indecisive

Lack of culturally appropriate eye contact
Nonassertive/passive
Overly conforming/dependent on others' opinions
Rationalizes away/minimizes positive feedback
Self-negating verbalizations

CONTRIBUTING FACTORS

Pathophysiological

None

Psychosociobehavioral

Chronic social rejection (prejudice; belittling based on handicap, disfigurement, or other differences)
Excessive self-expectations (perfectionistic ideal that is not realistically achievable)
Hypercritical input from significant others
Learned helplessness
Powerlessness
Long-standing relationships characterized by abuse (physical or emotional) or neglect

473

EXPECTED OUTCOMES

Client will accept and perceive self as a person of value/worth.

    Realistic strengths and personal assets are identified.

    Personal views and needs are asserted directly and appropriately .

    Feelings of competence in everyday living and work roles are expressed.

    Weaknesses or limitations which cannot be changed are accepted.

    Activities are planned and initiated that contribute to realistic self-growth or improvement
        goals.

INTERVENTIONS	RATIONALE
Universal	
Assess and validate the problem and its duration.	Differentiation of chronic low self-esteem from situational low self-esteem is important prior to undertaking specific interventions or referral for mental health therapy. Validation of the problem permits collaborative problem solving.
Assess whether clinical depression (loss of libido, changes in food intake and sleep patterns) or suicidal ideas/intent is present.	Suicidal intent would require continuous supervision and admission to a mental health facility.
Accept and respect as a unique, worthwhile person.	A hurried, impatient, and/or depersonalizing manner conveys disrespect, violates personal dignity, and serves to reinforce feelings of low self-esteem.
Permit choice and personal control in situations.	Provide adequate information and available choices to promote a sense of personal mastery and control in all situations possible.
Identify and reinforce strengths.	Genuine recognition of real assets and personal strengths on a consistent basis may assist in gradual changes in self-concept and subsequent feelings of self-worth. Reality-based opportunities to apply/demonstrate these strengths are essential in this process.
Take the initiative in making contacts.	Reluctance or unworthiness to express needs may inhibit contacts.

INTERVENTIONS	**R**ATIONALE
Promote and support personal care and grooming.	Self-neglect reinforces low self-esteem.
Explore perception of how low self-esteem interferes with life goals and interpersonal relationships. If willing, refer to community mental health center or qualified therapist.	This information addresses the need and motivation for mental health therapy.
Facilitate awareness of personal values and goals, promoting behavioral choices compatible with value system.	Failure to accommodate teaching and care regimens to values and life-style is likely to result in noncompliance, failure to achieve goals, and further undermining of self-esteem.

Psychiatric Inpatient

Convey genuineness, respect, acceptance, and empathy to provide climate for growth.	This communicates hope and the expectation that responsibility for own growth and behavior change will be assumed.
Point out negative and self-defeating thoughts and challenge them. Note how negative expectations inhibit positive actions and become self-reinforcing. Discourage negative self-evaluations and comparisons with others.	Cognitive approaches are effective in identifying and stopping self-negating thoughts, which reinforce low self-esteem and contribute to depression.
Conduct a positive asset search.	Client strengths, interests, and past accomplishments are basic to planning diverse tasks and activities to build confidence and self-esteem based on real achievements. This will gradually set realistic expectations for increased accomplishments and recognize these achievements.
Provide assertiveness training and opportunities to role play and rehearse anxiety-provoking interactions.	Improved self-assertion is likely to result in positive feedback and reinforce feelings of greater competence. Role-play techniques permit safe practice and rehearsal of approaches and build confidence.

INTERVENTIONS

RATIONALE

Community Health/ Home Care

Teach and promote a climate of nurturance and respect in the client's family by encouraging direct, open communication; tolerance and acceptance of individual differences; flexibility in rules; and strong mutual support.

The family system and environment are basic to enhancing or altering self-esteem.

REFERENCES/BIBLIOGRAPHY

Coopersmith, S. (1967). Antecedents of self-esteem. San Francisco: Freeman.

Crouch, M.A., & Staub, V. (1983). Enhancement of self-esteem in adults. **Family Community Health, 6,** 79–81.

Ellis, A., & Grieger, R. (1977). Handbook of rational-emotive therapy. New York: Springer.

Murphy, S. (1982). Learned helplessness: From concept to comprehension. **Perspectives in Psychiatric Care, 20,** 27–32.

Norris, Joan, & Kunes-Connell, Mary. (1985). Self-esteem disturbance. **Nursing Clinics of North America, 20**(4), 745–761.

North American Nursing Diagnosis Association. **Taxonomy I** (Rev. 1990). St. Louis: NANDA.

Satir, Virginia (1972). Peoplemaking. Palo Alto, CA: Science & Behavior Books.

Self-Esteem Disturbance: Situational Low

A state in which an individual has negative evaluation/feelings about the self, which develops in response to a loss or change in an individual who previously had a positive self-evaluation (NANDA, 1990, p. 90).

Joan Norris, R.N., Ph.D.

DEFINING CHARACTERISTICS

Difficulty making decisions
Episodic occurrence of negative self-appraisal in response to life events in a person with a previously positive self-evaluation
Evaluates self as unable to handle events or situations
Expresses shame or guilt
Self-negating verbalizations
Verbalizes negative feelings about the self or self capabilities (e.g., helplessness, uselessness)

CONTRIBUTING FACTORS

Pathophysiological

Changes in physical energy level or capabilities (e.g., from serious illness or sensory deficit), which interfere with ability to perform previously significant roles or functions
Loss of a body part or loss of sensation and/or voluntary control in a part of the body
Loss of significant cognitive abilities

Psychosociobehavioral

Behavior inconsistent with personal values
Disturbances in body image resulting from disfiguring scars; physical handicaps; rapid, large shifts in weight; changes of aging

477

Loss of emotional control related to overwhelming feelings of anxiety, grief, helplessness, or powerlessness

Perceived powerlessness to control personal situation or environment

EXPECTED OUTCOMES

Client will resolve the loss or change, and the previously positive self-evaluation/feelings will be restored.

Feelings of grief and loss are expressed.

A sense of personal control and mastery of the situation are attained.

Functioning in personally satisfying situations, activities, and social roles is achieved.

Focus is on total self rather than only on the missing or dysfunctional aspect.

INTERVENTIONS	RATIONALE
Universal	
Monitor for the presence of crisis through identification of perceptions, resources, coping strategies, and tension level. Explore possible suicidal ideas and intention.	Crisis is a state of disorganization, tension, anxiety, and heightened emotion in which coping with the demands of a precipitating event seems impossible. Customary coping strategies may have been unsuccessfully employed and assistance is welcomed. Crisis is time limited, lasting only four to six weeks.
Display active listening, acceptance, and empathy.	Exploration of perceptions and the meaning of the experience assists self-understanding. The nurse's understanding facilitates self-acceptance.
Recognize that adaptation will proceed at its own pace.	Months may be required to adapt to a significant change or loss. Pressure to accelerate or conceal the grief process inflicts additional feelings of isolation and inadequacy.
Employ generic crisis intervention techniques. Include the following: 1. Focus on understanding the crisis and its meaning to the client 2. Explore and promote expression of feelings 3. Reduce tension	Generic crisis intervention uses known tasks and patterns of coping with specific types of events to support and assist with coping.Information readily available in the literature (e.g., the grief process...) may be used by non-mental-health professionals. If resolution fails to occur or if symptoms of depression or dysfunctional grieving are present, referral to a mental health professional would be appropriate.

INTERVENTIONS	RATIONALE
4. Identify available resources and support systems 5. Mutually derive new alternatives for coping 6. Provide anticipatory guidance	
Inpatient	
Assign consistent care givers and permit client to control events and surroundings to the extent desired and possible.	Unpredictability, dependency, and lack of control increase feelings of inadequacy and powerlessness.
Model matter-of-fact acceptance and comfort in regard to alterations in function and/or appearance. Provide opportunities to talk with others who have successfully coped with the problem.	Models promote hope and self-acceptance.
Help those who have significant alterations in appearance or functioning to focus on the attributes of the total self, not just on the alteration or loss.	Nurses and family members can assist the client in regaining a sense of perspective on the self, rather than overemphasizing the negative effects of a specific deficit.
Teach the client (and family, as appropriate) to master a full understanding of the situation, appropriate resources available, and the related tasks associated with symptom control, treatment, and coping.	A sense of mastery and confidence is important to self-esteem and recovery.
Community Health/ Home Care	
Promote family-client communication to realistically plan for the future, accommodate changes into customary life-style, and assure meaningful activities and social roles.	The family system will be influenced by any significant losses or changes. Effective communication is necessary to renegotiate roles, realign tasks, and/or develop mutual understanding in order to promote effective functioning of the family as a unit and adequate social support to the client.

REFERENCES/BIBLIOGRAPHY

Aquillera, D. (1990). **Crisis intervention and methodology**. St. Louis: Mosby.

Berlinger, J.E. (1983). Coping tasks in critical care. **Dimensions of Critical Care Nursing, 2**, 80–89.

Engel, G.L. (September, 1964). Grief and grieving. **American Journal of Nursing, 64**(9), 93–98.

Geach, B. (1987). Coping with acute and chronic illness. In Norris, et al. (Eds.). **Mental-health psychiatric nursing: A continuum of care**. New York: Wiley.

Gillis, C.L. (1989). Why family health care? In Gillis, et al. (Eds.). **Toward a science of family nursing**. Menlo Park, CA: Addison-Wesley.

Mitchell, P.H. (1983). Crisis management for nurses coping with chronic illness. **Washington State Journal of Nursing, 54**, 2–8.

Moos, R.H., & TSU, V.D. (1977). **Coping with physical illness**. New York: Plenum.

Norris, J., & Kunes-Connell, M. (1985). Self-esteem disturbance. **Nursing Clinics of North America, 20**(4), 745–761.

North American Nursing Diagnosis Association (1990). **Taxonomy I** (Rev. ed.). St. Louis: NANDA.

Zisook, S., & DeVaul, R. (March, 1983). Grief, unresolved grief and depression. **Psychosomatics, 24**(3), 247–256.

Sensory Perception, Altered

A state in which an individual experiences temporary, nonpsychotic sensory or perceptual distortions ranging from mild (seeing colors, hearing sounds, experiencing body temperature changes) to severe (seeing objects , hearing voices). Distortions may be environmentally-, drug-, or other-induced.

Gladys Simandl, R.N., Ph.D.
Leona VandeVusse, R.N., C.N.M., M.S.

Note: Assessment for mild to severe alterations in behavior should be made on all clients. Unusual sensory experiences have been reported in many populations, including clients with restricted mobility, those following bilateral eye surgery, general surgery clients, and clients on general care units. Similar terms and phrases used in the literature and their definitions:

Hypovigilance: A disturbance in awareness affecting receptivity and reactivity (Meinhart, 1969).

ICU psychosis: A label applied to unusual sensory experiences reported by patients in intensive care units.

Indeterminate stimulus experience (ISE): Experiences of a patient for which there is no apparent appropriate stimulus within the patient's environment (Ellis, 1972).

Perceptual deprivation: Absence or reduction of stimulus variability. Perceptual deprivation occurs in an environment where sound is muffled, light is diffused, and bodily sensations are non-distinct. (Worrell, 1971).

Sensory deprivation: An absolute reduction in the variety and intensity of sensory input, with or without a change in pattern, e.g., an environment of silence and darkness would be considered an instance of sensory deprivation.

Sensory overload: A condition of highly intense stimulation that is not patterned (Bolin, 1974).

DEFINING CHARACTERISTICS

Agitation
Anxiety
Behavior changes, e.g., noncompliance,
          combativeness, disruptiveness
Catecholamine changes
Clouding of consciousness
Daydreaming
Delirium
Depression
Disorientation
Distortions in time sense
Electroencephalographic changes
Excitement
Fatigue
Fear

Galvanic skin response changes
Hallucinations
Illusions
Inability to think and reason
Inattentiveness
Incoherence
Mood changes
Paranoid delusions
Poor concentration
Reports feeling mild body changes
Reports feeling warmer or cooler
Reports hearing sounds
Reports seeing colors
Restlessness

CONTRIBUTING FACTORS

Pathophysiological

Age
Changes in usual life patterns, e.g., sleeping, exercise, eating, lighting
Medication effects
Normal response of the reticular activating system to cope with altered sensory experiences
Pain
Physiologic changes or abnormalities in body systems or sensory organs

Psychosociobehavioral

Excessive auditory, visual, or tactile stimuli,
          e.g., repetitive noises, blinking
          lights, excessive procedural touch-
          ing, monotonous environment
Immobility or change in mobility state
Institutionalization
Invasive procedures
Isolation

Lack of normal stimuli
Lack of privacy
Language/cultural barriers
Predisposing psychological disturbances/
          diagnoses
Situational, maturational stress
Substance abuse
Unfamiliar people or routines

EXPECTED OUTCOMES

Client will be oriented to time, place and person.
      Interactions with nurse are appropriate.
      Responses to questions of time, place, and person are appropriate.

Client will engage in meaningful conversations with nurse.
    Unusual experiences are shared with nurse.
    Factors contributing to sensory stimulation/deprivation are identified.
    Planning is participated in to remedy unusual sensory experiences.
Client will engage in meaningful living activities.
    Ambulation about environment is pursued.
    Involvement in diversional activities is initiated.
    Activities are changed as needed to avoid boredom.

INTERVENTIONS   RATIONALE

INTERVENTIONS	RATIONALE
Universal	
None	
Inpatient	
Orient to time, place, and person.	Orientation is cited frequently in the literature as a measure to reinforce reality.
Develop a personal relationship.	The relationship between the nurse and the client is critical in developing trust, maintaining communication, and providing familiarity in the client's environment.
Use presence.	Research has shown that clients who received a single preoperative interview intervention from a nurse experienced 50% less delirium experiences than those who received no interview intervention.
Alleviate fears; interpret unusual sensory experiences.	Informing a client that his/her unusual sensory experience is a transient, nonpsychotic and fairly common, although undesirable, occurrence helps alleviate fears. Informing that the unusual sensory experiences are avoidable helps with planning of daily activities.
Include sensations while explaining procedures that may be experienced and show equipment that will be encountered.	When technical and procedural information, as well as sensory information about impending procedures has been given, a better understanding of the events as well as less fear with the experience has been reported.

INTERVENTIONS	**R**ATIONALE
Engage in meaningful talk, rather than brief assessments.	Research has shown that clients who received reassurance, orientation, and explanations experienced fewer unusual sensory experiences than those who received routine surveillance, quick medication requests, and lights left on.
Inform about the unusual sensory experiences reported by others prior to technical procedures or surgery. Provide special attention to the sense-impaired or those who will be sense-impaired after certain interventions.	Research has demonstrated that clients who were informed prior to a surgical intervention were more likely to share their unusual sensory experiences and were less afraid of them.
Ask directly if unusual sensory experiences have occurred or are occurring. Describe in detail the experiences to elicit the client responses.	When nurses asked routine, general questions such as "How are you?" or "How was your night?", only 8% of clients surveyed reported their unusual sensory experiences. When nurses gave descriptive accounts of the types of unusual sensory experiences reported by others, 41% of the clients surveyed reported their unusual sensory experiences. Clients were relieved to know others had had similar experiences.
Relieve pain.	A client experiencing pain may focus attention on the pain and its relief. Pain relief measures are intended to facilitate normal responses to environmental stimuli.
Observe after administering pain medications for signs and symptoms of unusual sensory experiences.	Some medications potentiate untoward sensory experiences.
Encourage to use prosthetic devices.	Hearing aids, dentures, and similar devices that are a part of the client's daily life may help communication—using familiar means as well as maintenance of normalcy in daily living patterns.
Involve in decisions regarding care.	Research has shown that clients who were allowed greater personal control in activities of daily living (ADL) experienced less stress.

INTERVENTIONS	**RATIONALE**
Provide natural lighting when possible.	Delirium was found to be twice as frequent in windowless ICUs.
Provide uninterrupted rest periods.	Normal circadian rhythms will be promoted with uninterrupted rest.
Encourage ambulation if able. Change the position of a client on bedrest frequently; have client sit in chair, and change the viewing environment routinely.	Research has shown that subjects confined to bed experienced unusual visual, auditory, olfactory, and tactile experiences after two and one-half hours. Subjects who were confined to eight hours of restricted stimulation, combined with uncertainty about impending events, experienced dreams and images. Restricted movement increased the effects.
Reduce noise levels.	Noise levels produced by nurses and physicians are of a higher decibel range than those produced by machines. Noise reduces sleep ability. A quiet environment simulates normal daily experiences and decreases anxiety. A client learns the importance of the signals that indicate warnings or distress from machines that may contribute to sensory overload.
Simulate day and night experiences through the use of lighting.	This intervention is intended to promote normal circadian rhythms. Harsh or excessive lighting should be monitored and limited to short periods. Rest and sleep may be facilitated by low to no light.
Remove unnecessary equipment from client's room.	Patients and families associate the amount of equipment with the severity of the illness.
Limit the amount of nursing or medical jargon within hearing range.	Erroneous conclusions may be drawn about client's illness or prognosis based on language heard in the unit.
Alter the environment to simulate the client's usual environment by (1) eliminating or muffling monotonous noises, (2) using pictures or memoirs from the client's home, (3) using color, and (4) providing warmth and comfort measures.	These measures are intended to create a more home like environment and thereby reduce the monotony or over-stimulation of hospital-type environments.

INTERVENTIONS	RATIONALE
Provide special attention to the sensory needs of the elderly.	Sensory acuity in general decreases with age, leaving the elderly particularly vulnerable to changes in the environment that may potentiate unusual sensory experiences.
Schedule (increase or decrease) and pattern the number and quality of visitors according to the client's needs.	When unusual sensory experiences occur, the results may be under- or over-stimulation. Visits from friends or family may contribute to the unusual experiences or they may help mitigate them. Using assessment skills, the nurse determines if more or less visits are needed to maintain equilibrium in the client's daily routine.
Involve significant others in diversional activities.	Family and friends who know the client can provide meaningful stimulation, especially through reminiscing or recalling stories that involved the client.
Use diversional therapy.	Nurses have found the use of occupational or physical therapists or volunteers useful in providing reality orientation.
Use music therapy.	Playing familiar tunes, encouraging the client to sing along, or having the client beat rhythms can orient and soothe.
Place in room with other clients.	Communication will be increased among people, and monotony of the environment will be decreased.
Provide interpreter service.	Inability to communicate using a common language may contribute toward unusual sensory experiences.
Provide opportunities to talk to others about their unusual sensory experiences.	Clients learn that they are not alone. It also provides an opportunity to interpret and reorganize their experiences.
Community Health/ Home Care Assess the need for appropriate diversional therapy in the home.	Clients in diverse settings have experienced unusual sensory experiences.

INTERVENTIONS	**R**ATIONALE
Teach families and care givers about unusual sensory experiences and to be attentive to sensory stimulation and deprivation	Unusual sensory experiences in the home can be prevented through education.
Become involved in policy level interventions to enhance appropriate levels of stimulation (education, social interaction, recreation) in all communities.	Some causes of sensory stimulation and deprivation at the community level include overcrowding, poor sanitation, poverty, and unequal access to community resources. Efforts to alleviate the effects of such conditions may contribute toward a healthier people.

REFERENCES/BIBLIOGRAPHY

Ballard, K.S. (1981). Identification of environmental stressors for patients in a surgical intensive care unit. **Issues in Mental Health Nursing, 3**, 89–108.

Belitz, J. (1983). Minimizing the psychological complications of patients who require mechanical ventilation. **Critical Care Nurse, 3**(3), 42–46.

Bernardini, L. (1985). Effective communication as an intervention for sensory deprivation in the elderly client. **Topics in Clinical Nursing, 6**, 72–81.

Betz, C.L. (1982). Sensory disturbances among children in the ICU. **Dimensions of Critical Care Nursing, 1**(3), 145–151.

Bolin, R.H. (1974). Sensory deprivation: An overview. **Nursing Forum, 13**, 241–258.

Bulechek, G.M., & McCloskey, J.C. (Eds.). (1985). **Nursing interventions: Treatments for nursing diagnosis**. Toronto: Saunders.

* CURN Project. (1981). **Distress reduction through sensory preparation**. New York: Grune & Stratton.

* Easton, C., & MacKenzie, F. (1988). Sensory-perceptual alterations: Delirium in the intensive care unit. **Heart & Lung, 17**, 229–235.

* Ellis, R. (1972). Unusual sensory and thought disturbances after cardiac surgery. **American Journal of Nursing, 72**(11), 2022.

* Hansell, H.N. (1984). The behavioral effects of noise on man: The patient with intensive care unit psychosis. **Heart & Lung, 13**, 59–65.

* Helton, M.C., Gordon, S.H., & Nunnery, S.L. (1980). The correlation between sleep deprivation and the intensive care unit syndrome. **Heart & Lung, 9**, 464–469.

* Johnson, J.E. (1973). Effects of accurate expectations about sensations on the sensory and distress components of pain. **Journal of Personality and Social Psychology, 27**, 264–275.

* Johnson, J., & Levanthal, H. (1974). Effects of accurate expectations and behavioral instructions on reactions during a noxious medical examination. **Journal of Personality and Social Psychology, 29**, 710–718.

* Kallio, J.T., & Sime, A.M. (1980). The effect of induced control on the perceptions of control, mood state and quality of nursing care for clients in critical care unit. **Advances in Nursing Science, 2**(3), 105–107.

Kee, C.C. (1990). Sensory impairment: Factor X in providing nursing care to the older adult. **Journal of Community Health Nursing, 7**(1), 45–52.

* Keep, P., James, J., & Inman, M. (1980). Windows in the intensive therapy unit. **Anesthesia, 35,** 257–261.

* Kornfeld, D.S., Heller, S.S., Frank, K.A., & Moskowitz, R. (1974). Personality and psychological factors in postcardiotomy delirium. **Archives of General Psychiatry, 31,** 249–253.

* Lazarus, H.R., & Haggens, J.H. (1968). Prevention of psychosis following open heart surgery. **American Journal of Psychiatry, 124**(9), 76–81.

Meinhart, N.T., & Aspinall, N.J. (1969). Nursing interventions in hypovigilance. **American Journal of Nursing, 69**(5), 994–998.

Noble, M.A. (1979). Communication in the ICU: Therapeutic or disturbing? **Nursing Outlook, 27,** 195–199.

* Platzer, H. (1989). Post-operative confusion in the elderly: A literature review. **International Journal of Nursing Studies, 26,** 369–379.

Roberts, S. (1986). **Behavioral concepts and the critically ill patient**. Norwalk, CT: Appleton-Century-Crofts.

* Schnaper, N., & Cowley, R.A. (1976). Overview: Psychiatric sequelae to multiple trauma. **American Journal of Psychiatry, 133,** 883–890.

Schultz, D. (1965). **Sensory restriction: Effects on behavior**. New York: Academic Press.

* Sime, M., & Kelly, J.W. (1983). Lessening patient stress in the CCU. **Nursing Management, 14**(10), 24–26.

* Smith, M.J. (1975). Changes in judgment of duration: With different patterns of auditory information for individuals confined to bed. **Nursing Research, 24,** 93–98.

Snyder, M. (Ed.). (1985). **Independent nursing interventions**. New York: John Wiley.

* Stewart, N.J. (1986). Perceptual and behavioural effects of immobility and social isolation in hospitalized orthopedic patients. **Nursing Papers: The Canadian Journal of Nursing Research, 18**(3), 59–74.

* Wilson, L.M. (1972). Intensive care delirium. **Archives of Internal Medicine, 130,** 225–226.

Wolanin, M.O., & Phillips, L.R.F. (1981). **Confusion: Prevention and care**. St. Louis: Mosby.

Worrell, J. (1971). Nursing implications in the care of the patient experiencing sensory deprivation. **Advanced concepts in clinical nursing**. Philadelphia: Lippincott.

* Zuckerman, M., Persky, H.J., Link, K.E., & Basu, G.K. (1968). Responses to confinement: An investigation of sensory deprivation, social isolation, restriction of movement and set factors. **Perceptual and Motor Skills, 27,** 319–334.

Sensory Perception, Altered: Auditory

A state in which an individual experiences a change in the amount or patterning of oncoming auditory stimuli accompanied by a diminished, exaggerated, distorted, or impaired response to such stimuli (NANDA, 1990, p. 92) .

Carol Lewis Cullinan, R.N., C., M.S.N., F.N.P.
Janice K. Janken, R.N., Ph.D.

DEFINING CHARACTERISTICS

Advancing age
Altered communication patterns
Cerumen-occluded ear canals
Change in behavior pattern

Change in usual response to auditory stimuli
Reported or measured change in hearing acuity

OTHER POSSIBLE CHARACTERISTICS

Asking to have things repeated
Complaints of vertigo
Discharge or lesions in the auditory canals
Feelings of fullness in the ears
Hypersensitivity to high-intensity sounds
Inappropriate response to questions

Inattentiveness, unresponsiveness
Ringing, clicking, or rushing noise in one or both ears
Strained or intense facial expression during communication
Withdrawal from social activities

CONTRIBUTING FACTORS

Pathophysiological

Acoustic trauma
Eustation tube dysfunction
Impacted cerumen
Infection, upper respiratory or ear

Neoplasm
Ototoxic drugs
Presbycusis

Psychosociobehavioral

Excessive exposure to environmental noise
Hearing aid use

Solitary lifestyle
Use of cotton-tipped swabs

EXPECTED OUTCOMES

Client will achieve maximal use of residual hearing.
   Clean ear canals, unobstructed with cerumen, are maintained.
   Satisfactory communication is reported.

INTERVENTIONS	RATIONALE
Universal	
Assess understanding of what is said.	Due to poor discrimination, communication may not be comprehended.
Assess need for referral of client with unevaluated hearing deficits for audiologic testing.	Early detection can lead to proper treatment and often to prevention of severe disability.
Remove impacted cerumen by performing ear canal lavage.	Research has shown improved hearing scores were obtained in 75% of the ears after the impacted cerumen was removed.
Check the hearing aid battery to ensure proper working order.	A common problem among the elderly is forgetting to change hearing aid batteries.
Use techniques to maximize communication. Include the following: 1. Speak at a slower rate than usual	Research has shown that speech delivered at a rate of 125 words/min is more understandable to the hearing-impaired than speech delivered at 175 words/min.

INTERVENTIONS	RATIONALE
2. Eliminate background noises such as television, as much as possible, before trying to communicate	Distracting noises make auditory localization more difficult and increase difficulty in understanding by masking weaker speech sounds.
3. Gain attention before beginning to speak by using techniques such as turning the light on and off or touching the client	Getting attention is the first step in communication.
4. Face directly when speaking	Facing the client allows for visualization of mouth movements and facial expressions, providing added cues about what is being said.
5. Lower the pitch of voice	In progressive hearing loss, higher frequency tones are affected first and most severely, followed by middle and then lower frequency tone losses.
6. Supplement verbal communication with visual communication	Visual cues help improve communication.
7. Rephrase questions and thoughts, when there is not understanding, trying to use different words	Words that contain high-frequency consonants such as s, th, f, k, t, p, sh, c, ch, h, z, and w are often difficult to discriminate, and other words not using these high-pitched consonants may aid in comprehension.
8. Do not shout or speak loudly	Shouting obscures consonants and amplifies vowels, making words more difficult to understand.
Teach how to clean ear canal correctly to remove wax accumulations.	Being aware that wax accumulation can impair hearing and preventing this from occurring will allow better hearing; encourages follow through with the procedure.
1. Never use cotton-tipped swabs or other sharp objects to clean ears	Sharp objects are capable of harming the external auditory canal and tympanic membrane, as well as compacting the cerumen into the ear canal.
2. Suggest over-the-counter drugs available, such as Cerumex or Debrox, which soften cerumen and when followed by lavage assist in removing it	Increased knowledge of one's condition motivates the client to make necessary changes in life-style.

INTERVENTIONS

RATIONALE

Interventions	Rationale
Teach family/significant other adaptive strategies for communicating with the hearing impaired, such as not initiating conversations from other rooms.	Significant others need explanations of sensory loss and ways in which they can help the client better cope with the loss.
Inpatient None	
Community Health/ Home Care None	

REFERENCES/BIBLIOGRAPHY

* Cullinan, C.A., & Janken, J.K. (1990). Effect of cerumen removal on the hearing ability of geriatric patients. **Journal of Advanced Nursing, 15,** 594–600.

* Janken, J.K., & Cullinan, C. (In press). Auditory sensory/perceptual alteration: validation study suggests revisement of defining characteristics. **Nursing Diagnosis**.

McConnell, E.S. (1988). Nursing diagnoses related to physiological alteration. In M.A. Matteson, & E.S. McConnell (Eds.). **Gerontological nursing concepts and practice** (pp. 331–428). Philadelphia: Saunders.

North American Nursing Diagnosis Association. (1990). **Taxonomy I** (Rev. 1990). St. Louis: NANDA.

Stone, J.T. (1987). Interventions for psychosocial problems associated with sensory disabilities in old age. In B. Heller, L. Flohr, & L. Zegans (Eds.). **Psychosocial interventions with sensorially disabled persons** (pp. 243–259). New York: Grune & Stratton.

Sensory Perception, Altered: Touch

A state in which an individual of any age experiences tactile stimulation deprivation or lack of arousal of response perceptible as the sense of touch.

Gladys Simandl, R.N., Ph.D.
Leona VandeVusse, R.N., C.N.M., M.S.

DEFINING CHARACTERISTICS

Crying
Decreased activity
Emaciation
Failure to thrive
Inability to localize touch
Increased incidence of infection
Listlessness
Low IQ scores

Quietness
Pallor
Paresthesia
Poor nutrition
Relative immobility
Social isolation
Unresponsiveness to social stimuli
Verbalizes lack of meaningful relationships

CONTRIBUTING FACTORS

Pathophysiological

Neurological impairment
Physical anomalies

Restricted mobility
Specialized care provisions required

Psychosociobehavioral

Abuse
Family problems
Inadequate stimuli
Institutionalized living conditions
Lack of proximity of loving relationships

Limited access to social resources
Monotonous environment
Parental deprivation
Violence

EXPECTED OUTCOMES

Client will receive amount of human touch experiences appropriate to individual needs and
        development.
      Weight is gained.
      There is a decreased rate of infections.
      Meaningful relationships are developed.
      Desire for handholding, hugs is expressed.
      Normal growth and development patterns are resumed.
Client will remain in a safe environment, free from potential safety hazards, such as excessive
        heat or sharp objects.
      Ways to cope with paresthesia are verbalized.
      Safety hazards in living environment are recognized.
      Suggestions for the elimination of safety hazards in living environment are contributed.

INTERVENTIONS	RATIONALE
Universal	
Assess self-awareness of touch and how it is used in the individual nurse's practice.	Three types of touch (protective, task, and caring) were identified among a group of intensive care nurses (Estabrooks, 1989). Human touch experiences have had positive effects on various populations, including infants (Scarr-Salapetek, & Williams, 1973; Solkoff, Yaffe, Weintraub, & Blase, 1969), surgical patients (Tovar, & Cassmeyer, 1989), seriously ill patients (McCorkle, 1974), and the elderly (Burnside, 1973).
Assess need for touch, including whether the touch experiences are procedural or human, and the quality of touch such as the intensity, duration, type, and frequency.	A limited amount of affectional touch was found in neonatal intensive care units and intensive care units (Pohlman, & Beardslee, 1987; Schoenhofer, 1989).
Use touch as a means of communication.	Touch has been found to convey attitudes of caring, acceptance, support, clinical competence, and pain relief (Weaver, 1990). Touch has also been defined within a communication framework (Rubin, 1963; Barnett, 1972).

INTERVENTIONS	RATIONALE
Teach safe ways to cope with paresthesia, such as testing for hot surfaces with other body parts or using other senses to assess danger.	There are little empirical data to support nursing interventions in the perceptual touch area. This intervention is supported, however, by traditional teaching among nurses.
Inpatient Vary textures in the environment.	This intervention has been used effectively with infant and elderly populations to increase responses to perceptual touch deficits.
Schedule (increase or decrease) the amount of human and procedural touches appropriate to individual need. Cluster procedural touches.	Touch experiences, especially the procedural type, can be viewed as negative by the client. This intervention is suggested by numerous authors as a way to group task-oriented procedures so the client gains a sense of pattern about when to expect procedural and other types of touch.
Use volunteers to help program touch interventions.	Volunteers and grandmothers have been helpful in meeting the demands for touch with select client groups (Fritsch-deBruyn, Capalbo, Rea, & Siano, 1990; LaRossa, & Brown, 1982).
Use backrubs and massage to intervene therapeutically.	The effects of backrubs and massage remain to be explored, but they are generally believed to promote healing and comfort (White, 1988).
Encourage touch among parents, safe adults, and children.	Certain qualities of touch, such as strong intensity and contact over a large extent of a child's body, was related to the child's sophisticated body image (Weiss, 1984).
Design and implement group activities that promote social interaction and touching, such as dancing and handholding.	Noninteractive older adults have been found to touch and communicate with each other in meaningful human ways following group touch activities (Burnside, 1973).
Use contact or noncontact therapeutic touch (see Appendix A).	Therapeutic touch has had positive effects on various client populations, including infants (Leduc, 1989), rehabilitation clients (Payne, 1989), clients experiencing pain (Wright, 1987), persons with AIDS (Newshan, 1989), and anxiety (Heidt, 1981).

INTERVENTIONS

RATIONALE

Community Health/ Home Care

Teach clients, families, and communities the need for safe, meaningful touch in people's lives.

Numerous benefits (e.g., a sense of acceptance and connectedness as well as comfort and an expression of compassion) have been identified as outcomes of safe, meaningful touch.

REFERENCES/BIBLIOGRAPHY

* Barnett, K. (1972). A theoretical construct of the concepts of touch as they relate to nursing. **Nursing Research, 21**, 102–110.
* Beaver, P.K. (1987). Premature infants' response to touch and pain: Can nurses make a difference? **Neonatal Network, 6**(3), 13–17.
* Burnside, I.M. (1973). Caring for the aged: Touching is talking. **American Journal of Nursing, 73**, 2060–2063.
* Estabrooks, C.A. (1989). Touch: A nursing strategy in the intensive care unit. **Heart & Lung, 18**, 392–401.
  Fritsch-deBruyn, R., Capalbo, M., Rea, A., & Siano, B. (1990). Cuddler program provides soothing answers. **Neonatal Network, 8**(6), 45–49.
* Gunzenhauser, N. (Ed.). (1990). **Advances in touch: New implications in human development**. Skillman, NJ: Johnson & Johnson.
* Hasselmeyer, E.G. (1964). The premature neonate's response to handling. In American Nurses' Association, **ANA Clinical Sessions: Expanding Horizons in Knowledge: Implications For Nursing,** (pp. 15–22). New York: American Journal of Nursing.
  Klaus, M.H., & Kennell, J.H. (1976). **Maternal-infant bonding**. St. Louis: Mosby.
  Klaus, M.H., & Kennell, J.H. (1982). **Parent-infant bonding** (2nd ed.). St. Louis: Mosby.
* Kramer, M., Chamorro, I., Green, D., & Knudtson, F. (1975). Extra tactile stimulation of the premature infant. **Nursing Research, 24**, 324–334.
  LaRossa, M.M., & Brown, J.V. (1982). Foster grandmothers in the premature nursery. **American Journal of Nursing, 82**, 1834–1835.
* McCorkle, R. (1974). Effects of touch on seriously ill patients. **Nursing Research, 23**, 125–132.
* Medoff-Cooper. (1988). The effects of handling on preterm infants with bronchopulmonary dysplasia. **IMAGE: Journal of Nursing Scholarship, 20**, 132–134.
  Montague, A. (1978). **Touching: The human significance of the skin.** New York: Harper & Row.
* Pohlman, S., & Beardslee, C. (1987). Contacts experienced by neonates in intensive care units. **Maternal-Child Nursing Journal, 16**, 207–226.
* Rubin, R. (1963). Maternal touch. **Nursing Outlook, 2**, 828–831.
* Scarr-Salapatek, S., & Williams, M.L. (1973). The effects of early stimulation on low birth weight infants. **Child Development, 44**, 94–101.
* Schoenhofer, S.O. (1989). Affectional touch in critical care nursing: A descriptive study. **Heart & Lung, 18**, 146–154.

* Solkoff, N., Yaffe, S., Weintraub, D., & Blase, B. (1969). Effects of handling on the subsequent development of premature infants. **Developmental Psychology, 1**, 765–768.
* Tovar, M.K., & Cassmeyer, V.L. (1989). Touch: The beneficial effects for the surgical patient. **AORN Journal, 49**, 1356–1361.
* Weiss, S.J. (1984). Parental touch and the child's body image. In C. C. Brown (Ed.). **The many facets of touch**, (pp. 3–12). Skillman, NJ: Johnson & Johnson.
* Weiss, S.J. (1988). Touch. In J.J. Fitzpatrick, R.L. Taunton, & J.Q. Benoliel (Eds.). **Annual Review of Nursing Research, 6**, 3–27.
* Weaver, D.F. (1990). Nurses' views on the meaning of touch in obstetrical nursing practice. **Journal of Gynecological Nursing, 19**, 157–161.
  White, J.A. (1988). Touching with intent: Therapeutic massage. **Holistic Nursing Practice, 2**(3), 63–67.

APPENDIX A

Therapeutic Touch As Intervention

DEFINITION: A specific healing intervention that involves a secularized laying-on-of-hands. It is derived from Eastern traditions and requires additional educational preparation.

DATA

Overall efficacy: 40%

PROCESS

Centering: the nurses put themselves in the best state for healing
Assessment: the nurse assesses the client for fluctuations, decreases, increases, or changes in energy fields

---

498 SECTION TWO

Unruffling the field: the nurse disrupts the client's energy patterns to facilitate healing
Intervention: the nurse redistributes the client's energy patterns
Variations in technique

Expected Outcomes for Therapeutic Touch

Decreased anxiety and fear.
Decreased pulse and respiratory rate.
Decreased sense of loneliness.
Energy exchange.
Improved circulation and tissue perfusion.
Increased effectiveness and general coping skills.

Increased sense of belonging.
Increased sense of body-mind relaxation.
Increased sense of well-being.
Person-centeredness.
Requests future therapeutic touch sessions.

REFERENCES/BIBLIOGRAPHY

(for therapeutic touch)

Carlson, R., & Shield, B. (Eds.). (1989). **Healers on healing**. Los Angeles: Tarcher.

* Clark, P.E., & Clark, M.J. (1984). Therapeutic touch: Is there a scientific basis for the practice? **Nursing Research, 33**, 37–41.

Dossey, B.M., Keegan, L., Guzzetta, C.E., & Kolkmeier, L.G. (1988). **Holistic nursing: A handbook for practice**. Rockville, MD: Aspen.

* Heidt, P. (1981). Effect of therapeutic use of touch on anxiety level of hospitalized patients. **Nursing Research, 30**, 32–37.

* Krieger, D. (1975). Therapeutic touch: The imprimatur of nursing. **American Journal of Nursing, 75**, 784–787.

Krieger, D. (1979). Therapeutic touch: **How to use your hands to help or to heal**. Englewood Cliffs, NJ: Prentice-Hall.

* Krieger, D., Peper, E., & Ancoli, S. (1979). Therapeutic touch: Searching for evidence of physiologic change. **American Journal of Nursing, 79**, 660–662.

* Leduc, E. (1989). The healing touch. **Maternal Child Nursing, 14**(1), 41–43.

Macrae, J. (1987). **Therapeutic touch: A practical guide**. New York: Knopf.

* Newshan, G. (1989). Therapeutic touch for symptom control in persons with AIDS. **Holistic Nursing Practice, 3**(4), 45–51.

* Payne, M.B. (1989). The use of therapeutic touch with rehabilitation clients. **Rehabilitation Nursing, 14**, 69–72.

* Quinn, J.F. (1984). Therapeutic touch as energy exchange: Testing the theory. **Advances in Nursing Science, 6**(2), 42–49.

* Randolph, G.L. (1984). Therapeutic and physical touch: Physiological response to stressful stimuli. **Nursing Research, 33**, 33–36.

* Wright, S.M. (1987). The use of therapeutic touch in the management of pain. **Nursing Clinics of North America, 22**, 705–714.

Sexual Dysfunction

A state in which an individual experiences a disruption of satisfactory sexual activities.

Von Best Whitaker, R.N., Ph.D.

DEFINING CHARACTERISTICS

Confusion with gender identity and gender role behavior
Confusion with sexual preferences
Impaired interdependent relationship
Inability to achieve desired satisfaction
Inhibited sexual desire
Reports of pain
Verbalization of problem

RELATED FACTORS

Pathophysiological

Altered body structure or function, e.g., pregnancy, recent childbirth, drugs, surgery, anomalies, radiation
Decreased physiological drive (with aging)
Medical conditions, e.g., endocrine disorders, urological disorders, neuromuscular and skeletal disorders, trauma to genital area

Psychosociobehavioral

Agoraphobia
Conflicting values
Cultural conflict
Fear of nurturing or being nurtured
Fear of pregnancy
Fear of sexual failure
Grief (loss of home, limbs, significant other, death)
Impaired relationship with partner
Inability to express sexual feelings, (e.g., hugging, touching, kissing, handholding)
Lack of information
Lack of privacy
Legal constraints
Nonavailability of a partner
Poor appreciation of sexual feelings
Poor body image
Poor sense of self
Religious conflict
Stress (e.g., occupational, relocation, financial)

499

EXPECTED OUTCOMES

Client's anxiety about sexual activities will be decreased.

    Knowledge of cause for altered sexual activities is expressed.

    Factors contributing to altered sexual activity are identified, e.g., illness, lack of privacy, unwilling partner, pain.

    Specific target of grief or loss that is contributing to anxiety is identified, e.g., loss of home, body part, job; death; divorce.

Client's thoughts and feelings about altered sexual activities will be translated into words.

    Fear about normalcy and appropriateness of sexual behaviors is expressed.

Client will establish honesty and trustworthiness about sexual issues.

    Way in which sexual dysfunction is affecting daily functioning is identified and discussed with sensitivity.

Client will increase interpersonal skills.

    Verbal communication is increased, and environment for verbalization is seen as non-threatening.

Client's self-concept will be enhanced.

    Feelings and concerns are verbalized.

    Positive attributes are emphasized rather than negative ones.

    Self-awareness and mutual trust are increased. (Dolan, 1990).

Client will explore ways to enhance sexual satisfaction.

    Alternative ways of expressing sexual activities are identified, e.g., hugging, kissing, touching, massage, masturbation.

Client will resume previous satisfactory sexual activity.

    The integration of the sexual self into the total identity is exhibited.

Client's own sexual feelings will be identified and accepted.

    Self-acceptance is expressed.

INTERVENTIONS   RATIONALE

INTERVENTIONS	RATIONALE
Universal	
Assess perceptions of normalcy and appropriateness of sexual activities.	Taboo topics, such as sexual activity, are ripe for misinformation, myth, and anxiety.
Assess perceptions of body image.	A positive body image enhances sexuality.
Assess perceptions of how illness has altered body image.	Illness alters perceptions of body image in two ways: acute illness causes temporary changes in body image; and chronic illness results in dramatic permanent changes in body image. Surgeries associated with altered body image are, e.g., amputation, mastectomy, orchidectomy.

Interventions	Rationale
Assess ability to verbally communicate sexual concerns.	Verbally expressing sexual concerns assists in defining pertinent issues and solutions while letting the listener know concerns exist, which will lead to decreased anxiety.
Assess knowledge of cause(s) for altered sexual behavior.	Anxiety decreases if it is known that external factors can precipitate alteration in sexual activity. It is not unusual for an intervention to correct an underlying health problem to produce alterations in sexual functioning.
Assess changes in cognitive functioning.	Changes in cognitive functioning due to disease may contribute significantly to the loss of interest in intimate and sexual behavior.
Assess the need to grieve after loss of familiar sexual activities.	Grief due to a loss is within the range of normal human emotion.
Assess previous sexual activities.	Sexual activity during the mature years is highly associated with frequency and satisfaction of sexual behaviors during the younger years.
Assess presence of depression.	Clients with chronic illnesses are at high risk for the development of depression.
Assess the degree to which chronic illness alters life style.	Reactive depression (feelings of discontent, fatigue, anxiousness) is frequently manifested in individuals with chronic illness and, its intensity is influenced by the gravity of the loss caused by chronic illness.
Assess perception of the problem.	Verbal ventilation via semi-structured open-ended questions allows for guided questions and concern that openly address sexual problems.
Assess perception of sexual behavior.	Sexual behavior includes verbal and nonverbal expressions (i.e., words of caring, touching, hand-holding, etc.) and genital and nongenital activities.

INTERVENTIONS	**R**ATIONALE
Assess the influence of religion on sexual functioning.	Specific religious doctrines influence sexuality by prescribing or prohibiting certain behaviors, such as premarital intercourse or abortion; but in general, religion has an effect on sexuality by how it shapes a person's concept as a sexual being, e.g., as essentially good or bad.
Assess the influence of culture and society upon sexual function.	Culture is the map that directs the pace for the genesis of sexual development and expression within a society, i.e., sexuality is organized, defined, and policed via society.
Assess physical condition.	Changes in body systems (cardiorespiratory, musculoskeletal, etc.) may increase tiredness or decrease activity endurance, e.g., arthritis may impede movement and flexibility, thus necessitating an alteration in sexuality.
Assess age changes.	Body systems change with the maturational process.
Determine if the alteration of sexual activities is temporary.	The focus is on assisting the resumption of satisfactory sexual activity as quickly as possible if the alteration of sexual activities is temporary.
Determine if the alteration of sexual activities is permanent.	Discovering novel ways to achieve sexual satisfaction is essential to a return to sexual health if the alteration of sexuality is permanent.
Assess availability of privacy.	Alternative sexual activities, e.g., masturbation, may be inhibited if one does not have a personal location for activities to take place.
Monitor the presence of pain.	Chronic pain as well as medication for pain may decrease libido.
Monitor the level of energy.	Fatigue decreases the client's enthusiasm for participation in sexual activity.
Assess history of satisfying sexual activity prior to illness.	Having had satisfying sexual activity prior to illness increases the likelihood of seeking alternative strategies to reproduce this satisfaction.

INTERVENTIONS	RATIONALE
Strive to maintain a nonjudgmental interview milieu.	Perceptions of what rules should govern sexuality, sexual activities, and what is right and wrong abound and vary among individuals.
Conduct sexual assessment in privacy.	The provision of privacy helps to preserve dignity, increase verbal exchange, and decrease anxiety.
Include significant others as part of the therapeutic discussion of altered sexual activities.	Inclusion of significant other decreases anxiety by enhancing verbal exchange about the loss of familiar sexual activity.
Be an active listener.	The use of body language, e.g. facial expressions and encouraging words, demonstrates active listening and caring.
Use clear, simple, and specific language when discussing sexual concerns.	The use of clear, simple language assists in the stating of concerns while concomitantly decreasing anxiety. Also, verbal simplicity communicates an awareness and an understanding of issues of concern.
Identify acceptable sexual alternatives.	Discussion of acceptable alternatives decreases anxiety and demonstrates that the listener is concerned about clients' values and beliefs about sexuality.
Discuss alternative sexual activities that are compatible with life style, e.g., illness, living arrangement.	Knowledge that alternative sexual activities, such as hugging, kissing, massage, single or mutual masturbation, and sexual aids other than sexual intercourse are available helps to decrease anxiety and increase sexual satisfaction.
Provide anticipatory guidance about the impact of medical treatments upon sexual function.	Questions about secondary problems, e.g., sexual alterations, are seldom addressed; thus the effects of therapy on sexual behavior may be undiagnosed.
Teach about body changes related to gender and age.	Male and female body changes differ (e.g., males' experience may include erectile alterations, prostatectomy, circulation, etc.; and female experiences may include vaginal dryness, vaginal pain, etc.).
Increase knowledge base about sexuality and sexual functioning.	The dispelling of myths and preconceived ideas increases hope for satisfying sexual activities.

INTERVENTIONS	RATIONALE
Provide education addressing cultural and social diversity.	Social, cultural, and ethnic environments are the foundations that shape expectations of sexual behaviors and delineate boundaries for sanctioned expression of sexuality.
Provide education addressing ethnic and racial diversity.	Racial and ethnic factors are frequently stereotyped; and judgments about sexuality are not predicated upon presenting data and empirical evidence but upon prejudices, myths and social stereotypes.
Provide education addressing religious influence on sexuality.	Religion affects sexuality by influencing individual behavioral choices and perceptions of self.
Teach to increase knowledge of sexuality and sexual activities.	Information describing the effects that specific factors (age, pregnancy, and therapies) may have on sexuality and sexual functioning decreases feelings of powerlessness and anxiety.
Teach about alternative interventions to aid in sexual functioning.	Information addressing assistive devices (e.g., penile implants), modification in clothing that enhances self-image, changes in position for sexual intercourse, alternative sexual practices, and methods to increase energy levels—e.g., participation in sexual activities after resting—assists to promote sexual satisfaction.
Teach about possible rejection in social situations because of physical condition (e.g., paraplegic, mastectomy, etc.).	Discussions addressing fear of rejection help to prepare for fear or prejudice harbored by others.
Assist with locating appropriate sexual partners.	If socialization is to increase, potential places for socialization to occur must be identified.
Educate about factors that contribute to optimum sexual performance.	Knowing which factors increase sexual satisfaction prevents disillusionment, e.g., self-image, mood, consenting relationship, absence of anxiety, variability in sexual interest, arousal, and enjoyment and satisfaction.

INTERVENTIONS	RATIONALE
Inpatient	
Assess for opportunities for sexual expression.	Sexual opportunities require privacy, which is frequently lacking in an institution.
Assess ability to express sexual activities.	The institutionalized are frequently perceived as too frail, impaired, etc. to desire sexual activities.
Assess perceptions of the organizational structure of the institution.	Expressions of sexual activity as a basic human need are frequently not accepted. Clients are not provided a place to be alone or to meet alone with another.
Promote privacy for residents.	The placement of a Do Not Disturb sign on a closed door, or having roommate removed to another room when privacy is needed, promote the inclusion of sexual activities and an intimate relationship. Altered sexuality usually returns to normal when the client learns to interact within the inpatient environment.
Promote sexuality and sexual functioning through teaching.	Knowledge about factors which decrease sexual functioning, such as course of illness, medications, and perceptions of illness allays anxiety and promotes an early return to sexual health.
Assess knowledge concerning the actions and side effects of medication(s).	Knowledge of medication(s) assists in the observations of typical and atypical drug responses, e.g., decreased libido, impotence, irritability, fatigue.
Assess living arrangements, such as crowding.	Availability of privacy promotes sexual activities.
Community Health/ Home Care	
Assist in developing and using community support systems.	Awareness of support systems such as nurse, sex therapist, marriage and family counselor, physician, singles group, sex education, physical therapist, contraceptive counselor, etc., decreases anxiety by knowing that assistance is available. Support groups may assist in dispelling myths that are inhibiting sexual activities by promoting verbal communication between similar others.

INTERVENTIONS	**R**ATIONALE
Share the possible changes in life-style that are to occur as a result of alterations in sexual functioning.	Knowing what alterations in life-style might occur helps to prepare for such an occurrence and contributes to mutual problem solving with sig-nificant others—e.g., stress management, need for private time for intimacy, grieving for significant other, coping with illness or physical disability, acceptance of sexual orientation (homosexuality, transsexuality).

REFERENCES/BIBLIOGRAPHY

Annon, J.S. (1976). The PLISSIT Model: A proposed conceptual scheme for the behavioral treatment of sexual problems. **Journal of Sex Education and Therapy, 2**, 1–15.

Bancroft, J. (1989). **Human sexuality and its problems** (2nd ed.). New York: Churchill Livingstone.

* Boyer, G., & Boyer, J. (1982). Sexuality and aging. **Nursing Clinics of North America, 17**(3) 421–427.

Brusich, J. (1990). Religious influence and sexuality. In C. J. Fogel, & D. Laurer (Eds.). **Sexual health promotion** (pp. 160–178). Philadelphia: Saunders.

Buchaya, H. (1988). Dangerous obsession. **Nursing Times, 84**(35), 69–71.

Bullough, V., & Bullough, B. (1983). Childhood and family of male sexual minority groups. **High Values: Achieving High Level Wellness, 7**(4), 19–26.

Carpenito, L.J. (1987). **Nursing diagnosis: Application to clinical practice** (2nd ed.). Philadelphia: Lippincott.

Carter, M. (1990). Disturbances in sexuality. In C.I. Fogel, & D. Laurer (Eds.). **Sexual health promotion** (pp. 305–312). Philadelphia: Saunders.

Conine, T.A., & Evans, J.H. (1982). Sexual reactivation of chronically ill and disabled adults. **Journal of Allied Health, 11**, 261–270.

Davenport, W. H. (1977). Sex in a cross cultural perspective. In F. A. Beach (Ed.). **Human sexuality in four perspectives** (pp. 115-163). Baltimore: John Hopkins University Press.

Deakin, G. (1988). Male sexuality. **Nursing: The Journal of Clinical Practice, Education and Management, 3**(26), 961–962.

Dolan, M. (1990). Community and home health care plans. Springhouse, PA: Springhouse.

Fonseca, J.D. (1970). Sexuality—A quality of being human. **Nursing Outlook, 18**(11), 25.

Gordon, D. (1988). Male sexuality. **Nursing: The Journal of Clinical Practice, Education and Management, 3**(26), 961–962.

* Hogan, R.M. (1982). Influences of culture on sexuality. **Nursing Clinics of North America, 17**(3), 365–376.

Kaas, M. (1978). Sexual expression of the elderly in nursing homes. **Gerontologist, 18**, 372.

Kinsey, A., Pomeroy, W.B., & Martin, C.E. (1948). **Sexual behavior in the human male**. Philadelphia: Saunders.

Kinsey, A. Pomeroy, W.B., & Martin, C.E. (1952). **Sexual behavior in the human female**. Philadelphia: Saunders.

Kolaszynska-Carr, A.B. (1987). Prejudice, differences and deviation. **Nursing: The Journal of Clinical Practice, Education and Management, 3**(19), 715–717.

Kronberg, M.E. (1983). Nursing interventions in management of the assaultive patient. In J.R. Lion, & W.H. Reid (Eds.). **Assault within psychiatric facilities** (pp. 225–240). New York: Grune & Stratton.

LeLievre, J. (1986). When sex becomes a problem. **Nursing Times, 82**(21), 57–58.

Masters, W.H., & Johnson, V. (1970). **Human sexual inadequacy**. Boston: Little, Brown.

Miller, J.F. (1983). **Coping with chronic illness: Overcoming powerlessness**. Philadelphia: Davis.

Montagu, A. (1971). **Touching: The human significance of the skin**. New York: Columbia University Press.

Newman, G., & Nichols, C.R. (1969). Sexual activities and attitudes in older persons. **Journal of the American Medical Association, 73**(3), 226–229.

Pfeiffer, E., & Davis, G.C. (1972). Determinants of sexual behavior in middle and old age. **Journal of the American Geriatric Society, 20**, 151.

Renshaw, D.C. (1988). Sex and cognitively impaired patients. **Consultant, 28**(3), 133–137.

Shippee-Rice, R. (1990). Sexuality and aging. In C.I. Fogel, & D. Lauver (Eds.). **Sexual health promotion** (pp. 97–116). Philadelphia: Saunders.

Smith, L.S. (1990). Human sexuality from a cultural perspective. In C.I. Fogel, & D. Lauver (Eds.). **Sexual health promotion** (pp. 87–96). Philadelphia: Saunders.

Starr, B., & Weiner, M. B. (1981). **On sex and sexuality in the mature years**. New York: Stein & Day.

Zilbergeld, B. (1978). **Male sexuality: A guide to sexual fulfillment**. Boston: Little, Brown.

Sexuality Patterns, Altered

A state in which an individual indicates concern regarding his/her sexuality or sexual expression.

Leona VandeVusse, R.N., C.N.M., M.S.
Gladys Simandl, R.N., Ph.D.

DEFINING CHARACTERISTICS

Change of interest in self or other
Complaints of fatigue, weakness, or sleep disturbance
Complaints of pain
Reported conflicts involving values
Reported inability to achieve desired satisfaction
Seeking confirmation of desirability
Sleep disturbance
Statements of altered body image
Verbalization of problem
Verbalizes fear of incontinence
Verbalizes fear of pregnancy
Verbalizes limitation or change in sexual behavior or activities

CONTRIBUTING FACTORS

Pathophysiological

Altered body structure or function (pregnancy, recent childbirth, drugs, surgery, anomalies, disease process, trauma, or radiation)
Pain

Psychosociobehavioral

Alteration in self-concept
Alteration in self-esteem
Change in relationship with partner(s)
Cultural norms regarding gender roles
Decreased opportunities for socialization
Ineffectual or absent role models

508

Lack of privacy
Lack of significant others
Misinformation or lack of knowledge
Physical abuse
Poor communication with partner
Prescriptive religious beliefs

Psychosocial abuse, e.g., harmful
    relationships
Societal values of attractiveness,
    stigmatizing differences
Values conflict
Vulnerability

EXPECTED OUTCOMES

Client will express comfort with own sexuality.
    Understanding of own unique sexual response rather than comparison to norm is verbalized.
    Statements about others' responses to sexuality are made, but client is able to affirm own as positive.
    Self is viewed as a sexual person.
    Varied modes of sexual expression are verbalized, as well as satisfaction with them.
Client will verbalize ways to cope with alterations.
    Nature of sexual alteration is verbalized, including adverse effects of treatments, medications, and surgical alterations.
    Ways to enhance relaxation and reduce stress are verbalized.
Client will express comfort with own body image.
    Three self-affirming things about own body are stated.

INTERVENTIONS

RATIONALE

Interventions	Rationale
Universal	
Assure confidentiality.	Reassurance must be given that intimate details will not be shared with others in ways that could be identifiable.
Establish a therapeutic relationship, using oneself to convey genuineness, caring, empathy, and acceptance.	The interpersonal sensitivity of the nurse is important in expressing the value, worth, dignity, and uniqueness of each individual. In such a context, the client and nurse develop mutual respect and a trusting relationship.
Be attentive to own language use and be nonjudgmental to avoid imposing one's own values and preconceptions, making assumptions, or promoting stereotypes.	Sexuality is a sensitive and personal area. It is important that the nurse acknowledge many and varied expressions of people's sexuality. In order to not impose assumptions or stereotypes, the nurse needs to be aware of her or his personal values, sexuality, and a wide range of

INTERVENTIONS	RATIONALE
	human sexual behaviors. The more open the nurse, the more readily clients will share their unique selves without fear of being judged. By obtaining client data, the nurse can more readily diagnose and intervene appropriately with the client evidencing an alteration in sexuality.
Actively listen; listen attentively and respond, both verbally and nonverbally.	This conveys that the nurse is available to help. Also, by attending to what the individual shares, the nurse receives and interprets cues about concerns and needs for information about sexuality.
Draw sexual genogram to demonstrate diagrammatically the client's (and partner's) family patterns.	This three-generation diagram, using a family tree model, portrays the client's views of family members' sexual attitudes and practices. Past history may be helpful to the client in understanding her or his own sexual patterns, and in elucidating the influences of family history, attitudes, roles, and interactions.
Acknowledge that discussing sexuality can seem difficult in our culture.	By acknowledging this common difficulty in discussing sexuality openly, the nurse helps to place the client at ease.
Use presence.	By remaining in the room, engaged in sexual discussions—despite the difficulty of the subject matter—the nurse conveys her or his willingness to care for the client in a holistic manner.
Inform that expressing concerns and asking questions of the nurse can also help the client be more comfortable and open with others, such as partner, friends, family, and those in life situations similar to the client's.	During client-nurse interactions, the nurse models discussing sexuality in a matter-of-fact manner, using appropriate terminology, and evidencing a nonjudgmental approach. This can benefit clients' communication with significant others by enhancing clients' own clarity and comfort while discussing sexuality. Once freedom and openness in discussions occur, sharing information, preferences, and suggestions are facilitated and people generally express relief and greater satisfaction.

INTERVENTIONS	RATIONALE
Provide reassurance that (1) there are certain common human needs such as affection, touching, holding, and closeness; (2) people vary greatly in their personal choices and preferences for expressing these needs; (3) there are some general experiences that people share; and (4) there is some information, or at times misinformation, that is often commonly believed by people.	The purposes of these reassurances are to (1) allow the client to feel more at ease; (2) provide some basic information, without limiting the discussion to only culturally normative behaviors; (3) allow the client to counter commonly held opinions that do not fit personally; (4) inform the client that a wide range of human behavior exists; (5) acknowledge that there is a lack of complete knowledge about human sexuality; and (6) place the client in the position as the most knowledgeable person about his or her own sexuality.
Emphasize that the only standards for satisfaction of importance are those that meet that particular individual's (and partner's) needs.	Assuming a client-centered attitude helps the client trust the nurse and share vital sexual information that promotes problem solving.
Provide permission-giving for the client to explore personal needs and desires.	The nurse conveys openness and a willingness to facilitate discussion of concerns, indicates that sexuality is an appropriate topic of exploration, and conveys the message that flexibility and creativity are possible in meeting needs.
Teach that sexuality is a normal human response, involved in all human beings' relationships with people.	Human sexuality is not synonymous with any one sexual act, since it involves complex inter-relationships among one's self-concept, body image, personal history, family and cultural influences, and all interactions with others.
Teach that human skin is richly supplied with nerve endings and that there are many other ways to find pleasure than exclusively genital, coital stimulation.	The Western notion of sexuality is centered primarily in the belief that orgasm is the goal or end point. This may not be true for persons who have altered sexual responses nor for healthy persons or couples.
Discuss ways to accommodate the client's life style to physical, emotional, or spiritual changes.	In order for a person to cope, information on alterations that have permanent consequences for that person's life is essential. Matter-of-fact presentation of what is known, honest admission of what is not known, and encouragement for exploration of what is best for each client will facilitate the client's adjustment.

INTERVENTIONS	**R**ATIONALE
Discuss stressors and ways to lessen them.	Stress interferes with relaxation and the ability to enjoy the affection and sensations during sexual encounters.
Teach relaxation techniques, such as imagery, fantasy, massage, local warmth, warm bath, or shower.	These can increase comfort, feelings of calm, and promote mobility—while secondarily enhancing personal hygiene.
Teach to focus on pleasuring and sensual touching of all areas of the body, but only gradually incorporating genital touch.	Called "sensate focus," this involves nondemanding encounters to awaken and develop awareness of pleasure over more of the body surface. Initial discouragement of genital contact is to prolong the encounter and allow perception of sensations from all over the body.
Teach normalcy of masturbation.	It is important to dispel myths regarding untoward effects of masturbation for all clients, but in particular those who are coping with changing their sexual patterns due to illness, disease, or choice.
Teach alternative expressions of sexuality, using varied skin surfaces for caressing, fondling, nibbling, kissing, suckling, mutual masturbation, oral-genital stimulation—plus coital alternatives such as intrathigh, intramammary, and anal intercourse, as well as artificial aids.	Western notions of sexuality have emphasized the view that sexual expression is synonymous with penis-in-vagina intercourse. Human sexual behavior is much more varied and creative. Suggesting options and encouraging people to explore and discover what satisfies them can assist people to better meet their own needs.
Teach client who is experiencing changes in body processes (e.g., pregnancy, postpartum, postsurgery, altered mobility states) alternative positions to use. Teach adaptations to the major positions (facing each other with one partner above the other, side-lying, or rear approach).	Knowledge of alternative positions may enhance comfort. These adaptations, such as changing angles of approach or supporting furniture (e.g., table, bed, chair, wheelchair with arm rests removed, pillows, wall) can make a significant difference in people's ability to continue lovemaking. Showing pictures or diagrams of couples using varied positions conveys information that other people have explored alternatives and allows consideration of a wider range of possibilities.

INTERVENTIONS	RATIONALE
Teach about available sexual aids such as lubricants, scented oils, vibrators, prosthetic devices, erotic clothing or stories, as well as the beneficial effects of pubococcogeal muscle exercises (Kegel exercises).	These aids and exercises may enhance sensation or ability to engage in a variety of sexual activities.
Teach to empty bladder before sexual activity.	An empty bladder can increase comfort, promote bladder control, and decrease the chance of infection.
Teach methods of contraception if client is sexually active during childbearing years with partner(s) of the opposite sex. Include back-up methods and ways to discuss best methods between couples.	Education about contraceptive methods is imperative in preventing unwanted pregnancies.
Teach prevention of sexually transmitted diseases and the need for early recognition, diagnosis, and treatment.	Individuals may make informed decisions regarding their sexual choices.
Teach possible effects of treatment such as radiation therapy, medications, or surgery.	Knowledge of sexual alterations due to treatments or surgery helps the client cope with the changes in bodily functioning.
Encourage the use of personal affirmations every day.	It is important that self-affirmation be stated about one's body and functioning in order to promote self-esteem.
Use music therapy.	Music and its diverse rhythms can be used to calm people, increase stimulation and pleasure, decrease pain and anxiety, encourage movement, and enhance a sense of freedom. Personal preferences are important to assess. Encourage clients to participate, individually or with partners, by singing, humming, dancing, moving in time to the music, or beating out rhythms.

INTERVENTIONS	RATIONALE
Suggest a variety of readily available self-help books, pamphlets, and community resource groups.	These enable the expansion of knowledge through personal reading and the extension of support systems by meeting others in similar circumstances. These approaches may be more flexible and provide a valuable supplement to the exclusive use of one-to-one interaction with the nurse.
Refer to community resources for additional assistance, such as American Cancer Society, Reach for Recovery, United Ostomy Association, or many others.	These groups provide information, acceptance, models of others who are adjusting to various health challenges, and community building among people with similar experiences.
Refer for specialized help, such as sexual therapy, for premature ejaculation or vaginismus; refer for specialized help such as psychological therapy for long-term effects of abusive relationships. Inform clients of their right to treatment by nonjudgmental practitioners who will respect their individual needs, and clients' rights to change practitioners if desired.	Use available resources when a client requests and when the situation requires more knowledge, skill, or extensive care than the nurse can provide. It is important that the nurse suggest referrals to practitioners who will treat clients with respect, empathy, cooperation, and a nonjudgmental attitude when addressing their particular needs. These suggestions help clients make their own choices about their sexuality, place the nurse in a client advocacy role, and admit that the nurse does not know everything.
Inpatient Provide privacy. Use locked doors if possible when partner visits. Accept masturbation when done privately by individuals or consenting adults. In long-term situations, accept physical closeness among consenting residents; consider supplying rooms with double beds for couples.	Sexual expression is a normal human response. It is customary and acceptable to express one's sexuality privately.

INTERVENTIONS	RATIONALE
Encourage involvement, support, and visitation by the people the client indicates are close relationships, without exclusion based on nuclear family definitions.	In some instances, the family of origin or immediate family may be estranged or unavailable, and the client may have identified others whom the client considers as close, supportive partners or members of a family of choice. The client's needs and wishes are respected. The nurse supports these people as the client's family and utilizes them as vital components of the client's social support network when planning care.
Advocate for nonexclusionary visitation policies.	When visitation policies are restricted to legally recognized family members, some clients are separated from the people who comprise their family of choice. Such restrictive visitation policies contribute to stereotyping, do not recognize changing societal patterns in family composition, and eliminate a valuable resource for the client and nurse when planning care.
Community Health/ Home Care Contribute to a societal change about people who appear different or who have chosen alternative life styles through consciousness raising, advocacy, encouragement of the work of various community support groups, and promotion of legislation that is nondiscriminatory and increases access for all members of society.	Broad-scope nursing actions can contribute to lessening the impact of social stigmatizing of those who appear different, while affirming the worth of all individuals.

REFERENCES/BIBLIOGRAPHY

Allen, M.E. (1987). A holistic view of sexuality and the aged. **Holistic Nursing Practice, 1**(4), 76–83.
Bernhard, L.A., & Dan, A.J. (1986). Redefining sexuality from women's own experiences. **Nursing Clinics of North America, 21**, 125–136.
Bing, E., & Colman, L. (1977). **Making love during pregnancy**. New York: Bantam.
Blackmore, C. (1988). The impact of orchidectomy upon the sexuality of the man with testicular cancer. **Cancer Nursing, 11**, 33–40.

Brink, P.J. (1987). Cultural aspects of sexuality. **Holistic Nursing Practice, 1**(4), 12–20.

* Brunngraber, L.S. (1986). Father-daughter incest: Immediate and long-term effects of sexual abuse. **Advances in Nursing Science, 8**(4), 15–35.

Bulechek, G.M., & McCloskey, J.C. (Eds.). (1985). **Nursing interventions: Treatments for nursing diagnoses**. Philadelphia: Saunders.

Butler, R.N., & Lewis, M.J. (1987). Myths and realities of sex in the later years. **Provider, 13**(10), 11–13.

Carty, E.A., & Conine, T.A. (1988). Disability and pregnancy: A double dose of disequilibrium. **Rehabilitation Nursing, 13**, 85–87, 92.

Cooley, M.E., & Cobb, S.C. (1986). Sexual and reproductive issues for women with Hodgkin's disease: I. Overview of issues. **Cancer Nursing, 9**, 188–193.

Cooley, M.E., Yeomans, A.C., & Cobb, S.C. (1986). Sexual and reproductive issues for women with Hodgkin's disease: II. Application of PLISSIT model. **Cancer Nursing, 9**, 248–255.

Csesko, P.A. (1988). Sexuality and multiple sclerosis. **Journal of Neuroscience Nursing, 20**, 353–355.

* Ellis, D.J., & Hewat, R.J. (1985). Mothers' postpartum perceptions of spousal relationships. **Journal of Obstetric, Gynecologic, and Neonatal Nursing, 14**, 140–146.

* Fischman, S.H., Rankin, E.A., Soeken, K.L., & Lenz, E.R. (1986). Changes in sexual relationships in postpartum couples. **Journal of Obstetric, Gynecologic. and Neonatal Nursing, 15**, 58–63.

Fogel, C.I., & Lauver, D. (Eds.). (1990). **Sexual health promotion**. Philadelphia: Saunders.

Friend, R.A. (1987). Sexual identity and human diversity: Implications for nursing practice. **Holistic Nursing Practice, 1**(4), 21–41.

Goddard, L.R. (1988). Sexuality and spinal cord injury. **Journal of Neuroscience Nursing, 20**, 240–244.

Heinrich-Rynning, T. (1987). Prostatic cancer treatments and their effects on sexual functioning. **Oncology Nursing Forum, 14**(6), 37–41.

* Hirsch, A.M., & Hirsch, S.M. (1989). The effect of infertility on marriage and self-concept. **Journal of Obstetric, Gynecologic and Neonatal Nursing, 18**(4), 13–20.

Hogan, R.M. (1980). **Human sexuality: A nursing perspective**. New York: Appleton-Century-Crofts.

Julty, S. (1979). **Men's bodies, men's selves**. New York: Dell.

Kaplan, H.S. (1974). **The new sex therapy: Active treatment of sexual dysfunctions**. New York: Brunner/Mazel.

Kitzinger, S. (1983). **Woman's experience of sex**. New York: Putnam.

Kus, R.J. (1987). Sex, AIDS, and gay American men. **Holistic Nursing Practice, 1**(4), 42–51.

MacElveen-Hoehn, P., & McCorkle, R. (1985). Understanding sexuality in progressive cancer. **Seminars in Oncology Nursing, 1**(1), 56–62.

Malek, C.J., & Brower, S.A. (1984). Rheumatoid arthritis: How does it influence sexuality? **Rehabilitation Nursing, 9**(6), 26–28.

Masters, W. H., & Johnson, V. E. (1966). **Human sexual response**. Boston: Little, Brown.

McCormick, G.P., Riffer, D.J., & Thompson, M.M. (1986). Coital positioning for stroke afflicted couples. **Rehabilitation Nursing, 11**(2), 17–19.

* McCusker, J., Zapka, J.G., Stoddard, A.M., & Mayer, K.H. (1989). Responses to the AIDS epidemic among homosexually active men: Factors associated with preventive behavior. **Patient Education and Counseling, 13**(1), 15–30.

Metcalfe, M.C., & Fischman, S.H. (1985). Factors affecting the sexuality of patients with head and neck cancer. **Oncology Nursing Forum, 12**(2), 21–25.

Moore, D.S. (1984). A literature review on sexual abuse research. **Journal of Nurse-Midwifery, 29**, 395–398.

*Moore, D.S., & Erickson, P.I. (1985). Age, gender, and ethnic differences in sexual and contraceptive knowledge, attitudes, and behaviors. **Family and Community Health, 8**(3), 38–51.

Mueller, L.S. (1985). Pregnancy and sexuality. **Journal of Obstetric, Gynecologic, and Neonatal Nursing, 14**, 289–294.

North American Nursing Diagnosis Association. (1990). **Taxonomy I** (Rev. 1990). St. Louis: NANDA.

*Olshansky, E.F. (1988). Responses to high technology infertility treatment. **Image: Journal of Nursing Scholarship, 20**, 128–131.

Pervin-Dixon, L. (1988). Sexuality and the spinal cord injured. **Journal of Psychosocial Nursing and Mental Health Services, 26**(4), 31–34.

Poorman, S.G. (1988). **Human sexuality and the nursing process**. Norwalk, CT: Appleton & Lange.

*Rickus, M.A. (1987). Sexual concerns of the female patient: Research study and analysis, Part 3. **ANNA Journal, 14**, 192–195.

Rieve, J.E. (1989). Sexuality and the adult with acquired physical disability. **Nursing Clinics of North America, 24**, 265–276.

Saylor, C.R. (1990). The management of stigma: Redefinition and representation. **Holistic Nursing Practice, 5**(1), 45–53.

Schwarz-Appelbaum, J., Dedrick, J., Jusenius, K., & Kirchner, C.W. (1984). Nursing care plans: Sexuality and treatment of breast cancer. **Oncology Nursing Forum, 11**(6), 16–24.

Sheahan, S.L. (1989). Identifying female sexual dysfunctions. **Nurse Practitioner, 14**(2), 25–26, 28, 30, 32, 34.

Shipes, E. (1987). Sexual function following ostomy surgery. **Nursing Clinics of North America, 22**, 303–310.

Snyder, M. (Ed.). (1985). **Independent nursing interventions**. New York: Wiley.

Spica, M.M. (1989). Sexual counseling standards for the spinal-cord injured. **Journal of Neuroscience Nursing, 21**(1), 56–60.

*Stanley, M.J.B., & Frantz, R.A. (1988). Adjustment problems of spouses of patients undergoing coronary artery bypass graft surgery during early convalescence. **Heart and Lung, 17**, 677–682.

*Stevens, P.E., & Hall, J.M. (1988). Stigma, health beliefs and experiences with health care in lesbian women. **Image: Journal of Nursing Scholarship, 20**, 69–73.

*Swanson, J.M. (1988). The process of finding contraceptive options. **Western Journal of Nursing Research, 10**, 492-503.

Wabrek, A.J., & Gunn, J.L. (1984). Sexual and psychological implications of gynecologic malignancy. **Journal of Obstetric Gynecologic and Neonatal Nursing, 13**, 371–376.

*White, E.J. (1986). Appraising the need for altered sexuality information. **Rehabilitation Nursing, 11**(3), 6–9.

*Winter, L. (1988). The role of sexual self-concept in the use of contraceptives. **Family Planning Perspectives, 20**, 123–127.

Woods, N.F. (Ed.). (1984). **Human sexuality in health and illness** (3rd ed.). St. Louis: Mosby.

Woods, N.F. (1987). Toward a holistic perspective of human sexuality: Alterations in sexual health and nursing diagnoses. **Holistic Nursing Practice, 1**(4), 1–11.

*Zeidenstein, L. (1990). Gynecological and childbearing needs of lesbians. **Journal of Nurse-Midwifery, 35**, 10–18.

Skin Integrity, Impaired

A state in which an individual's skin continuity is disrupted.

Nancy A. Stotts, R.N., Ed.D.

DEFINING CHARACTERISTICS

Abrasion
Avulsion
Eruptions
Erythema
Excoriation
Exudate
Incision

Lesions
Necrotic tissue
Pain
Slow/no capillary refill
Subcutaneous tissue exposed
Tenderness
Ulceration

CONTRIBUTING FACTORS

Pathophysiological

Decreased sensation
Diabetes
Dry skin
Excess moisture
Hyperthermia
Hypothermia
Illness therapies
    Chemotherapy
    Radiation therapy
    Medications, e.g., steroids

Immunoincompetence
Impaired perfusion
Obesity
Pressure over a bony prominence
Starvation
Stressors
    Caffeine
    Pain
    Smoking
Trauma

Psychosociobehavioral

Psychological stress

518

EXPECTED OUTCOMES

Client will have completely healed skin.
  Epithelial cells on surface of wound are replaced.
  Dermal repair is characterized by healthy granulation tissue.
Client's epidermal and dermal tissue will remain intact.
Client can identify cause of disruption of skin integrity and propose methods to prevent or mitigate recurrence.

INTERVENTIONS

RATIONALE

Universal	
Monitor the skin for progress in repair or increased disruption characterized by increased inflammation, exudate, pus, formation of a scab, necrotic tissue.	Ongoing evaluation of status is the basis for determining whether the treatment is effective or whether the care needs to be changed.
Monitor systemic status to determine if factors present may contribute to delayed healing e.g. starvation, obesity, immunocompetence, impaired perfusion.	Same as above.
Evaluate the cause of the skin impairment and focus intervention on it to prevent recurrence.	The focus of the intervention must include the etiology in order to prevent exacerbation of the problem and support repair.
Keep the impaired skin in a moist physiological environment. 1. Remove exudate with dressings and irrigation; or treat the wound with antibacterial medications 2. Remove necrotic tissue by supporting autolytic processes, using enzymes, surgical excision, or dressings to debride the dead skin 3. Use a dressing that will keep the tissue moist	Repair occurs most rapidly in a physiologically moist environment. Debris delay healing and so must be removed. The treatment schedule (including dressing) must be selected considering the nature of the injury, knowledge of the treatments selected, and the physiological status.

INTERVENTIONS	RATIONALE
4. Establish a schedule for treatment of the impairment that is congruent with the severity of the wound, the overall physiological status, and the type of dressing selected	
Remove the cause of the skin impairment. If due to pressure over a bony prominence: 1. Put on regular and more frequent turning schedule 2. Consider the need for mattress overlays or specialty beds 3. Mitigate shearing when moving in bed If due to therapy: (e.g., surgery, intravenous therapy) 1. Treat symptomatically 2. Try to prevent recurrence	Tissue that has been injured is more fragile and susceptible to reinjury than is uninjured skin.
Keep intact skin surrounding the wound clean. 1. Establish a regular bathing schedule 2. Use skin oil to keep clean tissue moist 3. Bathe after excess perspiration, urinary, and fecal incontinence	Perspiration, urine, and feces are skin irritants and also change the pH of the skin, supporting growth of skin flora and increasing the possibility of infection.
Provide adequate nutrients for healing. 1. Provide a well-balanced diet, enteral feedings, or parenteral nutrition as needed 2. Record intake 3. Refer for dietary consultation if intake is not or will not be sufficient for 7–10 days	Nutrients are required for repair of tissue. Healing of minor injuries in healthy persons can occur without adequate intake. More severe or prolonged injuries in healthy persons or minor injuries in ill or debilitated persons require exogenous nutrients.

INTERVENTIONS	RATIONALE
Maintain normal glucose level in diabetics. 1. Balance activity, diet, and insulin to achieve normal blood glucose 2. Monitor blood glucose on a regular schedule, promptly reporting elevations or providing prescribed insulin	Increased glucose levels impair healing.
Provide sufficient fluid intake. 1. Encourage 1500-2000 cc/24 H in healthy persons 2. The required intake in those with renal or cardiovascular disease will be established by the physician based on the client's physiological ability and client losses 3. Consult with physician, if oral intake is not sufficient, for order for intravenous support	Water is critical to cell viability and hypovolemia is a serious threat to replacement of damaged skin.
Encourage optimal oxygenation to tissues. 1. Provide maximal inspiratory maneuvers 2. Establish a regular turning and positioning schedule for clients confined to bed 3. Establish a progressive ambulation and activity schedule for ambulatory clients	Oxygen is critical to cellular activity. Inspiratory maneuvers, changing position, ambulation, and activity all have been established as means to enhance ventilation and therefore oxygenation.
Inpatient Consider referral to centers where treatment such as hyperbaric oxygen, implantation with cultured keratinocytes, or growth factor	Persistent wounds require therapy that will lead to closure, as chronic open wounds disrupt lives, reduce ability to return to work or take part in daily activities, and may develop into cancerous lesions.

INTERVENTIONS	RATIONALE
therapy are available for chronic tissue impairment resistant to usual therapy.	
Teach signs and symptoms of healing, progression of tissue impairment, and when to call the wound care nurse or physician.	Self-care is based on understanding of what is expected and usual as well as when help from a professional is needed.
Prepare the client and significant other to provide wound care after inpatient discharge, as needed. 1. Provide a list of needed supplies 2. Teach the procedure for wound care and dressing removal 3. Encourage return demonstration of the technique	Same as above
Teach client, and significant other, ways to support repair by maintaining regimen for oxygenation and activity, nutrition, and, when needed, glucose control.	Same as above
Refer to home health care as needed for wound care.	Wounds require ongoing care. It is important to prospectively plan for needs so wounds are not neglected, which leads to increased possibility of infection.
Community Health/ Home Care None	

REFERENCES/BIBLIOGRAPHY

Alvarez, O., Rozint, J., & Meehan, M. (1990). Principles of moist wound healing: Indications for chronic wounds. In D. Krasner (Ed.). **Chronic wound care**. King of Prussia, PA: Health Management Publications.

Cuzzell, J.Z. (1990). Choosing a wound dressing: A systematic approach. **AACN Clinical Issues, 1**, 566–577.

Cuzzell, J.Z., & Stotts, N.A. (1990). Wound Care: Trial & error yields to knowledge. **American Journal of Nursing, 90**, 53–63.

DeWitt, S. (1990). Nursing assessment of the skin and dermatologic lesions. **Nursing Clinics of North America, 25**, 235–247.

Orgill, D., & Demling, R.H. (1988). Current concepts and approaches to wound healing. **Critical Care Medicine, 16**(9), 899–908.

Reed, B.R., & Clark, R.A. (1985). Cutaneous tissue repair: Practical implications of current knowledge. II. **Journal of American Academy of Dermatology, 13**(6), 919–941.

Rodheaver, G.T. (1990). Controversies in topical wound management: Wound cleansing and disinfection. In D. Krasner (Ed.). **Chronic wound care**. King of Prussia, PA: Health Management Publications.

Rosenberg, C.S. (1990). Wound healing in the patient with diabetes mellitus. **Nursing Clinics of North America, 25**, 247–261.

Stotts, N.A. (1986). Impaired wound healing. In V.K. Carrieri, A.M. Lindsey, & C.M. West (Eds.). **Pathophysiological phenomena in nursing** (pp. 343–366). Philadelphia: Saunders.

Wheeland, R.G. (1987). The newer surgical dressings and wound healing. **Dermatology Clinics, 5**(2), 393–407.

Witkowski, J.A., & Parish, L.C. (1986). Cutaneous ulcer therapy. **International Journal of Dermatology, 25**(7), 420–426.

Young, M.E. (1988). Malnutrition and wound healing. **Heart & Lung, 17**(1), 60–67.

Skin Integrity, Impaired: Risk

A state in which an individual's skin continuity is vulnerable to disruption.

Nancy A. Stotts, R.N., Ed.D.

RISK FACTORS

Pathophysiological

Decreased sensation
Diabetes
Dry skin
Edema
Hyperthermia
Hypothermia
Illness therapies
    Chemotherapy
    Intravascular lines
    Medications, e.g., steroids
    Radiation therapy

Immunoincompetence
Impaired perfusion
Obesity
Old age
Pressure over a bony prominence
Starvation
Stressors
    Caffeine
    Pain
    Smoking
Trauma

Psychosociobehavioral

Psychological stress

EXPECTED OUTCOMES

Client's skin will remain intact.
    No symptoms of skin trauma are experienced.
    All skin surfaces are intact, warm, and pink.
    Nutritional status meets body requirements.

INTERVENTIONS

RATIONALE

Universal Institute a regular and uniform method to evaluate skin integrity. 1. Determine whether the risk for impairment is due to local factors (e.g., excess pressure, dry skin, excessively moist skin) or systemic factors (e.g., starvation, impaired perfusion, immunoincompetence, obesity)	Prospective identification of skin disruption is important to prevent complications. Ongoing evaluation of status is the basis for determining whether prevention is effective or whether the interventions need to be changed.
Evaluate the cause of the risk for skin impairment and focus intervention on it. If due to pressure over a bony prominence: 1. Place on regular and more frequent turning schedule 2. Consider the need for mattress overlays or specialty beds 3. Mitigate shearing when moving in bed If due to therapy: (e.g., surgery, intravenous therapy) 1. Treat symptomatically 2. Try to prevent recurrence	The focus of the prevention must include the etiology in order to prevent the problem.
Keep skin at risk both clean and moist. 1. Establish a regular bathing schedule 2. Use skin oil to keep clean tissue moist 3. Bathe after excess perspiration and urinary and fecal incontinence	Epideral and dermal cell replacement occurs most optimally in a moist environment. Perspiration, urine, and feces are skin irritants and also change the pH of the skin, supporting growth of skin flora and increasing the possibility of infection.

INTERVENTIONS	RATIONALE
Provide adequate nutrients for skin cell replacement. 1. Provide a well-balanced diet, enteral feedings, or parenteral nutrition as needed 2. Record intake 3. Refer for dietary consultation if intake is not or will not be sufficient for 7-10 days	Nutrients are required for replacement of skin tissue.
Maintain normal glucose level in diabetics. 1. Balance activity, diet, and insulin to achieve normal blood glucose 2. Monitor blood glucose on a regular schedule, promptly reporting elevations or acting to provide prescribed insulin	Increased glucose levels impair cellular defenses and increase risk of skin disruption.
Provide sufficient fluid intake. 1. Encourage 1500–2000 cc/24 H in healthy persons 2. The required intake in those with renal or cardiovascular disease will be established by the physician based on the client's physiological ability and losses 3. Consult with physician, if oral intake is not sufficient, for order for intravenous support	Water is critical to cell viability.
Encourage optimal oxygenation to skin tissues. 1. Provide maximal inspiratory maneuvers 2. Establish a regular turning and positioning schedule for clients confined to bed	Oxygen is critical to cellular activity. Inspiratory maneuvers, changing position, ambulation, and activity all have been established as means to enhance oxygenation.

INTERVENTIONS	RATIONALE
3. Establish a progressive ambulation and activity schedule for ambulatory clients	
Teach signs and symptoms of skin impairment that require attention from a wound care nurse or physician.	Self-care is based on an understanding of what is expected and usual and when help from a professional is needed.
Teach the client and significant other ways to prevent breakdown by maintaining regimen for oxygenation and activity, nutrition, and, as appropriate, glucose control.	Same as above.
Inpatient None	
Community Health/ Home Care None	

REFERENCES/BIBLIOGRAPHY

Colburn, L. Early intervention for the prevention of pressure ulcers. In D. Krasner (Ed.). **Chronic wound care,** pp. 78–88. King of Prussia, PA: Health Management Publications.

Cuzzell, J.Z., & Stotts, N.A. (1990). Wound care: Trial & error yields to knowledge. **American Journal of Nursing, 90,** 53–63.

DeWitt, S. (1990). Nursing assessment of the skin and dermatologic lesions. **Nursing Clinics of North America, 25,** 235–247.

Sleep Pattern Disturbance

A state in which an individual experiences disruption in the quality or quantity of sleep

Kathleen Beyerman, R.N., Ed.D.

. . . .

DEFINING CHARACTERISTICS

Awakening early and not being able to fall
      back to sleep
Dark circles under eyes
Disorientation
Expressionless face
Fatigue
Frequent yawning
Inability to concentrate
Midsleep awakening, interrupted sleep
Mild, fleeting nystagmus

Postdormital confusion ("sleep drunkenness")
Posture changes
Ptosis
Restlessness
Sleep latency
Slight hand tremor
Thick speech with mispronunciation and
      incorrect words

CONTRIBUTING FACTORS

Pathophysiological

Dementia
Depression
Functional hypersomnia
Illness symptoms: cough, dyspnea, fever, immobility, nocturia, pain, pruritus
Illness therapies
      Medications: diuretics, antihypertensives, beta blockers, corticosteroids, histamine antag-
          onists, anti-inflammatory agents, antineoplastics, anticonvulsants, sympathomimetics
      Procedures: monitoring, treatments
Klein-Levine syndrome
Narcolepsy

Neurological disorders: brain tumors, head trauma, infections, spinal cord lesions
Nocturnal myoclonus
Pickwickian syndrome
Pregnancy and postpartum hormonal disorders
Pulmonary compromise
Restless-legs syndrome
Sleep apnea
Thyroid disfunction
Uremia

Psychosociobehavioral

Abuse of CNS stimulants
Alcohol ingestion
Anxiety
Boredom
Caffeine ingestion
Chronic alcoholism
Circadian rhythm changes
Daytime napping
Depression
Discomfort: bed, room temperature, pillow, position, therapeutic devices
Disruption of sleep to fulfill responsibilities: family, work
Disruptions in life routines and habits due to imposed hospital routine
Environmental change
Environmental stimuli
Excessive use of hypnotics and/or tranquilizers
Fear
Fewer than 5 hours of sleep every 24 hours
Inability to relax

Invasive procedures
Jet lag
Lack of exercise
Light
Living alone
Nasal obstruction
Negative expectations about sleep
Noise: patients, staff, environment
Psychiatric disorders: personality disorders, affective disorders, functional psychoses
REM sleep interruptions
Sleep/wake reversal
Sleeping in a strange place
Stress
Thinking about home
Weight loss
Withdrawal from CNS depressants
Worry about diagnosis, family, health, job, tests, dislodging tubing, and attached equipment

EXPECTED OUTCOMES

Client will report feeling rested after waking.
  Sleep occurs within 20 minutes of going to bed.
  Ability to fall back to sleep prior to rising time occurs within five minutes after waking.
Client will remain asleep until desired or planned waking time.
  Sleep disturbers are identified and strategies are developed to diminish or eliminate them.

INTERVENTIONS	**R**ATIONALE
Universal Ascertain the cause(s) of the sleep pattern disturbance. Refer to the physician for medical or psychiatric problems.	The focus of the interventions must be on the etiologies of the problem in order to adequately treat.
Monitor sleeping pattern.	Continued evaluation of the efficacy of interventions will help the nurse develop a plan which works.
Teach good sleep hygiene 1. Maintain regular sleep hours 2. Develop bedtime routines such as reading, snacking, listening to music 3. Follow a bedtime preparation routine of settling activities: bathing, brushing teeth, tidying room, straightening bed, dimming or eliminating light	Sleep hygiene stimulates an expectation of rest and sleep prior to bedtime. These routines help people to wind down. A set rising and retiring time (without napping during the day) helps the body maintain a regular sleep/wake rhythm.
Teach relaxation strategies such as medication, imaging, progressive muscle relaxation, and self-hypnosis (positive thinking).	Relaxation techniques can substantially decrease sleep latency and improve the perception of the quality of sleep.
Teach the avoidance of bedtime drinking and to keep a commode, bedpan, or urinal near the bed if nocturia is a problem.	Decreased fluid intake will reduce urinary output. Tea, colas, coffee, cocoa have both stimulant and diuretic properties. Falling back to sleep is easier if one spends less time out of bed.
Teach sidelying sleeping positions.	Poor sleepers are more likely to spend prolonged periods on their backs with their head straight than are good sleepers.
Teach those with sleep apnea to reduce their weight and to wear a collar around their neck during sleep.	Weight reduction decreases the incidence of sleep apnea in those who are obese. A neck collar prevents neck flexion and maintains the airway while sleeping.

INTERVENTIONS	**RATIONALE**
Teach to void just prior to retiring.	Proprioreceptors are activated when the bladder fills; this leads to awakening with the sensation of urgency.
Teach to avoid large meals, caffeine, and nicotine for several hours prior to bedtime.	Stimulants interfere with sleep. It takes about eight hours to metabolize these stimulants.
Inpatient Assess for pain, pruritus, or any other discomforts; treat and/or medicate accordingly prior to bedtime.	Discomfort will interfere with sleep.
Reduce environmental noise by assessing the environment, and eliminate unnecessary noise.	The auditory awakening threshold is decreased with age and in strange environments.
Provide comfort measures before bedtime such as conversation and the offer of a backrub.	The security of knowing that nurses are available promotes sleep. Backrubs foster muscle relaxation and sleep.
Administer prescribed tranquilizers or hypnotics *only* if other sleep-promoting interventions have failed.	Unwanted daytime effects from sleep medications may be experienced.
Community Health/ Home Care Teach the importance of moderate and regular exercise more than two hours prior to bedtime.	Moderate exercise can increase the perception of tranquility, well-being, and sleepiness. Strenuous exercise may be stimulating.
Teach to avoid the prolonged use of hypnotics and/or to seek assistance for supervised drug withdrawal after taking hypnotics for four to six months.	Hypnotics lose sleep-promoting effects after two to three weeks of continuous use. Increased dosage for effect leads to residual daytime effects of sluggishness, poor coordination, and depression. Rebound insomnia may occur as a result of withdrawal of some hypnotics.

INTERVENTIONS	**R**ATIONALE
Teach avoidance of alcohol.	Alcohol may cause sleepiness for a few hours after ingestion, but it interferes with REM sleep, causes early morning awakening, and accentuates daytime sleepiness.
Teach the value of not going to bed too soon and the importance of getting up and going into another room until feeling sleepy if awake 15 minutes after going to bed.	Some fatigue is necessary to sleep. Returning to bed reactivates the stimulus/response of sleepiness by associating the bed with falling asleep quickly.
Teach to arrange for respite (periodic uninterrupted sleep) if necessary sleep is consistently interrupted due to responsibilities of work or family care.	A long night of uninterrupted sleep may lessen the deleterious effects of sleep loss.
Teach that as one ages, there are normal changes in sleep architecture.	Aging leads to increased time spent sleeping, increased sleep latency, increased night awakenings, a marked decrease in stage four, and a shortened REM.
Teach the use of ear plugs, white noise, quiet music, or to move to a quiet room if noise interferes with sleep.	Ear plugs will block sounds. White noise such as a white-noise machine, radio tuned between two stations, air conditioner, or fan will diminish the perception of sound. A bedroom away from the front of the house/apartment will have less street noise.
Teach to stay in bed only as long as sleep is needed—no longer.	Remaining in bed too long results in shallow and fragmented sleep with many awakenings.
Teach the benefit of a light bedtime snack.	Digestive hormones may have a sedative effect. Tryptophan in the snack may stimulate the production of serotonin.

REFERENCES/BIBLIOGRAPHY

Erma, K.L., & Herrera, C.O. (1989, September). When your patient tells you he can't sleep. **RN,** 79–84.

* Fontaine, D.K. (1989). Measurement of nocturnal sleep patterns in trauma patients. **Heart & Lung, 18**(4), 402–410.

Fredrickson, P.A., Richardson, J.W., Esther, M.S., & Lin, S. (1990). Sleep disorders in psychiatric practice. **Mayo Clinic Proceedings, 65,** 861–868.

Gottlieb, G.L. (1990). Sleep disorders and their management: Special considerations in the elderly. **The American Journal of Medicine, 88** (Suppl. 3A), 29–33.

Hauri, P.J., & Esther, M.S. (1990). Insomnia. **Mayo Clinic Proceedings, 65,** 869–882.

* Kao LoC., & Kim, M.J. (1986). Construct validity of sleep pattern disturbance: A methodological approach. In M.E. Hurley (Ed.). **Classification of Nursing Diagnoses: Proceedings of the Sixth Conference**. (pp. 197–206). St. Louis: Mosby.

* Kinney, M., & Guzzetta, C.E. (1989). Identifying critical defining characteristics of nursing diagnoses using magnitude estimation scaling. **Research in Nursing & Health, 12,** 373–380.

Mendelson, W.B. (1987). **Human sleep: Research and clinical care**. New York: Plenum.

Morgan, K. (1987). **Sleep and aging: A research based guide to sleep in later life**. Baltimore: Johns Hopkins University Press.

Muncy, J.H. (1986). Measures to rid sleeplessness: 10 points to enhance sleep. **Journal of Gerontological Nursing, 12**(8), 6–11.

* Reimer, M. (1987). Sleep disturbance: Nursing interventions perceived by patients and their nurses as facilitating nocturnal sleep in hospitals. In A. McLane (Ed.). **Classification of Nursing Diagnoses: Proceedings of the Seventh Conference** (pp. 372–376). St. Louis: Mosby.

Social Interaction, Impaired

A state in which an individual participates in an insufficient or excessive quantity or ineffective quality of social exchange (NANDA, 1990, p. 51).

Patricia Danaher-Dunn, R.N., M.S.

DEFINING CHARACTERISTICS

Subjective Reports

Dysfunctional interaction with peers, family, and/or others
Inability to form a satisfying intimate relationship with another person
Verbalized discomfort in social situations
Verbalized inability to receive or communicate a satisfying sense of belonging, caring, interest, or shared history

Objective Observations

Dysfunctional interaction with peers, family and/or others
Family report of change of style or pattern of interaction
Inability to care for self
Observed discomfort in social situations
Observed inability to receive or communicate a satisfying sense of belonging, caring, interest, or shared history
Observed use of unsuccessful social interaction behaviors

CONTRIBUTING FACTORS

Pathophysiological

Altered physical appearance	Communicable diseases	Sensory deficits
Altered thought processes	Limited physical mobility	Substance abuse
Chronic illness	Mental retardation	Terminal illness

Psychosociobehavioral

Absence of available significant others or peers
Alternating clinging and distancing behaviors
Communication barriers
Distractibility/inability to concentrate
Divorce/death of a spouse
Emotional barriers
Exploitation of others for personal gratification
Hopelessness
Institutionalization
Knowledge/skill deficit about ways to enhance mutuality

Lack of vocational skills
Language barriers
Low self-esteem
Physical or verbal aggression toward others when one's own wishes are thwarted
Poor impulse control
Severe anxiety
Sociocultural dissonance
Therapeutic isolation

EXPECTED OUTCOMES

Client will acknowledge impairment in social interaction and explore the nature of relationships with others.

Thoughts and feelings related to existing inability to form close interpersonal relationships with others are verbalized.

Previous or current relationships with others are discussed, exploring patterns of communication and behavior which enhance or inhibit these relationships.

A desire for change in the quality of interaction with others in the future is expressed.

Client will develop a plan to improve social interaction.

Behavioral goals for change are identified.

Realistic time frames for achieving goals are identified.

Skill development is practiced, specifically addressing areas of deficit.

Behavior consistent with behavioral goals is demonstrated.

Barriers to goal attainment are anticipated and alternative actions are planned.

Client will interact with others in a mutually satisfying fashion.

Social interaction with others is sought.

Existing strengths are used and newly acquired skills are applied to social interaction.

Feedback from others about newly acquired behaviors is sought.

Improved self-esteem is verbalized and demonstrated.

INTERVENTIONS

RATIONALE

Universal

Interventions	Rationale
Assess for prexisting mental health problem which may be ameliorated by psychotherapeutic or psychopharmacological intervention.	This may need to precede intervention dealing with social interaction.

INTERVENTIONS	RATIONALE
Observe current social interactions including existing social skills, risk-taking behaviors, self-disclosure patterns, coping skills, self-defeating behaviors, and ability to empathize with others.	Knowledge of baseline behavior is necessary when assisting in setting realistic goals.
Explore feelings related to interacting with others, including fears, anxieties, and desires.	Sensitivity to feelings enhances development of a therapeutic relationship, promotes self-esteem, and facilitates examination of the experience.
Explore the interpretation of interactions with others including distortions, automatic thoughts, and assumptions.	This assists with discovery of inconsistencies in assumptions and alternative interpretations that may have been overlooked.
Encourage the development of specific goals for behavioral change to clearly identify the types of interactions to be improved and with whom.	Client involvement in the problem-solving process is critical if behavioral change is to occur.
Provide for the development of interactive skills through modeling, education, practice, interaction, and feedback.	Development of alternative behavior and interactive skills will enhance relationship building. Positive feedback improves self-esteem and reinforces behavioral change.
Inpatient Observe behavior and interaction patterns with others on the unit, including avoidance, splitting, clinging, and projection as well as effective coping skills.	Observation of behavior and interaction patterns provides identification of areas of impairment as well as coping skills upon which to expand.
Explore feelings and thoughts related to interaction with others on the unit.	Sensitivity to feelings facilitates a trusting therapeutic relationship. Exploration of thoughts related to interaction with others on the unit provides an opportunity to assess interpretations and assumptions. Focusing on the here and now provides an opportunity for immediate feedback.

INTERVENTIONS	RATIONALE
Assist with establishment of reasonable goals and clear behavioral objectives for improving social interaction during inpatient hospitalization.	Change is more likely to occur if there is involvement in the problem-solving process, and goals are based upon client wishes. Focus in inpatient period keeps objectives within a reasonable time frame and allows opportunity for immediate feedback.
Provide unit activities which address the needs of individuals with impaired social interaction, including daily community meetings, group therapy, social skills training, and shyness groups.	Activities of varying types, size, and intensities offer opportunities for practicing new behaviors and developing potential for growth.
Provide recognition and positive reinforcement for risk-taking and improvement in behavior, appearance, and interaction.	Recognition promotes self-esteem, and positive reinforcement encourages repetition of behavior.
Encourage involvement of significant others in treatment on the unit.	Involvement of significant others emphasizes their importance. This provides an opportunity to further explore problem areas and reinforce new learning.
Develop a discharge plan which addresses continued need for development or maintenance of improved social interaction, e.g., day hospital, self-help groups.	Appropriate social interaction is reinforced, and continued growth is facilitated.
Community Health/ Home Care Explore community resources which address the needs of individuals with impaired social interaction, including community mental health centers, psychotherapy agencies, day treatment programs, self-help groups, community support programs, etc. and refer as appropriate.	Knowledge of an array of services promotes selection of the best resource.

Interventions	Rationale
Attempt to provide resources necessary to access community services, including financial, transportation, communication, and advocacy.	Ease of access to service facilitates compliance with treatment.
With permission, facilitate communication among significant others as well as agencies and systems.	Open dialogue avoids confusion and promotes a consistent approach among those involved. It also emphasizes the value of following through with treatment.
Teach use and side effects of psychoactive medication as well as other symptom management strategies. Monitor medication if necessary.	Relapse of symptoms and hospitalization may be avoided. Medication compliance improves when there is a clear understanding of the indication and management of side effects.

REFERENCES/BIBLIOGRAPHY

Carpenito, L.J. (1989). **Nursing diagnosis: Application to clinical practice**. Philadelphia: Lippincott.

Liberman, R.P., & Engel, J. (1990). Rehabilitation of the seriously mentally ill. **Directions in Psychiatry, 9**(4), 1–8.

Liberman, R.P., et al. (1986). Training skills in the psychiatrically disabled: Learning, coping and competence . **Schizophrenia Bulletin, 12**(4), 632–647.

McFarland, G.K., & McFarlane, E.A. (1989). **Nursing diagnosis and intervention**. St. Louis: Mosby.

McLane, A.M. (Ed.). (1987). **Classification of Nursing Diagnoses: Proceedings of the Seventh Conference**. St Louis: Mosby.

North American Nursing Diagnosis Association. (1990). **Taxonomy I** (Rev. 1990). St. Louis: NANDA.

Peplau, A.L., & Perlman, D. (1982). **Loneliness: A sourcebook of current theory, research and therapy**. New York: Wiley.

Schwartz, M.F. (1989). Social isolation. In J.M. Thompson, G.K. McFarland, J.E. Hirsch, S.M. Tucker, & A.C. Bowers (Eds.). **Mosby's manual of clinical nursing** (pp. 1769–1770). St. Louis: Mosby.

Tilden, V.P., & Weinert, C. (1987). Social support and the chronically ill individual. **Nursing Clinics of North America, 22**(3), 613–620.

Torrey, E.F. (1988). **Surviving schizophrenia: A family manual**. New York: Harper & Row.

Townsend, M.C. (1988). **Nursing diagnosis in psychiatric nursing: A pocket guide for care plan construction**. Philadelphia: Davis.

* Vaglum, P., et al. (1990). Treatment response of severe and nonsevere personality disorders in a therapeutic community day unit. **Journal of Personality Disorders, 4**(2), 161–172.

Social Isolation

A state in which an individual experiences aloneness and perceives it as imposed by others and as a negative or threatening state (NANDA, 1990, p. 52).

Patricia Danaher-Dunn, R.N., M.S.

. . . .

Note: Social isolation is a subjective experience and therefore must be validated with the individual before the diagnosis can be made.

DEFINING CHARACTERISTICS

Subjective Reports

Difficulty establishing or maintaining relationships with others
Expressed values unaccepted by the dominant cultural group
Feeling of aloneness imposed by others and/or desire for more contact with people
Feelings of rejection, uselessness, or difference from others
Inability to meet expectations of others
Inadequacy in or absence of significant purpose in life
Insecurity in social situations

Objective Observations

Absence of supportive significant others
Alteration in physical or emotional health
Altered thought processes (hallucinations, delusions, confusion)
Developmental behavior inconsistent with age level
Disregard for social customs relating to interactions
Exhibited behavior unaccepted by dominant cultural group
Hostility or violence in voice or behavior
Preoccupation with own thoughts, repetitive meaningless actions
Sad, dull affect
Uncommunicative/withdrawn behavior

CONTRIBUTING FACTORS

Pathophysiological

Alterations in mental status
Alterations in physical appearance
Chronic illness
Communicable diseases
Developmental disabilities
Drug or alcohol addiction

Incontinence
Nervous system alteration
Obesity
Physical handicaps
Sensory losses

Psychosociobehavioral

Crisis—maturational or situational
Death of a significant other
Divorce
Emotional disorders
Hospitalization
Immature interests
Inability to engage in satisfying personal
   relationships
Inadequate personal resources
Inadequate support system
Living alone

Living within a subculture
Loss of transportation
Mental illness
Move to another culture
Poverty
Recent or frequent change of residence
Recent retirement
Stress
Unaccepted social behavior
Unaccepted social values

EXPECTED OUTCOMES

Client will acknowledge social isolation and verbalize a desire and willingness to be involved with
      others.
   Feelings associated with social isolation are expressed.
   Information is disclosed about the nature and extent of social isolation.
   Expectations of self and others within relationships are explored.
Client will identify factors which contribute to social isolation.
   Previous relationships with others are discussed, exploring patterns of difficulty in
      maintaining or reestablishing these relationships.
   Areas of skill or resource development necessary for establishing new relationships are
      identified.
Client will develop a plan to become more involved with others.
   Available options for interaction with others are explored and selected.
   Resource base is expanded and skills necessary for improved interaction with others are
      developed.
   Realistic behavioral goals are set.
   Realistic time frames for achieving goals are identified.
   Concerns about risk-taking are expressed and explored.
   Barriers are anticipated and alternative actions are planned.

Client will become actively involved with others.

> Effective mechanisms to deal with anxiety are used.
> Increasing comfort with interactions and desire to continue involvement with others is reported.
> Factors which have contributed to success are identified.
> Increased self-esteem is reported.

INTERVENTIONS	**R**ATIONALE
Universal	
Explore perception of social isolation.	Examination of client perceptions serves to promote understanding and validation of feelings.
Examine specific causes of social isolation.	Understanding client-specific causes of social isolation will provide direction for planning interventions.
Engage in active listening, maintaining eye contact. When appropriate, use touch as a means of contact and comfort.	An accepting attitude conveys positive regard and promotes trust.
Explore relationship between behavior and alleviation of social isolation.	This exploration will initiate the problem-solving process. Specific behavioral goals may then be identified.
Explore available activities which promote social interaction.	Discovering available activities opens up an array of options for selection.
Encourage the development of realistic time frames for achievement of goals.	Realistic time frames promote interest and involvement in the process.
Positively reinforce active involvement with others.	Positive reinforcement enhances self-esteem and encourages maintenance of behavior.
Explore possible barriers to social interaction and teach skills necessary to overcome these barriers.	Anticipating inhibiting factors and developing skills necessary to overcome them promotes successful outcome.
Examine elements which have contributed or inhibited successful outcome.	This reinforces new knowledge and promotes continued success.

INTERVENTIONS	RATIONALE
Inpatient	
Observe behavior and interaction patterns on the unit. Explore concerns and feelings related to interaction with others.	Knowledge of baseline behavior and sensitivity to concerns and feelings promotes appropriate joint goal setting and intervention.
Make frequent contacts, orient to the unit, and assist with physical needs.	Frequent contact and attending to basic needs promote relationship building. Orientation to unit facilitates connection with the environment.
Provide feedback about withdrawn or alienating behaviors.	Demonstration of appropriate behavior will promote acceptance of others.
Provide unit activities which support various opportunities for interaction.	Activities and groups of varying types, sizes, and intensities offer opportunities for continued growth.
Give recognition and positive reinforcement for voluntary attendance at unit activities.	Recognition promotes self-esteem, and positive reinforcement encourages repetition of activity.
Encourage family members or significant others in the client's life to be involved in treatment planning on the unit.	Involvement of significant others in unit activities reinforces their importance in the client's life.
Develop discharge plan to address need for socialization upon return home from the institution.	Addressing the need for socialization upon return home emphasizes the importance of transferring new skills to the real world.
Identify physical and sensory impairments which affect communication and body image and teach compensatory strategies.	Compensating for physical or sensory impairment can reduce social isolation.
Teach recognition of signs of increasing anxiety and techniques with which to manage anxiety.	Management of anxiety will promote interaction with others.
Provide educational opportunities to enhance skill development (communication, social skills, assertiveness, ADL, etc.).	Enhancement of interactive skills promotes confidence when interacting with others.

INTERVENTIONS	**R**ATIONALE
Community Health/ Home Care	
Identify the range of resources available (people, agencies, financial, transportation, etc.).	Knowledge of existing resources may promote mobilization of support for resocialization.
Identify underlying causes of social isolation (physical, sensory, mental, financial, recent losses). Identify activities of interest.	Understanding underlying causes of social isolation and activities of interest will promote realistic goal setting, intervention attempts, and engagement in the problem-solving process.
Explore support groups available in the community for individuals isolated because of physical or mental disabilities. Provide interpreters to non-English speaking. Explore support groups available in the community for individuals isolated because of recent loss of a loved one.	Sensitivity to specific needs may promote involvement with others in similar situation.
Determine available transportation options.	Access to transportation may enhance opportunities for socialization.
Explore volunteer activities available in the community.	Volunteering may increase involvement with others and a sense of self-worth. Volunteer organizations may provide support necessary to enable access to other resources.
Explore financial and physical resources available to care givers. Explore community respite services available to care givers.	Support given to primary care givers promotes their continued involvement.
Assist with development of alternative means of communication for persons with compromised sensory ability. Explore literacy programs for persons unable to read or write.	Enhanced communication skills reduce isolation.

REFERENCES/BIBLIOGRAPHY

Carpenito, L.J. (1989). **Nursing diagnosis: Application to clinical practice**. Philadelphia: Lippincott.

* Cox, C.L., Spiro, M., & Sullivan, J.A. (1988). Social risk factors: Impact on elders' perceived health status. **Journal of Community Health Nursing, 5**(1), 59–73.

* Foxall, M.J., & Ekberg, J.Y. (1989). Loneliness of chronically ill adults and their spouses. **Issues in Mental Health Nursing, 10**, 149–167.

McFarland, G.K., & McFarlane, E.A. (1989). **Nursing diagnosis and intervention**. St. Louis: Mosby.

McFarland, G.K., & Wasli, E.L. (1986). **Nursing diagnosis and process in psychiatric mental health nursing**. Philadelphia: Lippincott.

McLane, A.M. (Ed.). (1987). **Classification of Nursing Diagnoses: Proceedings of the Seventh Conference**. St Louis: Mosby

North American Nursing Diagnosis Association. (1990). **Taxonomy I** (Rev. 1990). St. Louis: NANDA.

Schwartz, M.F. (1989). Social isolation. In J.M. Thompson, G.K. McFarland, J.E. Hirsch, S.M. Tucker, & A.C. Bowers (Eds.). **Mosby's manual of clinical nursing** (pp. 1766–1769). St. Louis: Mosby.

Tilden, V.P., & Weinert, C. (1987). Social support and the chronically ill individual. **Nursing Clinics of North America, 22**(3), 613–620.

Townsend, M.C. (1988). **Nursing diagnosis in psychiatric nursing: A pocket guide for care plan construction.** Philadelphia: Davis.

Spiritual Distress

A state in which an individual experiences a disruption in the life principle which pervades a person's entire being and which integrates and transcends one's biological and psychosocial nature (NANDA, 1990, p. 60).

Leona VandeVusse, R.N., C.N.M., M.S.
Gladys Simandl, R.N., Ph.D.

• • • • • • • • • • • •

DEFINING CHARACTERISTICS

Alterations in mood/behavior evidenced by anger, crying, withdrawal, preoccupation, anxiety, hostility, apathy, etc.
Alterations in sleep patterns
Anger toward God
Asks for space to set up shrine for religious observance
Asks for special dietary provisions
Asks nurse about his/her religious beliefs
Asks nurse to baptize child or perform other religious function
Asks to talk to clergy person
Description of nightmares/sleep disturbances
Displacement of anger toward religious representatives
Expresses concern with meaning of life/death and/or belief systems
Gallows humor
Inability to participate in usual religious practices
Questions meaning of own existence
Questions meaning of suffering
Questions moral/ethical implications of therapeutic regimen
Restlessness
Seeks spiritual assistance
Social isolation
Verbalizes concern about relationship with deity

Verbalizes fears of future, e.g., course of illness
Verbalizes inner conflict about beliefs

Contributing factors

Pathophysiological

Changes in patterns of structure or functions of body
New disease diagnosis
Terminal diagnosis or poor diagnosis

Psychosociobehavioral

Challenged belief and value system, (e.g., due to moral/ethical implications of therapy, due to
 intense suffering)
Separation from religious/cultural ties

Expected outcomes

Client will verbalize a sense of tranquility, peace, and restored integrity.
 Growth toward spiritual goals is verbalized.
 Views of how to cope with spiritual issues are discussed.
 A personal sense of meaning and purpose of life is shared.
 Statement of self-awareness of difficult life events is verbalized.

Interventions	Rationale
Universal	
Assess for substantive spiritual issues.	A person may respond more readily to general questions than to specific and direct questions about the meaning of life; their values; and their spiritual, ethical, philosophical beliefs about illness or their life situations.
Listen actively for cues as to what gives the person meaning and purpose in life.	Listening attentively and responding, both verbally and nonverbally, can indicate that the nurse is available to help. By attending to what the individual shares as personally meaningful, the nurse receives cues to that individual's spiritual state.

INTERVENTIONS	**R**ATIONALE
Clarify any desire for designation of specific religious affiliation, including any special dietary provisions and any special space or time adjustments needed for religious observances.	Institutionalized religion and its observances frequently provide comfort. There are many varied religions and clients' unique faith expressions should be respected and facilitated.
Assess the environmental context and its compatibility with the spiritual needs.	Advocating for changes in the immediate environment may need to be made in order to facilitate the client's spiritual observances, for example, designating a specific time and a separate area for prayer. Such advocacy affirms the particular spiritual needs and facilitates trust with the nurse.
Use cultural brokerage.	Cultural brokerage involves translating between the care provider's and the client's cultures when there is misunderstanding. It involves listening closely for different beliefs and values between the involved parties and recognizing the different perspectives of the people. Flexibility of the nurse is important. Sometimes respectful listening is sufficient; sometimes supporting the differing belief systems, providing information and time for its assimilation—while creatively seeking ways to accommodate both viewpoints—is crucial. At other times the client's belief system does not allow adaptations, and then the client must decide the health care that is personally acceptable, and providers must cope with understanding that person and that cultural environment.
Use self therapeutically.	It is important that the nurse engages honestly with the client in discussions to develop rapport, so that the client can know and trust the nurse.
Use presence.	Being present and "being there" with the client, offering help and a gift of the self, promotes mutual sharing and demonstrates the nurses's commitment.

INTERVENTIONS	RATIONALE
Admit that no one has answers.	Clients can find reassurance in hearing that no human being has found all the answers to life's deep questions, though they share a common search with many other humans. Affirming their personal searchings as important can provide freedom to continue exploring openly rather than inhibiting themselves out of a sense of inadequacy.
Assume a nonjudgmental attitude.	Spirituality is a sensitive and personal area. It is important that the nurse acknowledge many and varied expressions of people's spirituality. The more open the nurse, the more readily clients will share their unique beliefs without fear of being judged, and the more readily the nurse can diagnose and intervene appropriately with the client evidencing spiritual distress.
Support venting of difficult emotions.	Emotional release can be cathartic, which can promote healing of someone experiencing spiritual distress.
Share silence.	Being together in silence can help the client face some of the blankness or sense of meaninglessness that may be part of her or his spiritual distress.
Use touch.	Touch is used to enhance a sense of acceptance and connectedness with a client and to bring comfort and express compassion.
Use therapeutic touch.	Therapeutic touch may be used to relieve pain or congestion in an area in order to restore the energy levels and promote further healing.
Use relaxation techniques, including rhythmic deep breathing, meditation, etc.	There are a variety of relaxation techniques which generally include a quiet environment, a comfortable position, a repetitive sound or phrase, and adopting a passive attitude—accompanied by loose muscles and slowed, deeper breathing. These techniques are used to elicit the relaxation response which decreases sympathetic nervous system arousal, with accompanying decrease in heart rate, respiratory rate, blood pressure, oxygen

INTERVENTIONS	RATIONALE
	consumption, and anxiety. With practice, relaxation techniques contribute to feelings of peace, well-being, and a decrease in stress-related symptoms.
Use guided imagery.	Nurses can suggest that a client imagine a healing scene and process during a relaxed state. This can promote decreased stress and pain and help redirect the client toward healthy functioning as a desired effect. A suggestion can be made that the person imagine a meeting with a spiritual advisor or a personal source of spiritual strength during imagery and relate to that image.
Use prayer.	Many have expressed the helpfulness of prayer, especially in times of crisis. Nurses may be requested to pray with, pray for, or remain with a client during a prayer.
Encourage creative outlets such as journaling, poetry writing, drawing, painting.	Creative expressions can release feelings, help explore the meaning of experiences, promote hope and strength, and assist communication with spiritual source.
Encourage reminiscence and life review.	Through reminiscing and life review, "persons remember and often resolve or understand old pain and conflicts from a new perspective. . . make decisions, and reframe events. Life review may be an opportunity to 'let go' of aspects of one's self and to grieve for losses" (Burkhardt & Nagai-Jacobson, 1985, p. 196).
Use cognitive restructuring.	This is suggested for use after patterns of relaxation and meditation are well established and client is in a relaxed state. It involves the use of personal affirmations as positive thoughts to replace negative thoughts. The positive attitude promotes healing through clients' verbal declarations and repetitions of positive statements about themselves.
Use music therapy.	Music can be used to calm people, and decrease pain and anxiety, as well as provide stimulation and orientation. Personal preferences are important to assess. Specific religious music is only one

INTERVENTIONS	RATIONALE
	possible type of music to consider. It may be useful to people expressing dismay at being unable to attend their usual spiritual observances. Also helpful might be music popular in previous eras, to promote reminiscing, or any music the person finds soothing or otherwise pleasing to hear. Encouragement can be given for the person to participate through singing, humming, dancing, moving in time to the music, or beating out rhythms.
Coordinate support groups.	Groups that come together for mutual support as they face common concerns and challenges can be beneficial for clients experiencing spiritual distress. Support groups can promote a sense of personal worth for members. Altruistic (unselfish) helping of other members can also instill hope that problems are resolvable, thus feelings of belonging, attachment, and acceptance through group cohesiveness are possible. Meanwhile, alternative responses are presented, with members sharing their difficulties, hopes, and strengths, while drawing on each other and being nurtured in the process.
Refer for clergy assistance as appropriate.	Utilize available clergy resources when requested and when the situation requires more in-depth or long-term follow-up than the nurse can provide.
Teach to assure client that every individual responds uniquely to health, illness, and prognostic data.	Clients may need to hear permission to express their unique beliefs and concerns. Reassurance that every person is different and responds uniquely can free the client to share openly with the nurse, which can promote their mutual understanding of the client's spiritual distress.
Inpatient None	
Community Health/ Home Care None	

REFERENCES/BIBLIOGRAPHY

Belcher, A.E., Dettmore, D., & Holzemer, S.P. (1989). Spirituality and sense of well-being in persons with AIDS. **Holistic Nursing Practice, 3**(4), 16–25.

Buckwalter, K.C., Hartsock, J., & Gaffney, J. (1985). Music therapy. In G.M. Bulechek, & J.C. McCloskey (Eds.). **Nursing interventions: Treatments for nursing diagnoses** (pp. 58–74). Philadelphia: Saunders.

Burkhardt, M.A., & Nagai-Jacobson, M.G. (1985). Dealing with spiritual concerns of clients in the community. **Journal of Community Health Nursing, 2**, 191–198.

Burnard, P. (1987). Spiritual distress and the nursing response: Theoretical considerations and counselling skills. **Journal of Advanced Nursing, 12**, 377–382.

Carson, V.B. (1989). **Spiritual dimensions of nursing practice**. Philadelphia: Saunders.

Dickinson, C. (1975). The search for spiritual meaning. **American Journal of Nursing, 75**, 1789–1793.

* Francis, M.R. (1986). Concerns of terminally ill adult Hindu cancer patients. **Cancer Nursing, 9**, 164–171.

Gardner, D.L. (1985). Presence. In G.M. Bulechek, & J.C. McCloskey (Eds.). **Nursing interventions: Treatments for nursing diagnoses** (pp. 316–324). Philadelphia: Saunders.

Granstrom, S.L. (1985). Spiritual nursing care for oncology patients. **Topics in Clinical Nursing, 7**(1), 39–45.

Henderson, V., & Nite, G. (Eds.). (1978). **Principles and practice of nursing** (6th ed.). New York: MacMillan.

Highfield, M.F., & Cason, C. (1983). Spiritual needs of patients: Are they recognized? **Cancer Nursing, 6**, 187–192.

Hover, M. (1986). If a patient asks you to pray with him. **RN, 49**(4), 17–18.

Hover-Kramer, D. (1989). Creating a context for self-healing: The transpersonal perspective. **Holistic Nursing Practice, 3**(3), 27–34.

Kinney, C.K.D., Mannetter, R., & Carpenter, M. (1985). Support groups. In G.M. Bulechek, & J.C. McCloskey (Eds.). **Nursing interventions: Treatments for nursing diagnoses** (pp. 185–197). Philadelphia: Saunders.

Labun, E. (1988). Spiritual care: An element in nursing care planning. **Journal of Advanced Nursing, 13**, 314–320.

Nagai-Jacobson, M.G., & Burkhardt, M.A. (1989). Spirituality: Cornerstone of holistic nursing practice. **Holistic Nursing Practice, 3**(3), 18–26.

North American Nursing Diagnosis Association (1990). **Taxonomy I** (Rev. 1990). St. Louis: NANDA.

Peterson, E.A. (1985). The physical . . . the spiritual . . . can you meet all of your patient's needs? **Journal of Gerontological Nursing, 11**, (10), 23–27.

Richardson, G.E., & Noland, M.P. (1984). Treating the spiritual dimension through educational imagery. **Health Values: Achieving High Level Wellness, 8**(6), 25–30.

Ruffing-Rahal, M.A. (1984). The spiritual dimension of well-being implications for the elderly. **Home Healthcare Nurse, 2**(2), 12–13, 16.

Snyder, M. (1985). Music. In M. Snyder, **Independent nursing interventions** (pp. 211–223). New York: Wiley.

Sodergren, K.M. (1985). Guided imagery. In M. Snyder, **Independent nursing interventions** (pp. 103–124). New York: Wiley.

* Sodestrom, K.E., & Martinson, I.M. (1987). Patients' spiritual coping strategies: A study of nurse and patient perspectives. **Oncology Nursing Forum, 14**(2), 41–46.

Stuart, E.M., Deckro, J.P., & Mandle, C.L. (1989). Spirituality in health and healing: A clinical program. **Holistic Nursing Practice, 3**(3), 35–46.

Titlebaum, H.M. (1988). Relaxation. **Holistic Nursing Practice, 2**(3), 17–25.

Tripp-Reimer, T., & Brink, P.J. (1985). Culture brokerage. In G.M. Bulechek, & J.C. McCloskey (Eds.). **Nursing interventions: Treatments for nursing diagnoses** (pp. 352–364). Philadelphia: Saunders.

Vines, S.W. (1988). The therapeutics of guided imagery. **Holistic Nursing Practice, 2**(3), 34–44.

*Warner-Robbins, C.G., & Christiana, N.M. (1989). The spiritual needs of persons with AIDS. **Family and Community Health, 12**(2), 43–51.

Suffocation: Risk

A state in which an individual is at risk
for inadequate air supply to the lungs

Georgene C. Siemsen, M.S., R.N., C.S.

RISK FACTORS

Internal

Chest trauma
Cognitive impairment: judgment, percep-
        tion, and ability to interpret the
        environment
Decreased olfactory sense
Decreased oral sensation
Depression with suicidal tendencies
Developmental disability

Facial trauma
History of drug abuse
Infection of the upper airway
Neck surgery
Neck trauma
Reduced motor ability
Tracheostomy

External

Lack of awareness of hazards in the environment
Lack of safety education or precautions
Workplace presents potential exposure to suffocation risk from noxious gases, suffocating
        materials, or enclosed spaces

EXPECTED OUTCOMES

Client will identify internal and external factors that increase the potential for suffocation.
        Internal and external risk factors for suffocation are listed.
        Internal and external risk factors are determined as risks are evaluated.
        Level of risk for suffocation is identified.
Client will describe actions or resources for addressing established internal and external risk factors.
        Changes in physical status that indicate a need to seek follow-up care are described.
        Procedures for the management of risk factors are applied.
        Resources for addressing environmental safety needs are identified.

Client will remain free from episodes of suffocation.

Procedures for the management of established risk factors are applied.

Appropriate follow-up is sought during early signs of inadequate air availability.

Emergency procedures are developed and followed when indicated.

INTERVENTIONS	RATIONALE
Universal	
Evaluate attitudes and knowledge regarding personal safety.	Perception and knowledge of self-risk determine needs related to education on risk factors.
Evaluate cognitive status.	The cognitively impaired individual's perception and interpretation of the environment may be inaccurate, resulting in a need to modify the environment.
Evaluate depression and suicide risk.	Individuals at risk for suicide need protection from self-inflicted injury.
Evaluate for choking.	Inability to masticate and swallow food results in a risk of mechanical air blockage from a food bolus.
Modify environment to eliminate hazards that may cause strangulation or choking in the cognitively impaired client—eliminate hanging cords or activities involving materials with small pieces that may be put in mouth.	Loss of cognitive function leads to misinterpretation of the environment. Motor abilities may be affected as well, resulting in the inability to safely manipulate the environment. A curtain cord can be wrapped around the neck, resulting in strangulation.
Develop alternative strategies to physical restraint.	A restraint used as a safety device may strangulate in the event of a fall resulting from an attempt to get free.
Teach risk factors for suffocation.	Prevention of suffocation is crucial as it may result in permanent disability or death.
Inpatient	
Monitor vital signs, breathing pattern, and temperature/color of skin.	Signs of hypoxemia include dyspnea, shallow respirations, use of accessory muscles, tachycardia, tachypnea, cyanosis, and cool clammy skin.

INTERVENTIONS	**R**ATIONALE
Insure that the mechanically ventilated client is free of airway obstruction. 1. Monitor for an increase in peak airway pressure 2. Suction 3. Request further evaluation of placement and function of the tracheostomy tube and balloon by the registered respiratory therapist or physician to determine cause of obstruction	Acute airway obstruction may result from a displaced tube, herniation, or overinflation of the balloon. An x-ray may be indicated to determine tube placement.
Elevate head of the bed for edema of the face, head, or neck.	Elevation of the head decreases edema in the traumatized area, decreasing obstruction to air flow. This intervention is contraindicated in hypotension.
Community Health/ Home Care Evaluate ability to comply with dietary and feeding guidelines.	Specialized feeding practices result in a need to change life-long habits. Observe mealtimes to determine follow-through.
Teach food and fluid preparation for providing the recommended texture.	The need for mechanical soft or pureed foods, or thickened liquids, is determined by the nature of the swallowing deficit or ability to protect the airway.
Teach signs of inadequate air availability and the need to seek follow-up care or resources.	Early detection of hypoxemia is imperative to prevent long-term complications and initiate safety measures.
Teach potential causes of suffocation in the work place.	Deaths from suffocation in the work place have resulted from multiple causes. These include asphyxiation from gas (propane, methane, argon, nitrogen, and carbon dioxide), mechanical asphyxiation (grain bins, storage bins, sand hoppers) or confined spaces where oxygen deficiency can develop.

INTERVENTIONS	RATIONALE
Advocate for community support of safety practices in the workplace to prevent suffocation. These include functional safety equipment (such as respirators) and protection from falls resulting in suffocation.	Accidents in the work place resulting in suffocation are preventable when safety measures are enforced and utilized.

REFERENCES/BIBLIOGRAPHY

* Asuruda, J.A. (1989). Deaths from asphyxiation and poisoning at work in the United States 1984–1986. **British Journal of Industrial Medicine, 46,** 541–546.

Barker-Stotts, K. (1989). Strangulation. **Nursing 89, 19**(3), 33.

* Cain, W.S., Leaderer, B.P., Cannon, L., Tosun, T., & Hanah, I. (1987). Odorization of inert gas for occupational safety: Psychosocial considerations. **American Industrial Hygiene Association Journal, 48**(1), 47–55

Lockhart, J.S., Griffin, C. (1987). Post thyroidectomy respiratory distress. **Nursing 87, 17**(7), 33.

McFarland, G.K., & McFarlane, E.A. (1989). Potential for injury, potential for trauma; potential for poisoning, potential for suffocation. **Nursing Diagnosis and Intervention** (pp. 62, 75, 79–81). Philadelphia: Mosby.

North American Nursing Diagnosis Association. **Taxonomy I** (Rev. 1990). St. Louis: NANDA.

Newquist, M.J., & Sobel, R.M. (1990). Traumatic asphyxia: An indication of significant pulmonary injury. **American Journal of Emergency Medicine, 8**(3), 212–215.

Peterson, P.J. (1988). Respiratory distress after facial trauma, **Nursing 88, 18**(1), 33.

Sinfield, A., DiVito, J., & Brandstetter, R.D.(1989). Airway obstruction from overinflation and herniation of tracheostomy tube balloon. **Heart and Lung, 18**(3), 260–262.

Stevens, SA., & Becker, K.L. (1988).How to perform picture-perfect respiratory assessment. **Nursing 88, 18**(10), 57–58, 74–75.

Swallowing, Impaired

A state in which an individual has decreased ability to voluntarily pass fluids/solids from the mouth to the stomach (NANDA, 1990, p. 80).

Phyllis Cerone, R.N., B.S.N., C.C.R.N.
• • • • • • • • • • • • • •

DEFINING CHARACTERISTICS

Avoidance of solid foods
Complaint of "I can't chew or swallow"
Complaint of pain when swallowing
Decreased gag reflex
Decreased strength or movement of muscles involved in mastication
Dehydration
Dry mouth
Excessive coughing/choking

Facial paralysis, facial drooping, drooling
Inability to swallow liquids
Perceptual impairment
Pocketing of food on flaccid side of mouth
Regurgitation of fluids/solids through mouth or nose
Sores in mouth
Weight loss

CONTRIBUTING FACTORS

Pathophysiological

Decreased level of consciousness, as in head injury or in states induced by medications or postanesthesia
Decreased salivation, as in radiation therapy
Mechanical obstruction caused by:
    Edema of the oropharygeal cavity
    Hiatal hernia

Ill-fitting dentures or missing teeth
Inadequate neck posturing, as in cervical arthritis or kyphosis
Inability to hold up head
Tracheostomy tube
Tumors of the esophagus
Wired jaw

Neuromuscular impairment related to:
> Disease, i.e., amyotrophic lateral sclerosis; advanced Alzheimer's; Guillain-Barré; Parkinson's edema; bleeding; manipulation around glossopharyngeal and vagus nerves—as in post-extubation; postoperative swelling, trauma

Paresis involving muscles and cranial nerves needed for chewing or swallowing as in:
> Brain tumors/aneurysms
> CVA or head injury

Stomatitis from radiation therapy

Psychosociobehavioral

Excessive alcohol ingestion
Fear of swallowing from impaired swallowing
Rapid eating

EXPECTED OUTCOMES

Client will have adequate nutrition through oral intake.
> Weight and hydration status are maintained.
> Swallowing without difficulty occurs.
> Aspiration is not experienced.
> Knowledge of feeding techniques is demonstrated if necessary.

INTERVENTIONS — RATIONALE

Interventions	Rationale
Universal	
Assess swallowing ability and causative factors of impaired swallowing.	Assessment of present ability and causative factors provides the basis for determination of intervention.
Assess for alertness and responsiveness.	Drowsiness causes increased risk for aspiration.
Assess motor function and muscle strength around the jaw and tongue. Assess facial symmetry.	Weakness of facial, oral, or tongue muscle strength causes difficulty in swallowing and chewing. Cranial nerves V, VII, IX, X, XI, and XII control facial, oral, and tongue muscles.
Assess for cough reflex.	The cough reflex keeps food and fluid from entering the upper respiratory tract. An impaired cough reflex leads to choking while eating or drinking and inhibits the ability to clear the airway.

INTERVENTIONS	RATIONALE
Assess for swallowing reflex by asking to swallow 4–5 ml of water.	The ability to swallow is a measure of whether or not the cortical and brainstem swallowing centers are intact.
Assess for gag reflex by stimulation at back of throat.	The gag reflex protects the airway and pharynx when a bolus is too large to swallow safely.
When feeding: 1. Have suction equipment available	The potential for aspiration is significant in the presence of swallowing difficulties.
2. Position the client correctly: High Fowler's position (60–90° elevation) Head flexed forward at midline and pointed down toward chest If neurologically impaired, support in this position	An upright position enhances alignment of the alimentary tract and assists the esophagus to be patent. Aspiration is more likely to occur if the head is tilted backward, as this opens the airway.
3. Provide pleasant, quiet environment	Complete clearing of the pharyngeal tract is facilitated by keeping distractions to a minimum, maintaining calmness and not rushing, and focusing on eating.
4. Feed in small portions	Small portions are more easily handled and less easily aspirated.
5. Select foods and fluids that can be accommodated, .i.e., thick fluids or semisolid foods. Avoid sticky, mucous-forming foods. Consult with dietitian for selections, if necessary.	Semisolid foods of medium consistency are easiest to swallow and moist enough not to crumble. Thin fluids are most difficult to control during swallowing. Sticky foods such as white bread and peanut butter are difficult to swallow.
6. Avoid milk products and chocolate	Milk products and chocolate thicken secretions, causing difficulty swallowing. They are, however, better tolerated after they have been cooked.
7. Provide foods with appealing taste, temperature, and texture	Appearance, texture, and odor of food have a direct effect on the ability and desire to swallow. Sweet, sour, and salty foods stimulate salivation and potentiate the swallowing reflex.

INTERVENTIONS	**R**ATIONALE
8. Moisten dry foods with liquids, sauces, or gravies	Swallowing is enhanced by moist foods.
9. Provide high protein, high calorie supplements, as necessary	The impaired ability to swallow leads to decreased nutritional status.
10. For excessive salivation, suction the mouth and swab with a small amount of meat tenderizer made from papaya	Papaya helps liquify secretions and makes mucus less thick and tenacious. Thick and tenacious secretions cause increased risk for choking.
11. Place food in back of mouth and on unaffected side, if applicable	Placing food in the back of the mouth facilitates swallowing.
12. Gently massage the throat and use unaffected side, if applicable	Gentle massage of the laryngopharyngeal musculature stimulates swallowing.
13. Provide a straw for drinking liquids, if appropriate	Using a straw requires less energy, decreases the risk of choking, and strengthens facial and swallowing muscles.
14. Keep positioned upright for 45–60 min after meals	An upright position enhances digestion and reduces the risk of aspiration.
15. Instruct to swallow twice after each bite, and feed slowly	Clearing of the pharyangeal tract is facilitated by eating slowly and swallowing enough to insure that the food has passed.
Consult with a speech pathologist for assistance with swallowing difficulties.	A speech pathologist is skilled in exercising and strengthening the muscles involved in chewing and swallowing.
Instruct client/significant other in specific feeding techniques.	Compliance is enhanced and risk reduced when the client is independent in self-care techniques.
Inpatient None	
Community Health/ Home Care Assess dietary intake by utilizing daily diary of all foods and liquids consumed.	Daily intake, when analyzed, provides information for the adequacy of nutritional needs. An inadequate diet easily ensues when experiencing difficulty swallowing.

INTERVENTIONS	RATIONALE
Assess medications being taken.	Some drugs cause lethargy, depression, or dry mouth, and these symptoms interfere with swallowing.
Weigh weekly.	Body weight gain or loss is an indication of whether or not metabolic and nutritional needs are met.
Teach about the signs and symptoms of aspiration.	Knowledge enhances appropriate compliance. Early recognition and treatment minimize risks associated with aspiration.

REFERENCES/BIBLIOGRAPHY

Carpenito, L.J. (1990). **Nursing diagnosis: Application to clinical practice**. Philadelphia: Lippincott.

DiIorio, C., & Price, M. (1990). Swallowing: An assessment guide. **American Journal of Nursing. 7**, 38–41.

Gettrust, K.V., Ryan S.C., & Engelman, D.S. (Eds.). (1985). **Applied nursing diagnosis: Guides for comprehensive care planning**. Albany, NY: Delmar.

North American Nursing Diagnosis Association. **Taxonomy I** (Rev. 1990). St. Louis: NANDA.

Price, M., & DiIorio, C. (1990). Swallowing: A practice guide. **American Journal of Nursing, 7**, 42–46.

Ulrich, S.P., Canale, S.W., & Wendall, S.A. (1986). **Nursing care planning guides: A nursing diagnosis approach**. Philadelphia: Saunders.

Thermoregulation, Impaired

A state in which an individual's temperature fluctuates between hypothermia and hyperthermia (NANDA, 1990, p. 17).

Jenny A. Zaker, R.N., M.Ed., C.C.R.N.

DEFINING CHARACTERISTICS

BP alterations
Cardiac dysrhythmias
Feeling hot or cold
Hyperthermia:
  Chills and shivering
  Confusion
  Convulsions
  Dehydration and thirst
  Diaphoresis
  Flushed skin
  Headache
Hypermetabolic state
Lack of diaphoresis/pallor
Rapid pulse and respirations
Warm skin
Hypothermia:
  Cold skin
  Coma
  Drowsiness
  Frostbite
  Pallor
  Slow pulse and respirations

CONTRIBUTING FACTORS

Pathophysiological

Adverse effects of chemotherapy/anesthesia
Illness states, e.g., brain tumor with pressure on the hypothalamus, CNS damage
Infections, e.g., meningitis, myocardial tissue necrosis, septicemia, pneumonia, pericarditis
Low birth weight or prematurity
Stages of development, e.g., newborn or old age
Trauma as in burns, cerebral injury, spinal cord injury
Vigorous activity

Psychosociobehavioral

Accidental misuse of drugs

562

Inappropriate clothing
Intentional exposure to heat or cold
Intentional ingestion of toxic drugs or substances
Intentional trauma

EXPECTED OUTCOMES

Client will have restoration of normal body temperature.
> There are no temperature fluctuations.
> Skin is warm and dry.
> Body temperature will be approximately 98.6°F or 37°C.

INTERVENTIONS / RATIONALE

INTERVENTIONS	RATIONALE
Universal	
Assess temperature.	Body temperature indicates effectiveness of the thermoregulatory mechanism in the hypothalamus.
Assess for clinical characteristics of hyper- or hypothermia (see defining characteristics).	Early recognition of key characteristics of thermal alterations facilitates prompt treatment and prevention of life-threatening symptoms.
Assess for signs of physiologic stability such as warm, dry skin.	Signs of physiologic stability indicate a return to homeostasis.
Assess for source of thermal alteration.	Identification of the source of the problem directs intervention and treatment modalities.
Assess: 1. BP; pulse for rate, rhythm, and volume; respirations for rate, effort, and rhythm 2. Lung sounds for presence of rales, rhonchi, or wheezes 3. Heart sounds to identify arrhythmias 4. Level of consciousness (LOC), orientation to time, person, place, and arousability 5. Peripheral pulses for presence and quality	Impaired thermoregulation is reflected in changes from the norm as the body struggles to reach homeostasis. Shivering raises the rate of respiration and heart beat to shunt more blood and nutrients to vital areas and to warm the body by increasing muscle activity. The presence of adventitious lung sounds can be an indicator of infection. Mental function decreases in extreme changes of body temperature as the vital centers respond to less than adequate oxygen and nutrition.

INTERVENTIONS	**R**ATIONALE
Monitor oral or rectal temperature at regularly scheduled intervals.	Temperature readings indicate the degree of thermoregulatory control from the hypothalamus. Thermoregulation instability represents an unstable body temperature, which indicates an imbalance between heat production and heat loss. Verifying temperature at regular intervals isolates trends in thermal changes and facilitates intervention.
Weigh on a regular basis.	Insensible fluid loss through lungs and skin is not reflected by intake and output, and yet these losses contribute to dehydration. Weight is a more accurate check on fluid loss.
If a spinal cord injury is present: 1. Ascertain the presence of poikilothermia	Poikilothermia occurs with a lesion above T_6 (The literature states this phenomenon is found at this level, but clinical experience has shown that poikilothermia can occur with lesions above T_8) and causes the client to assume the temperature of the environment related to spinal reflex uninhibited by higher centers. This lesion causes increased susceptibility to temperatures related to a loss in the ability to conserve or lower body heat and to shiver or perspire below the level of the lesion.
2. Provide consistent environment	Protecting from drafts, providing extra blankets or removing blankets as required, regulating the room temperature, etc., prevent the occurrence of symptoms related to poikilothermia.
Avoid exposing body parts during intervention.	Inability to internally regulate body temperature leads to assuming the ambient temperature, which must be constant and conducive to the maintenance of a body core temperature of 98.6°F or 37°C.
Provide a quiet, pleasant environment.	A calm environment decreases demands on vital centers and metabolic rate, which are already overtaxed as the body attempts to reach homeostasis.

INTERVENTIONS	RATIONALE
Keep client warm and dry and facilitate rest periods by grouping care needs.	The provision of comfort measures enhances healing and prevents loss of heat through evaporation.
Consult with physician regarding status and intervention changes.	Collaborative planning facilitates timely intervention.
Instruct to report feelings of very hot or very cold.	Impaired thermoregulation causes the body temperature to fluctuate between hypo- and hyperthemia. When alert, the client can assist in providing information about changes in condition.
Teach causes of impaired thermoregulation.	Knowledge facilitates acceptance and enhances timely intervention.
Inpatient Record intake and output.	Intake and output reflect hydration, which is affected when the body temperature fluctuates.
Have blood and other fluid cultures drawn, as necessary.	Cultures provide necessary information when a pathogen is suspected as the cause of impaired thermoregulation.
Administer oxygen as required.	Fever is catabolic in nature and consumes calories, oxygen, and water in the process of providing heat.
Administer and maintain IV fluids at the prescribed rate.	Body fluid lost as a result of diaphoresis, increased respiration, evaporation, and increased metabolic activity requires replacement.
Place on an automatic thermal regulatory blanket. 1. Place a sheet between mattress and client 2. Do not set unit below 72°F 3. Place one cover on top of client 4. Check skin every two hours 5. Teach about equipment, functioning, and sensations perceived	An automatic thermal regulatory blanket promotes rapid response to changes in body temperature by monitoring and automatically adjusting to temperature fluctuations. During use, however, the skin is susceptible to damage from local vasoconstriction. Setting the unit below 72°F causes shivering, which increases metabolic demands. Body heat is allowed to escape, thus causing cooling when the use of excessive covering is eliminated. Knowledge allays fear.

INTERVENTIONS   RATIONALE

Community Health/Home Health	
Assess ability to take and interpret temperature and when to seek medical attention.	Knowledge allays fear and promotes self-care and confidence.
Review key characteristics of impaired thermoregulation and intervention.	Recognition of signs, symptoms, and care facilitates prompt intervention and safe administration of care.
Teach to use air conditioning, fans, or heat as needed. Teach to avoid drafts.	Inability to internally regulate body temperature leads to the assumption of ambient conditions, which must be kept constant and conducive to the maintenance of a body core temperature of 98.6°F or 37°C.

(Note: This care plan centers on interventions aimed at fluctuating body temperatures. For interventions aimed specifically at hypothermia or hyperthermia, see those care planning guides.)

REFERENCES/BIBLIOGRAPHY

Alspach, J.G. (1991). **Core curriculum for critical care nursing**. Philadelphia: Saunders.

Berk, J.L., & Sampliner, J.E. (1990). **Handbook of critical care** (3rd ed.). Boston: Little, Brown.

Johanson, B.C., Wells, S.J., Hoffmeister, D., & Dungea, C.U. (1988). **Standards for critical care** (3rd ed.). St. Louis: Mosby.

Kirby, R.R., Taylor, R.W., & Siretta, J.M. (1990). **Pocket companion of critical care: Immediate concerns**. Philadelphia: Lippincott.

North American Nursing Diagnosis Association. (1990). **Taxonomy I** (Rev. 1990). St. Louis: NANDA.

Sommers, M.S. (1989). **Difficult diagnosis in critical care nursing**. Rockville, MD: Aspen.

Swearingen, P.L., Sommers, M.S., & Miller, K. (1988). **Manual of critical care**. St. Louis: Mosby.

Thought Processes, Altered

A state in which an individual experiences thought processes not based in reality and/or disruptions in conscious thought, conceptualization, problem solving, judgment, comprehension, or recall.

Laina M. Gerace, R.N., Ph.D.
Jill Anderson, R.N., M.S.N.

DEFINING CHARACTERISTICS

Altered abstract thinking
Cognitive dissonance
Confusion
Delusions
Distractibility
Egocentricity
Excessive indecisiveness
Grandiosity
Hallucinations

Hyper- or hypovigilance
Inaccurate interpretation of environment
Intrusive thoughts
Memory deficit/problems
Racing thoughts
Regression into fantasy
Slowed thinking
Suspiciousness

CONTRIBUTING FACTORS

Pathophysiological

Anxiety and related disorders
Chemical factors:
    Drug interactions
    Drug toxicity
    Substance abuse
    Withdrawal from substances

Major mental illnesses:
    Depression
    Manic-depressive illness
    Schizophrenia
Organic brain syndromes

Psychosociobehavioral

High- or low-panic level anxiety
Isolation
Low self-esteem
Sensory overload or deprivation

EXPECTED OUTCOMES

(Note: Outcomes will vary according to contributing factors and severity or progressive nature of the illness.)

Client will experience adequate concentration and reality orientation needed for activities of daily living (ADL) and interpersonal relations at the level of functional ability.

Situations that increase difficulties in evaluating reality and increase disrupted thoughts are identified.

Ability to differentiate between reality and thoughts not based in reality and disrupted thoughts is learned.

Ability to refrain from responding to thoughts not based in reality and disrupted thoughts is learned.

A health care professional is contacted when changes in thought processes occur.

Compliance with psychotropic medications given to manage thought disruptions is maintained.

Substances (alcohol and other drugs) that contribute to thought disruptions are avoided.

INTERVENTIONS

RATIONALE

Universal	
Monitor for changes in thought processes and precipitating events that increase altered thinking.	Avoidance or elimination of stressors that increase altered thought processes is enhanced by the determination of precipitants and the provision of feedback.
Convey acceptance of altered thought processes, but do not agree or argue.	Acceptance conveys that altered thought processes are real to the client. Not agreeing with impaired thoughts reinforces reality, but arguing with disrupted thoughts causes fright or accelerates delusional thinking. Reassurance rather than confrontation elicits a positive response when memory impairment is present.

INTERVENTIONS	RATIONALE
Interact on the basis of reality; do not dwell on disrupted thinking processes.	The separation of thoughts from reality is assisted when the attention is directed away from the altered thoughts. Focusing on reality, i.e., environmental events, distracts from disordered thoughts. In memory impairment, confusion decreases with frequent orientation to name, time, day, and place.
Protect from physical harm and embarrassing situations when behavior is inappropriate.	Altered thought processes can be frightening and may cause behavior which is inappropriate, dangerous, or embarrassing. The creation of a safe, non-threatening environment is essential to the protection of all involved.
Initiate and maintain a therapeutic relationship by being trustworthy, conveying interest, and initiating brief and frequent contacts.	Establishing a trusting relationship helps to reduce anxiety and provide security. A supportive relationship diminishes disordered thinking and enhances the effectiveness of intervention.
Provide reality orientation and keep communication simple, concrete, and direct.	Simple environmental tasks and concrete messages focus on reality. Communication which is clear enhances concentration and response formation.
Provide psychotropic medications and relevant teaching about medication compliance.	Psychotropic medications improve thought processes by altering neurotransmitters that affect thinking processes. Often long-term medication management is necessary for functioning.
Teach to differentiate altered thoughts from reality.	Greater control is felt if signs of thought disorders can be identified as part of illness. When this is gained, the individual is capable of assisting in illness assessment and contacting a health professional when altered thoughts increase.

Inpatient

Assess and document thought processes and behavior.	Altered thought processes vary with situations, underlying pathophysiology, and medical management. Assessment provides data for the care plan and for judging effectiveness of intervention.
Provide a structured environment which is safe.	Altered thought processes affect judgment, leading to inappropriate and unsafe behavior. Structure provides consistency, decreases stimuli, and provides memory cues for the memory impaired.

INTERVENTIONS	**R**ATIONALE
Gear activities to functional ability.	Expectations too great for functional ability cause stress.
Assist in ADL.	When self-care deficits are present, participating with the client in ADL establishes contact with reality and shows interest and concern.
Assist in and support attempts to communicate. If sentences do not make sense, ask for clarification. Listen for themes and emotional tone and respond to these.	Disrupted thoughts affect communication. Communication is enhanced when therapeutic strategies include orientation to emotions and accurate interpretation of meaning.
Teach to place memory cues within the environment when memory impairment is present.	Memory cues serve as stimuli which elicit familiarity responses and add to feelings of well-being.
Community Health/ Home Care Assess educational needs and support systems.	Thought disorders are often chronic or degenerative. A supportive and participative community which provides for on-going maintenance or growth enhances the quality of life and provides needed social support.
Acknowledge and encourage the family's participation in care.	Thought disorders are often chronic and degenerative. A supportive and participative family facilitates quality of life and provides needed social support.
Promote compliance with long-term treatment plan, i.e., medication management, and environmental modifications of decreasing stimuli or providing memory cues.	Unpleasant side effects, memory loss, or paranoia may lead to noncompliance with medications.
Assist in the use of environmental strategies that promote clear thinking, i.e., calendar, name tags, photographs, seasonal and holiday themes, reminder notes.	While the ability for improvement will vary according to underlying pathophysiology, environmental modifications which simplify and clarify facilitate improvement. A complex environment leads to feelings of being overwhelmed.

INTERVENTIONS	**R**ATIONALE
Encourage privacy and interpersonal space for paranoid clients.	Interpersonal closeness increases feelings of mistrust in paranoid persons.

REFERENCES/BIBLIOGRAPHY

Carpenito, L.J. (1985). Altered thoughts or altered perceptions? **American Journal of Nursing, 85**, 1283.

Chesla, C. (1988). Clients with schizophrenia and other psychotic disorders. In H.S. Wilson, & C.R. Kneisl (Eds.). **Psychiatric Nursing**. Menlo Park, CA: Addison-Wesley.

North American Nursing Diagnosis Association. **Taxonomy I** (Rev. 1990). St. Louis: NANDA.

O'Toole, A.W., & Loomis, M.E. (1990). Revision of the phenomena of concern for psychiatric mental health nursing. **Archives of Psychiatric Nursing, 3**, 288–299.

* Thomas, M.D., Sanger, E., Wolf-Wilets, V., & Whitney, J.D. (1988). Nursing diagnosis of patients with manic and thought disorders. **Archives of Psychiatric Nursing, 2**(6), 339–344.

Tissue Integrity, Altered

A state in which an individual's tissue continuity is disrupted. Tissue may include skin, fat, muscle, fascia, organs, and bone.

Nancy A. Stotts, R.N., Ed.D.

DEFINING CHARACTERISTICS

Abrasion
Avulsion
Bone exposure
Eruptions
Erythema
Excoriation
Exudate
Fat exposure
Impaired capillary refill

Incision
Lesions
Muscle visibility
Necrotic tissue
Organ(s) visibility
Pain
Tenderness
Ulceration

CONTRIBUTING FACTORS

Pathophysiological

Diabetes
Extremes of body temperature
Extremes of skin moisture
Illness therapies
    Chemotherapy
    Medications, e.g., steroids, anticoagulants
    Radiation therapy

Immunoincompetence
Impaired perfusion
Obesity
Pressure over a bony prominence
Starvation
Trauma

Psychosociobehavioral

None

572

Expected Outcomes

Client's healing process will be complete.
>   There is evidence of tissue regeneration.
>   Adequate circulation is achieved.
>   Nutritional needs meet body requirements.

Interventions   Rationale

Interventions	Rationale
Universal	
Monitor the wound closed by primary intention for presence of inflammation, drainage from incision, approximation of wound edges, and presence of healing ridge by seventh to ninth day.	Ongoing evaluation of status is the basis for determining whether the treatment is effective or whether the care needs to be changed.
Monitor the wound closed by secondary intention for new epithelial and granulation tissue, exudate, pus, and necrotic tissue.	Same as above.
Monitor area around wound for contributing factors to delayed healing (e.g., scar tissue, redness, edema, bruising).	Same as above.
Monitor systemic status to determine if factors present may contribute to delayed healing, e.g., starvation, obesity, immunoincompetence, impaired perfusion.	Same as above.
Evaluate the cause of the tissue impairment and focus intervention on it to prevent recurrence.	The focus of the intervention must include the etiology, in order to prevent exacerbation of the problem and support repair.
Keep the impaired tissue in a moist physiological environment. 1. Remove exudate with dressings and irrigation, or treat the wound with antibacterial medications	Repair occurs most rapidly in a physiologically moist environment. Debris delay healing and so must be removed. The treatment schedule (including dressing) must be selected considering the nature of the injury, knowledge of the treatments selected, and the physiological status.

INTERVENTIONS	**R**ATIONALE
2. Remove necrotic tissue by supporting autolytic processes, using enzymes, surgical excision, or dressings to debride the dead skin 3. Use a dressing that will keep the tissue moist 4. Establish a schedule for treatment of the impairment that is congruent with the goal of therapy, the overall physiological status, and the treatment being implemented	
Remove the cause of the tissue impairment. If due to pressure over a bony prominence: 1. Place on regular and more frequent turning schedule 2. Consider the need for mattress overlays or specialty beds 3. Mitigate shearing when moving in bed If due to therapy: (e.g., surgery, intravenous therapy) 1. Treat symptomatically 2. Try to prevent recurrence	Tissue that has been injured is more fragile and susceptible to reinjury than is uninjured skin.
Keep intact skin and tissue surrounding the wound clean. 1. Establish a regular bathing schedule 2. Use skin oil to keep clean tissue moist 3. Bathe after excess perspiration, and urinary and fecal incontinence	Perspiration, urine, and feces are skin irritants and also change the pH of the skin, supporting growth of skin flora and increasing the possibility of infection.

INTERVENTIONS	RATIONALE
Provide adequate nutrients for healing. 1. Provide a well-balanced diet, enteral feedings, or parenteral nutrition as needed 2. Record intake 3. Refer for dietary consultation if intake is not or will not be sufficient for 7–10 days	Nutrients are required for repair of tissue. Healing of minor injuries in healthy persons can occur without adequate intake. More severe or prolonged injuries in healthy persons or minor injuries in ill or debilitated persons require exogenous nutrients.
Maintain normal glucose level in diabetics. 1. Balance activity, diet, and insulin to achieve normal blood glucose 2. Monitor blood glucose on a regular schedule, promptly reporting elevations, or providing prescribed insulin	Increased glucose levels impair healing.
Provide sufficient fluid intake. 1. Encourage 1500–2000 cc/24 H in healthy persons 2. The required intake in those with renal or cardiovascular disease will be established by the physician, based on the client's physiological ability and client losses 3. If oral intake is not sufficient, consult with physician for order for intravenous support	Water is critical to cell viability, and hypovolemia is a serious threat to replacement of damaged skin.
Encourage optimal oxygenation to tissues. 1. Provide maximal inspiratory maneuvers 2. Establish a regular turning and positioning schedule for clients confined to bed	Oxygen is critical to cellular activity. Inspiratory maneuvers, changing position, ambulation, and activity all have been established as means to enhance ventilation and therefore oxygenation.

INTERVENTIONS	**R**ATIONALE
3. Establish a progressive ambulation and activity schedule for ambulatory clients	
Inpatient Consider referral to centers where treatment such as hyperbaric oxygen, implantation with cultured keratinocytes, or growth factor therapy are available for chronic tissue impairment resistant to usual therapy.	Persistent wounds require therapy that will lead to closure as chronic open wounds disrupt lives, reduce ability to return to work, or take part in daily activities and may develop into cancerous lesions.
Teach signs and symptoms of healing, progression of tissue impairment, and when to call the wound care nurse or physician.	Self-care is based on understanding of what is expected and usual as well as when help from a professional is needed.
Prepare the client and significant other to provide wound care after inpatient discharge, as needed. 1. Provide a list of needed supplies 2. Teach the procedure for wound care and dressing removal 3. Encourage return demonstration of the technique	Same as above.
Teach the client and significant other ways to support repair by maintaining regimen for oxygenation and activity, nutrition, and, when needed, glucose control.	Same as above.
Refer to home health care as needed for wound care.	Wounds require ongoing care. It is important to prospectively plan for needs so wounds are not neglected, which leads to increased possibility of infection.
Community Health/ Home Care None	

REFERENCES/BIBLIOGRAPHY

Alvarez, O., Rozint, J., & Meehan, M. (1990). Principles of moist wound healing: Indications for chronic wounds. In D. Krasner (Ed.). **Chronic wound care**, (pp. 266–281). King of Prussia, PA: Health Management Publications.

Cuzzell, J.Z. (1990). Choosing a wound dressing: A systematic approach. **AACN Clinical Issues, 1**, 566–577.

Cuzzell, J.Z., & Stotts, N.A. (1990). Wound Care: Trial & error yields to knowledge. **American Journal of Nursing, 90**, (October), 53–63.

Hudson-Goodman, P., Girard, N., & Jones, N.B. (1990). Wound repair and the potential use of growth factors. **Heart & Lung, 19**, 379–384.

Orgill, D., & Demling, R.H. (1988). Current concepts and approaches to wound healing. **Critical Care Medicine, 16**(9), 899–908.

Rodheaver, G.T. (1990). Controversies in topical wound management: Wound cleansing and disinfection. In D. Krasner. (Ed.). **Chronic wound care**, (pp. 282–289). King of Prussia, PA: Health Management Publications.

Rosenberg, C.S. (1990). Wound healing in the patient with diabetes mellitus. **Nursing Clinics of North America, 25**, 247–261.

Stotts, N.A. (1986). In V.K. Carrieri, A.M. Lindsey, & C.M. West (Eds.). **Pathological phenomena in nursing** (pp 343–366). Philadelphia: Saunders.

Wheeland, R.G. (1987). The newer surgical dressings and wound healing. **Dermatology Clinics, 5**(2), 393–407.

Witkowski, J.A., & Parish, L.C. (1986). Cutaneous ulcer therapy. **International Journal of Dermatology, 25** (7), 420–426.

Young, M.E. (1988). Malnutrition and wound healing. **Heart & Lung, 17**(1), 60–67.

Tissue Perfusion, Altered Peripheral

A state in which an individual experiences a decrease in nutrition and oxygenation at the cellular level due to a decrease in capillary blood supply (NANDA, 1990, p. 31).

Colleen Creamer-Bauer, R.N., M.S., C.C.R.N.

DEFINING CHARACTERISTICS

Aching pain
Atrophic skin changes (dry skin, thick nails)
Atrophy of leg muscles
Bruits
Burning
Capillary refill less than three seconds
             (arterial)
Cramping
Cyanosis
Darkly pigmented area of skin
Decreased blood pressure (arterial)
Dependent rubor
Dilation or prominence of superficial veins
Edema (venous)
Erythema
Gangrene
Hair loss (lower leg, dorsum of feet, toes)
Impotence
Increased tissue turgor with swelling
Inflammation
Lack of lanugo

Loss of motor function (arterial)
Mottling
Numbness
Pain on dorsiflexion of foot (Homans' sign)
Pale extremities on elevation: color does
             not return on lowering leg
Pallor (arterial)
Paresthesia
Reactive hyperemia
Redness
Rest pain
Skin temperature changes
       Cooler sensation (arterial)
       Warmer sensation (venous)
Shiny skin
Slow healing of lesions
Tenderness
Tingling
Trophic tissue changes
Ulceration

CONTRIBUTING FACTORS

Pathophysiological

Altered transport (e.g., low hemoglobin, blood dyscrasia)
Atherosclerosis
Disruption of arterial flow (e.g., thrombosis, acute)
Disruption of venous flow (e.g., thrombophlebitis)
Hypervolemia (e.g., congestive heart failure, renal failure, decreased blood flow)
Hypovolemia (e.g., hemorrhage, dehydration, shock)
Inadequate exchange (e.g., hypothermia, immobility)
Invasive lines (e.g., intra-aortic balloon pump)
Medications (e.g., vasoactive drugs, anesthesia)
Obstruction (e.g., cancer, tumor, edema)
Pregnancy
Pressure sites (e.g., positioning, casts)
Reduced arterial flow (e.g., aneurysm, hypertension)
Reduced venous flow (e.g., varicosities)
Spasm (e.g., Raynaud's Disease)
Vasoconstriction (e.g., hypothermia, stress)
Ventilation/perfusion disorders (e.g., pulmonary emboli, pneumonia)

Psychosociobehavioral

Exercise
Heredity (e.g., primary hyperlipidemia, diabetes)
Malnutrition
Obesity
Stress
Substance abuse (e.g., cigarette smoking)

EXPECTED OUTCOMES

Client will have adequate perfusion to the extremity as evidenced by presence of peripheral pulses, warm extremities, normal sensation and movement, and uncompromised skin integrity.
Circulation is supported by maintaining adequate position.
An acceptable level of comfort is reported.
Extremity is free of edema, ulcerations, and skin lesions.
Peripheral pulses are present and strong.
Neurovascular status is intact as evidenced by adequate sensation and movement.
Activities are engaged in to enhance circulation.
Evidence of new signs and symptoms to be reported to the physician are verbalized.
Anxiety and fear are reported to be lessened.
Extremities remain clean and free from all pressure areas.
Anticoagulant regime is maintained within therapeutic range.
Exercise program is established and maintained.

INTERVENTIONS	RATIONALE
Universal	
Assess the presence of pain.	Clients with venous disease will complain of aching, cramping discomfort in their legs when standing, that may accompany night cramps and/or swelling. This discomfort can be relieved by elevation of the legs above the heart. The client with arterial disease will complain of cramping muscle pain brought on by walking a predictable distance and relieved by periods of rest. This pain is called "claudication," and indicates inadequate arterial blood supply to contracting muscles. The client with arterial disease who has rest pain, describes pain in the toes, metatarsal head area, or heel when the extremity is resting in a horizontal position. This discomfort can be relieved when the foot is placed in a dependent position. This is a dire symptom and indicates a failure of collateral vessels to perfuse adequately and maintain basic nutritional needs of the extremity.
Check peripheral pulses.	Accurate assessment is essential. Pulses should always be palpated bilaterally and simultaneously. They should be compared for rate, rhythm, and quality. Pulses are often graded on a scale of zero to four, but documentation of their presence is important. Palpable, strong peripheral pulses indicate good arterial blood flow. It is considered an emergency when there are no palpable pulses in an extremity. It may be difficult at times to assess pulses secondary to clinical situations of hypothermic vasoconstriction or preexisting disease. Establishing a baseline assessment is crucial for comparison.
Assess skin integrity (color, texture, turgor, temperature).	Color of the extremities indicates cellular function and should be evaluated in different positions: elevate legs 30–45°. Pallor indicates that the arterial system cannot pump adequate blood into the capillary system against gravity through arterial blockages. Lower the extremity in the dependent position. If a deep red color develops (dependent rubor), it represents chronic vasodilation secondary

INTERVENTIONS	RATIONALE
	to the accumulation of cellular metabolites (e.g., lactic acid). Brawny discoloration or hyperpigmentation occur in venous disease. They are a result of breakdown of red blood cells into deposits of hemosiderin that stains the tissues. Normal tissue is a healthy, pink color that reflects adequate tissue metabolism. Note the turgor of the extremity. Turgor refers to the normal tension found in the skin. Dry, dehydrated skin is loose and easily lifted off the extremity. Taut, shiny skin indicates edema. Measure edema by the amount of depression that occurs during application of pressure (cm), and by the circumference of the limb by a tape measure. Note any difference in skin temperature from one side of the body to the other. Skin temperature can provide a clue to the site of the occlusion.
Assess for capillary refill.	Capillary refill indicates the perfusion time in the capillary beds. Press on the tips of the toes or soles of the foot with a finger and then release pressure. Normal refill time should occur within seconds when tactile pressure is released.
Inspect for trophic changes.	Trophic changes occur from tissue malnutrition or decreased blood flow. They include hair loss on the affected extremity; thick, brittle nails; thin, smooth, shiny skin; ulceration; or gangrene. Ulcerations usually occur over pressure points—heels, toes, dorsum of foot, metatarsal heads, bony prominences. Document size, depth, color, presence of drainage or odor. If gangrene has set in, note if it is dry and mummified or moist and draining.
Evaluate the presence of skin lesions.	The presence of varicosities, angiomas, petechiae, or other lesions is important. Cherry angioma is a bright red lesion and turns brownish with age. It is 1–3 mm in diameter, usually round in shape, has no pulsations, and has little clinical significance. The spider angioma is fiery red, usually smaller than 2 cc in size, and has a central body that occasionally is raised and surrounded by erythema and radiating legs. Pulsations may be

INTERVENTIONS	RATIONALE
	visible in the body of the lesion. These angiomas are usually distributed on the face and upper extremities and trunk. The venous star is bluish in color, varies in size from small to several inches, and is irregular in shape. It has no pulsations and is distributed on the legs and the anterior chest.
Evaluate circumferential measurements of the extremity.	A tape measure is an accurate, inexpensive method of evaluating size of a limb. Evidence of swelling, edema, or atrophy of a limb may provide a specific clue to a current diagnosis.
Inspect the extremity for size and symmetry.	Sensory function can be assessed by touch or pressure. Note if numbness or tingling are present. Acute arterial ischemia takes six hours before nerve tissue is affected. Movement is one of the most important parameters in the assessment. The ability of the client to dorsiflex and plantarflex the foot and wiggle the toes is an indication of intact motor nerve function. If ischemia progresses to muscle necrosis, the muscle may acquire a firm, doughy consistency.
Auscultate over pulse sites.	Listen with a stethoscope over the pulse sites for bruits, hums, or any abnormal sounds. These abnormal sounds indicate tumultuous blood flow in the arteries. Listen over the abdominal aorta. Compare blood pressure readings in the upper and lower extremities and compare the arms and legs for differences. Report these to the doctor. These changes may represent obstruction to blood flow.
Assess risk factors.	Clients usually have one or more of the following risk factors. Cigarette smoking is a single, independent risk factor most closely associated with atherosclerosis. Nicotine has a potent and lasting vasoconstrictive effect. Smoking exerts an adverse effect on platelet function, resulting in increased adhesiveness and thrombus formation. Hypertension has a detrimental effect by damaging the intimal endothelium and making it more permeable to lipid penetration and plaque formation. Hyperlipidemia has been associated with a marked increase in atherosclerotic lesions.

INTERVENTIONS	**RATIONALE**
Asses exercise pattern.	Exercise is an important adjunct to management of peripheral vascular disease (PVD). Those clients with claudication should be encouraged to walk several times daily to the point of discomfort; rest; and continue walking. This consistent demand for increased blood flow is thought to promote the development of collateral circulation.
Monitor laboratory data.	Anticoagulant therapy requires careful observation of bleeding profile. Monitor prothrombin time (PT) and partial thromboplastin time (PTT). Be aware that diet, alcohol, and medications may affect the anticoagulant doses. Observe for subjective and objective signs of bleeding and hemorrhage. Anticoagulant therapy may cause thrombocytopenia.
Asses sexual function.	Impotence may be a symptom of extensive aortoiliac disease or a complication of major vascular surgery. Establishing a baseline provides a means of comparison.
Place extremity in position of comfort.	If arterial insufficiency exists, place bed in arterial position (reverse Trendelenburg's) to increase gravitational blood flow. Proper positioning is mandatory to optimize tissue perfusion. If venous disease exists, elevate extremity above the level of the heart. The recumbent position promotes venous drainage. These measures will optimize blood flow and may provide relief of discomfort in the affected extremity. Avoid the use of the knee gatch in bed, or pillows under the knees. These measures constrict circulation and cause blood to pool.
Avoid graft pressure.	When upper and lower extremity revascularization occurs, grafts usually lie in subcutaneous tissue, and special precautions must be taken. Avoid severe flexion at the groin or knee and avoid crossing the legs. Bedrest is usually maintained 24–48 H postoperatively. Avoid lying or positioning on the side of the operative graft. The strength and character of the graft and pulse should be assessed every 2–4 H. Flexion of a graft site may cause blood pooling and thrombus formation.

INTERVENTIONS	RATIONALE
Maintain warmth of the extremity. 1. Keep room temperature between 72–74°F 2. Have the client wear socks/protective covering when walking or in bed 3. Avoid the use of hot water bottles or heating pads	Maintaining warmth of the extremity encourages vasodilation of the vessel and thus improves blood flow. Care must be taken to avoid tissue injury. Ischemic tissue is at much greater risk of injury from externally applied heat than nonischemic tissue.
Provide adequate hydration.	Hydration is essential to sustain the cardiac output, maintain peripheral blood flow, and decrease blood viscosity.
Provide foot and skin care.	Meticulous skin care daily provides a method of inspection, screening for abnormalities, and thereby reducing tissue damage and preventing injury and infection.
Avoid friction, pressure, accidental injury, and trauma to the extremities.	The use of a sheepskin under the feet and legs reduces friction and promotes warmth and comfort. Floating heels and heel protectors can be used to prevent development of pressure sores. Lambswool between the toes is used to prevent injury or pressure from adjoining toes. Use of padded board, footboard, or bed cradle keeps the linen off the toes. Bed cradles must be used with caution. Pad edges to prevent injury.
Apply support stockings.	These promote circulation to lower extremities by compressing superficial veins and encouraging blood flow through the deeper veins. Elastic compression garments are easier to put on in the morning before rising.
Avoid calf massage.	This may lead to clot fragmentation and possible embolism.
Prevent bleeding complications.	Avoid trauma while anticoagulation is necessary by using soft bristle toothbrushes, electric razors, avoid multiple venipunctures, and hold pressure on arterial wound sites.

INTERVENTIONS	RATIONALE
Administer prescribed analgesics and monitor effectiveness.	Evaluation of the effectiveness of pain medication is necessary so that use of the client's limb can be encouraged when reasonably comfortable.
Instruct in use of medications.	Understanding the purpose of the medication and the way in which it is to be taken can increase compliance and early detection of side effects.
Teach the importance of foot/extremity care.	Avoid crossing the legs and wearing constrictive clothing. This behavior physically constricts the blood vessels. Changing positions frequently and moving avoids pooling of blood.
This care includes: 1. Well-fitting shoes 2. Daily inspection 3. Wearing cotton hose 4. Washing with tepid water 5. Cutting nails straight 6. Use of lanolin and lambswool	Regular consultation with a podiatrist will ensure early prevention and detection of damage to skin.
Explain the importance of daily exercise.	Walking regularly and through the pain helps stimulate formation of collateral vessels in the extremity. It is crucial that regular walking be incorporated into a daily routine.
Instruct in smoking cessation.	Smoking causes vasoconstriction, which decreases blood flow. Nicotine irritates the arterial blood vessel structure and promotes atherosclerosis. A higher incidence of graft failure occurs in smokers.
Identify available community resources.	Support groups for risk factor modification, clinics for treatment of ulcers, support hose clinics, and exercise programs can be excellent resources.
Instruct in weight loss and dietary restrictions.	Keeping weight within normal range reduces an excess burden on the heart and blood vessels. A lower fat diet discourages the formation of artherosclerotic lesions. Diabetics have an accelerated process of atherosclerosis. Dietary management can promote healthy life-styles.

INTERVENTIONS	RATIONALE
Inpatient Perform or assist in diagnostic procedures.	Doppler ultrasound, plethysmography, and segmental limb pressures are techniques in diagnostic testing used to determine the presence and degree of blood flow. These measurements are used to quantify and diagnose disease. Interpretation of these results will aid in the understanding of the disease process.
Provide information regarding diagnostic and treatment procedures.	Explain purpose of testing and intervention, ask questions, and repeat information at frequent intervals to confirm understanding. Provide information regarding the sensations that will be experienced. Two major needs during hospitalization are a need for information and a need for support. A rehearsal of what was taught is a good way to measure level of understanding.
Community Health/ Home Care None	

REFERENCES/BIBLIOGRAPHY

Appleton, D., & LaQuaglia, J.D. (1985). Vascular disease and postoperative nursing management. **Critical Care Nurse, 5**(5), 34–42.

Beasley-Dixon, M., & Nunnelee, J. (1987). Arterial reconstruction for atherosclerotic occlusive disease. **Journal of Cardiovascular Nursing, 1**(2), 36–49.

Blank, C., & Irwin, G. (1990). Peripheral vascular disorders assessment and intervention. **Nursing Clinics of North America, 25**(4), 777–794.

Carpenito, L.J. (1989). **Nursing diagnosis—Application to clinical practice**. Philadelphia: Lippincott.

Carpenito, L.J. (1991). **Nursing care plans and documentation. Nursing Diagnoses and Collaborative Problems**. Philadelphia: Lippincott.

Gulanick, M., et al. (1990). **Nursing Care Plans, Nursing Diagnosis and Interventions**. Philadelphia: Mosby.

Herman, J. (1986). Nursing assessment and nursing diagnosis in patients with peripheral vascular disease. **Nursing Clinics of North America, 21**(2), 219–232.

Holter, A. (1987). Preventing cardiovascular complications following AAA surgery. **Dimensions in Critical Care Nursing, 6**, 10–18.

Hubner, C. (1988). Nursing management of the patient with an ischemic limb. **Progress in Cardiovascular Nursing, 3**, 115–121.

Jurgens, J.L., et. al. (1980). **Peripheral vascular diseases**. Philadelphia: Saunders.

Kim, M.J. (1984). Physiologic nursing diagnosis: Its role and place in nursing taxonomy. In Kim, M.J., McFarland, G.K., & McLane, A.M. (Eds.). **Classification of Nursing Diagnosis: Proceedings of the Fifth National Conference** (pp. 60–61). St. Louis: Mosby.

Kim, M.J., Amoroso-Seritella, R., & Gulanick, M., et al. (1984). Clinical validation of cardiovascular nursing diagnoses. In Kim, M.J., McFarland, G.K., & McLane, A.M. (Eds.). **Classification of Nursing Diagnosis: Proceedings of the Fifth National Conference** (pp. 128–137). St. Louis: Mosby.

Larson, M., Leigh, J., & Wilson, L.R. (1986). Detecting compartmental syndrome using continuous pressure monitoring. **Focus on Critical Care, 13**, 51–56.

Lederer, J., Marculescu, G., Moznik, B., & Seaby, N. (1988). **Care Planning Pocket Guide: A Nursing Diagnosis Approach**. Menlo Park, CA: Addison-Wesley.

Leech, J. (1982). Psychosocial and physiologic needs of patients with arterial occlusive disease during the preoperative phase of hospitalization. **Heart & Lung, 11**(5), 442–448.

North American Nursing Diagnosis Association. **Taxonomy I** (Rev. 1990). St. Louis: NANDA.

Roberts, S. (1987). **Nursing Diagnosis and the Critically Ill Patient**. Norwalk, CT: Appleton-Century-Crofts.

Turner, J. (1986). Nursing Interventions in patients with peripheral vascular disease. **Nursing Clinics of North America, 21**(2), 233–240.

Wagner, M.M. (1986). Pathophysiology related to peripheral vascular disease. **Nursing Clinics of North America, 21**(2), 195–206.

Warbinsk, E., & Wyness, A. (1986). Peripheral arterial occlusive disease: Part II. Nursing assessment and standard care plans. **Cardiovascular Nurse, 22**, 6–11.

Toileting Deficit

A state in which an individual experiences an impaired ability to perform or complete toileting activities for oneself (NANDA, 1990, p. 85).

Suellyn Ellerbe, R.N., M.N.
Carol Dickel, R.N.
Peg. A. Mehmert, R.N., C., M.S.N.
Rosemary J. McKeighen, R.N., Ph.D., F.A.A.N.
Diane C. Kolb, R.N., B.A.

DEFINING CHARACTERISTICS

Unable to carry out proper toilet hygiene
Unable to flush toilet or commode
Unable to get to toilet or commode
Unable to manipulate clothing for toileting
Unable to sit on or rise from toilet or commode

CONTRIBUTING FACTORS

Pathophysiological

Activity intolerance
Decreased strength and endurance
Discomfort
Impaired mobility

Impaired transfer ability
Musculoskeletal impairment
Neuromuscular impairment
Pain

Psychosociobehavioral

Anxiety, severe
Depression

Perceptual or cognitive impairment

EXPECTED OUTCOMES

Client will achieve maximum level of independence in toileting.
    Ability to transfer/ambulate to toilet/commode with assistance is demonstrated.
    Ability to transfer/ambulate to toilet/commode independently in a safe manner is
        demonstrated.
    Ability to manipulate clothing for toileting activity is demonstrated.
    Ability to maintain toilet hygiene is demonstrated.
    Knowledge of rationale for frequent waste disposal is communicated.
    Ability to empty toilet/commode with assistance is demonstrated.
    Ability to empty toilet/commode independently in a safe manner is demonstrated.

INTERVENTIONS	RATIONALE
Universal	
Assess current ability for independence in toileting activities.	Acute or chronic health problems may decrease ability to access toileting facilities.
Assess availability of significant other(s) for support/assistance, as necessary.	Resources for clients not achieving/maintaining maximum functional level are provided.
Monitor and document progress in attaining maximum level of functional ability in toileting.	Documentation provides a measurement level for evaluation of progress towards independence.
Establish maximum potential for independence in performing toileting activities.	The alleviation of current health problems may restore the level of functional ability.
Monitor for feelings of anger, depression, fatigue, frustration, and intolerance of limitations in independence. Provide an opportunity for discussion of feelings.	The expression of feelings allows an opportunity for discussion in a nonjudgmental environment. The provision of input may enhance self-esteem and self-confidence.
Establish goals for achievement of maximum functional level in toileting activities.	Mutual planning of the nurse and client enhances motivation for participation in activities and the achievement of outcomes.
Establish schedule for toileting with clients that is congruent with their personal needs and preferences.	Collaboration respects the ethical principle of autonomy and increases the client's self-control, thus decreasing feelings of powerlessness.

INTERVENTIONS	RATIONALE
Provide positive reinforcement for advancement in toileting activity.	Self-esteem, self-confidence, and motivation towards achievement of maximum level of independence are reinforced.
Use consistent language for verbal prompts when encouraging/monitoring independence in toileting.	Uniform directives enhance comprehension in the presence of decreased cognition.
Place mobility/visual aids/adaptive devices within easy reach of bed/chair.	Independent functioning is promoted. The risk for falls/injury is reduced.
Provide clear, unobstructed pathway to toileting facilities.	Independent functioning is increased. The risk for falls/injury is reduced
Provide partial or total assistance with transfer/ambulation to toileting facilities.	The risk for falls/injury is reduced.
Provide privacy for toileting activities.	Embarrassment is impeded during performance of bodily functions.
Collaborate with physician on need for physical therapy referral.	Interdisciplinary interventions may be required to achieve maximum functional level.
Initiate teaching regarding self-toileting when capability and readiness to learn are demonstrated.	Decreased cognition and/or neuromuscular/musculoskeletal status may impinge on the ability to learn.
Instruct on: 1. Use of mobility (e.g., cane, walker, wheelchair) and adaptive devices (e.g., toilet riser, commode, support rails)	The correct use of devices enhances independence and mobility.
2. The use of supportive measures that provide self and/or environmental stability during toileting activities	Risk of fall/injury is reduced.
3. Maintaining clear, unobstructed pathway to toileting facilities	Risk of fall/injury is reduced.

INTERVENTIONS	RATIONALE
4. Use of clothing that is loose fitting with easy-access closures	Independence is increased and chances of accidental soiling and embarrassment are decreased.
5. Pacing activity to allow adequate time for gaining access to toileting facility	Energy level to access resources is sustained and the risk of fall/injury is minimized.
Inpatient None	
Community Health/ Home Care Assess environment for safety and/or risk factors (e.g., stairs, throw rugs, pets).	Risk for injury is reduced.
Instruct on methods for reducing environmental hazards that are within clients socioeconomic means.	The use of available material and economic resources promotes safety and decreases financial burden.
Instruct on the necessity for timely waste disposal.	Contaminants create adverse health conditions/ hazards.

REFERENCES/BIBLIOGRAPHY

See References/Bibliography for "Feeding Deficit."

Trauma: Risk

A state in which an individual is at risk for tissue injury as a result of internal and external environmental factors interacting with individual adapting and defensive resources (NANDA, 1990, pp. 39, 42).

Colleen Lucas, R.N., M.N., C.S.

RISK FACTORS

Internal

Agitation
Altered sense of position
Altered speech patterns
Balancing difficulties
Decreased level of consciousness
Disorientation
Fatigue
Gait disturbance
Hallucinations
History of previous falls or other traumas
Impaired judgment
Incoordination

Lack of safety education
Language and communication barriers
Medication effects
Memory deficits
Motor deficits
Muscle or general weakness
Paralysis
Postural hypotension
Restlessness
Seizures
Sensory perceptual alterations
Tremors

External

Absent or unsteady handrails
Bathtub or shower without secured handgrip and antislip device
Contact with rapidly moving machines or conveyor belts
Defective equipment
Driving at excessive speeds or in unsafe conditions

Excessive grease build-up on cooking utensils or appliances
Failure to comply with safety rules when participating in sports
Failure to comply with safety rules when using machinery or electrical devices
Faulty electrical appliances
Floors made slippery with wax, liquid, oil
Frayed or ungrounded electrical cords
Gas leaks or faulty pilot lights
Ice-slickened walkways, stairs, streets
Improper storage of chemicals or combustibles
Inaccessible toileting facilities.
Inadequate lighting
Lack of communication aides
Lack of necessary ambulation or transportation aides
Lack of restraint use in automobiles
Moving unstable or unsecured loads
Obstructed passageways and floors
Operating automobiles, other moving devices, or machinery under the influence of alcohol or mind-altering drugs
Overexposure to the sun, sunlamps, or radiation therapy
Overloaded electrical circuits, outlets, fusebox
Pot handles facing the front of the stove
Safety equipment unavailable or not in use
Slick soles of shoes
Sliding over rough surfaces
Structural hazards
Uneven or slippery ground and rock surfaces
Unscreened fireplaces or heaters
Unsecured electrical cords
Unstable ladder or other equipment used in reaching high places
Using mechanically unsafe equipment or automobiles
Wearing highly inflammable or flowing clothing around open fires or when cooking
Working in or near the pathway of moving vehicles

EXPECTED OUTCOMES

Client will identify factors that increase the risk for trauma.
> Internal and external factors that place an individual or groups at risk for trauma are listed.
> Internal and external factors placing self or others at risk for trauma are assessed.
> Level of risk is related to available adaptive and defensive resources.
Client will apply safety precautions to self, others, and environment in reducing the risk for trauma.
> Measures that increase safety are identified.
> Structural changes in reducing the risk for trauma are made, e.g., lighting is added; defective equipment is replaced; handrails, grips, antislip devices are added; obstructions of passageways or floors are cleared.

Safe practices are incorporated into activities of daily living, e.g., ambulation and transportation aides are used; non-slip shoes are worn; communication and visual aides are used as necessary; safe clothing is worn while cooking or around open fires.

Safety orientation is completed prior to using machinery or electrical appliances; safety rules are followed during equipment use.

Safety orientation is completed prior to participating in individual or team sporting events.

A safe environment is maintained.

Client will remain free of bodily injury.

Correct fall and recovery techniques are demonstrated.

There is an absence of falls, moving vehicle accidents, and overexposure to ultraviolet light.

INTERVENTIONS

RATIONALE

Interventions	Rationale
Universal	
Monitor safety requirements.	Safety requirements change based upon orientation, physical abilities, sensory function, medications, and environment.
Provide night lighting and adequate day lighting, especially on stairs and changes in ground elevations.	With changes in vision and with decreased light, clear demarcation of one step from another or one elevation from another is difficult to ascertain. Falls are more likely to occur if lighting is not adequate.
Clearly mark edges of steps, changes in elevations.	Painting the edge of the step assists the visually impaired to see where one step begins and the previous step ends. Similarly, marking curb elevations and handicapped access ramps visually alerts the client to adjust gait.
Provide well-secured handrails, visually distinct in color from the wall, in all designated handicapped areas and stairwells.	Handrails painted a color different from the wall are easily seen, and when properly secured, offer balance and support during position changes.
Provide or request client to wear proper footwear.	Slick-soled shoes increase the risk of falling when walking on hard, waxed floors; open-toed shoes expose the foot to trauma; some rubber-soled shoes can stick to carpet or floors, causing a fall.

INTERVENTIONS	RATIONALE
Provide a safe, supervised, smoking environment away from flammable materials.	Altered judgment, memory, and sensory function affect the ability to handle smoking materials safely, necessitating supervision of smokers. Some environments contain highly combustible materials; thus areas away from these materials are designated for smoking.
Advocate for gun control, seatbelt and helmet use laws, and workplace environmental safety.	Nurses are leaders in health care and through a collective voice, shape state and national health policy as well as setting safety standards.
Assist client in developing environmental assessments for self-monitoring of risks.	Self-evaluation plans increase control of the environment.
Teach internal and external factors that place individual or groups at risk.	Knowledge of risk factors is a prerequisite to behavior change.
Teach methods of modifying the environment to reduce risk.	Information empowers intervention and risk reduction.
Teach measures to be taken in reducing the risk for injury from moving vehicles and machinery: 1. Refrain from operating moving vehicles or machinery after using alcohol, sedatives, hypnotics, and other drugs which alter judgment or attention span 2. Develop, implement, and complete training programs for safe equipment usage 3. Provide routine safety inspections and maintenance	Machinery and automobiles in good working order and users understanding their rights and responsibilities prevent injury.

INTERVENTIONS	RATIONALE
Teach safe medication usage: 1. Prescribed therapeutic dose and frequency 2. Anticipated effects 3. Side effects 4. Precautions and follow-up should side effects occur	Many drugs affect thought processes and judgment, while others may affect the response to trauma. Advanced warning of these effects allows for the implementation of safety precautions (e.g., have someone else drive; carry a medic alert card or bracelet; have another person supervise activities).
Teach to change positions slowly; sit briefly; then stand briefly before walking.	Gradual change in position decreases the effects of orthostatic hypotension and decreases the risk of falling.
Teach and evaluate use of the emergency response system (i.e., 911, emergency call light, Lifeline).	Skillful use of the emergency response system is necessary to obtain immediate and early assistance should trauma occur.
Inpatient Monitor risk for trauma throughout hospitalization.	Level of risk for trauma changes are based on the interaction of the environment with fluctuations in physical, emotional, and cognitive status. Changes in environment, such as transfer from one unit or room to another, affects orientation cues and sensory stimulation. Other examples of changes affecting mental status and orientation are biochemical, metabolic, and comfort stimuli.
Assess environment frequently. Keep personal items (glasses, hearing aid, etc.) and phone within reach.	Easy access to personal items that enhance sensory input aids orientation.
Evaluate voiding patterns. Develop voiding schedule and assist with voiding consistent with usual patterns, i.e., if client usually gets up during night to void, anticipate assisting client with this. Keep bedpan, urinal, and commode within easy reach.	Many falls occur at night when there is a need to void and the surroundings are unfamiliar. Evaluating voiding patterns helps to anticipate when assistance is needed.

INTERVENTIONS	RATIONALE
Obtain assistance and use turn sheets or flotation devices to reposition immobile clients.	Skin trauma is reduced when there is a decrease in gravitational resistance (i.e., flotation devices), an increase in energy efficiency, and a lessening of the shearing and friction on the skin.
Observe frequently.	Frequent observation is necessary in evaluating the effectiveness of actions, changes in condition, and to avoid trauma.
Use siderails and nurse alert devices.	In unfamiliar surroundings and in the presence of restlessness, confusion, sedation, obesity, or altered judgment, there may not be recognition of environmental risks for injury. Siderails act as a barrier, making it more difficult for ambulating without assistance. Alert devices cue the nurse that the client is attempting ambulation unaided. Both siderails and alert devices serve as a reminder to the client to call for assistance before ambulating.
Pad siderails.	Padded siderails absorb body impact, preventing injury during restlessness or seizures.
Remove rollers from bed or lock wheels.	Preventing the bed or chair from rolling provides a steady base during transfers.
Maintain the bed in low position.	The lower position of the bed makes it easier to get in and out of bed and simultaneously maintain balance. Injury is less likely to occur if balance is maintained and is less severe if a fall occurs.
Remove unnecessary furniture and equipment and provide a clear pathway between the bed and bathroom.	Balance is more easily maintained in a clear path versus stepping over or around furniture.
Orient to environment and collaborate with client in meeting activity restrictions.	Setting clear expectations assures that welfare is of concern and assistance is available. Information and mutual goal setting enhance compliance.

INTERVENTIONS	RATIONALE
Develop written plan of care that communicates to other care givers approaches to follow and anticipated outcomes.	A consistent, client-centered approach to care increases the likelihood of achieving target goals.
Orient to person, place, and time; reorient to activity plan.	Reorientation decreases confusion. A calendar, clock, or television enhances contact with the surroundings.
Assist with transfers and ambulation.	Assistance provides an opportunity for cueing and reorientation and provides increased balance and support, thus preventing falls.
Apply, monitor, and remove restraints in accordance with institutional policy. Vest and belt restraints allow some freedom of movement. Mitt restraints allow free arm movement but restrict use of hands. Wrist restraints restrict arm movement and often leave the client feeling helpless, increasing fear and agitation.	Frequent monitoring provides information about the response to restraints, adverse effects of restraints, and the feasibility of other approaches. Restraints can result in increased agitation. Close supervision, frequent removal of restraints, and reapplication are essential in preventing circulatory and integumentary damage.
Advocate for an institutional policy on the use of chemical and physical restraints, which provides guidelines for when to use, for the management of the restrained client, for alternative approaches to be tried, and for how restraints are used.	Several ethical principles are challenged when the decision to use restraints is made. Autonomy without constraint is challenged by the care giver's duty to do good and the duty to do no harm. A well-written institutional policy helps in determining what is right or best when this difficult situation occurs.
Instruct in correct use of assistive devices.	When correctly used, assistive devices promote balance when changing positions, steady the gait, and support weakened muscles. Incorrect usage results in muscle fatigue and injury.

INTERVENTIONS	**R**ATIONALE
Community Health/ Home Care	
Teach constant supervision of those with impaired judgment.	Supervision and intervention prevent follow-through on unsafe decisions.
Teach use of assistive devices in reaching items on upper shelves; assist in placing frequently used items within easy reach.	Assistive long-handled devices maintain balance and gait more so than using step ladders and stools.
Review assistive devices available for improving safety in the bathroom: 1. Raised toilet seat; grip bars by toilet 2. Grip bars attached to tub side or anchored on tub wall or shower 3. Emergency call system 4. Antislip device in tub, shower 5. Bath stool for placing in tub or shower	Assistive devices provide stable support when changing positions, especially when balance is altered. An emergency call system via an internal alarm or external phone system alerts others that help is needed. Early response is essential in minimizing the trauma.
Teach safety measures to be followed in the kitchen: 1. Keep pot handles facing the back of the stove 2. Use electrical appliances which are in good working order, have been maintained and have non-frayed cords 3. Immediately notify gas company of suspected leaks, faulty pilot lights 4. Select close-fitting clothing to wear while cooking	Pot handles facing the front of the stove may be jarred or bumped, causing contents to splash forward and burn. Faulty electrical appliances gas leaks, and wearing flowing clothing can all result in burns.

INTERVENTIONS	**R**ATIONALE
Teach other safety precautions to follow throughout the home and work setting.	Fireplace screens keep burning embers contained and off flammable objects. Maintaining clear passageways and floors assists to maintain balance and use assistive devices without interference from obstructions. Abrasive strips on steps provide traction for shoes and prevent slippage.
1. Keep fireplace screens in place and dampers open while the fireplace is in use	
2. Clear obstructions from passageways and floors	
3. Secure electrical cords; keep out of traffic area	
4. Clean up spills and post signs as necessary; avoid waxing floors	
5. Use non-skid mats or abrasive strips on walking surfaces that are likely to get wet, such as outdoor walkways and steps	
6. Anchor or remove loose carpets, rugs	
Teach activity abilities and limitations in accordance with physical and mental status. Reinforce frequently.	Knowing limitations **and** abilities focuses on what **can** be done, developing a positive outlook.
Teach correct use of cane, walking stick, or walker to be used on unfamiliar or uneven ground.	Assistive devices help maintain balance.
Teach correct fall and recovery technique.	Learning how to fall can minimize the injury incurred.

REFERENCES/BIBLIOGRAPHY

Blakeslee, J.A. (1988). Speaking out: Untie the elderly. **American Journal of Nursing**, 88(6), 833–834.

Dallaire, L.B., & Burke, E.V. (1989). A new program for reducing patient falls. **Nursing 89**, 19(6), 6–7.

Escher, J.E., O'Dell, C., & Gambert, S.R. (1989). Typical geriatric accidents and how to prevent them. **Geriatrics**, 44(5), 54–56, 66–69.

*Garcia, R.M., Reed, M., Taylor, P.V., Sloan, G., & Beran, N. (1988). Relationship between falls and patient attempts to satisfy elimination needs. **Nursing Management (Long-term care edition), 19**(7), 80v–80x.

Berryman, E., Gaskin, D., Jones, A., Tolley, J., & MacMullen, J. (1989). Point by point: Predicting elders' falls. **Geriatric Nursing**, July/August, 199–201.

*Byers, V., Arrington, M.E., & Finstuen, K. (1990). Predictive risk factors associated with stroke patient falls in acute care settings. **Journal of Neuroscience Nursing**, 22(3), 147–154.

Gettrust, K.V., Ryan, S.C., & Engelmon, D.S. (Eds.). (1985). **Applied nursing diagnosis: Guides for comprehensive planning** (pp. 105–108). Albany, NY: Delmar.

*Grant, J.S., & Hamilton, S. (1987). Falls in a rehabilitation center: A retrospective and comparative analysis. **Rehabilitation Nursing, 12**(2), 74–76.

*Hernandez, M., & Miller, J. (1986). How to reduce falls. **Geriatric Nursing,** March/April, 97–102.

*Hill, B.A., Johnson, R., & Garrett, B.J. (1988). Reducing the incidence of falls in high risk patients. **Journal of Nursing Administration,** 18(7, 8), 24–28.

*Janken, J.K., Reynolds, B.A., & Swiech, K. (1986). Patient falls in the acute care setting: Identifying risk factors. **Nursing Research,** 35(4), 215–219.

Kim, M.J., McFarland, G.K., & McLane, A.M. (1989). **Pocket guide to nursing diagnoses,** St. Louis: Mosby.

McFarland, G.K., & McFarlane, E.A. (1989). **Nursing diagnosis and intervention: Planning for patient care.** St. Louis: Mosby.

*Mion, L.C., et al. (1989). Falls in the rehabilitation setting: Incidence and characteristics. **Rehabilitation Nursing, 14**(1), 17–22.

Morton, D. (1989). Five years of fewer falls. **American Journal of Nursing,** 89(2), 204–205.

National Institute on Aging and National Osteoporosis Foundation (1987). Age page: Preventing falls and fractures. (1988). (pp. 195–375). U.S. Department of Health and Human Services, Washington DC: U.S. Government Printing Office.

North American Nursing Diagnosis Association. **Taxonomy I** (Rev. 1990). St. Louis: NANDA.

Rose, J. (1987). When the care plan says restrain. **Geriatric Nursing,** January/February, 20–21.

Schulman, B.K., & Acquaviva, T. (1987). Falls in the elderly. **Nurse Practitioner,** 12 (11), 30–38.

Spellbring, A.M., Gannon, M.E., Kleckner, T., & Conway, K. (1988). Improving safety for hospitalized elderly. **Journal of Gerontological Nursing,** 14(2), 31–37.

*Tack, K.A., Ulrich, B., & Kehr, C. (1987). Patient falls: Profile for prevention. **Journal of Neuroscience Nursing, 19**(2), 83–89.

Tideiksaar, R. (1989). Geriatric falls: Assessing the cause, preventing recurrence. **Geriatrics, 44**(7), 57–61.

Tobis, J., Block, M., Steinhaus-Donham, C., Reinsch, S., Tamaru, K., & Weil, D. (1990). Falling among the sensorially impaired elderly. **Archives of Physical Medicine and Rehabilitation,** 71, February, 144–147.

*Whedon, M.B., & Shedd, P. (1989). State of the science: Prediction and prevention of patient falls. **IMAGE: Journal of Nursing Scholarship,** 21(2), 108–114.

Yorker, B.C. (1988). The nurse's use of restraint with a neurologically impaired patient. **Journal of Neuroscience Nursing,** 20(6), 390–392.

Unilateral Neglect

A state in which an individual is perceptually unaware of and inattentive to one side of the body.

Jan A. Sheldon, R.N., M.S., C.C.R.N.

DEFINING CHARACTERISTICS

Actual injury to the affected side
Constant unfamiliarity with the environment
Does not look to the affected side

Inability to locate the affected side
Inattention to stimuli on affected side
Incomplete self-care on affected side

CONTRIBUTING FACTORS

Pathophysiological

Brain injury or trauma
Brain tumor with hemispheric tissue death
Cerebral vascular accident
Hemianopsia

Hemispheric neurological illness
Ruptured cerebral aneurysm
Unilateral blindness
Unilateral changes in sensation

Psychosociobehavioral

None

EXPECTED OUTCOMES

Client will attend to neglected side of body with minimal cues.
    All body parts are free of injury.
    Scanning techniques are learned.
    Decreasing reliance on verbal/tactile stimuli to locate neglected side of body is seen.
    Some personal care of neglected side is completed.

INTERVENTIONS	RATIONALE
Universal Assess awareness of total body. 1. Ask to locate unaffected and affected side 2. Approach from unaffected side, midline, and affected side 3. Observe position of affected side 4. Observe self-care activities on affected side 5. Observe direction of head and visual field 6. Ask to locate items on unaffected side and affected side 7. Observe for statements about inability to make sense of the environment	Focusing the interventions on the nature and presentation of the neglect enhances the opportunity for the client to respond to teaching that is focused directly on the presentation of the neglect.
Increase awareness of neglected body parts through systematic and consistent cueing. 1. Approach on unaffected side; gradually move toward midline and then affected side 2. Place affected side so client can find it and gradually move affected side to normal body position while client observes placement 3. Use tactile stimuli (i.e., distinguishable texture like rough fabric) on affected side to help client maintain awareness	Using the same consistent approach to increasing awareness of the affected side increases the likelihood that the client will respond to cueing. The impaired brain is most likely to process information that is presented through repetition.
Orient to environment with every contact.	Since the neglect may be due to a visual field loss, i.e., hemianopsia, it is necessary to point out landmarks in the environment to decrease confusion.

INTERVENTIONS	RATIONALE
Teach client and significant others about neglect deficits.	Informed significant others can facilitate learning with the client and assist in coping with the deficits. The client may respond to the assistance of familiar people and benefit from the support of loved ones. Involvement in care enhances feelings of being valued.
Teach scanning techniques. 1. Place all items in visual field 2. Gradually move items toward midline and then onto neglected side 3. Orient to environment by use of visual landmarks	Consistent cueing and systematic teaching provide feedback that decreases neglect deficits and increases the visual field.
Inpatient Assess extent of neglect. 1. Observe for incomplete attempts at activities of daily living (ADL). 2. Monitor dietary intake and position of meal tray 3. Observe for continual requests for items located on neglected side 4. Monitor position of affected side, i.e., placement of leg on wheelchair leg rest or arm position on lap board	Focusing interventions on the nature and presentation of the neglect enhances the opportunity for success in mastering deficits.
Avoid room changes; and position in room so that non-neglected side is toward the center of activity.	To begin orientation to the environment, a commitment to one room is essential to allow for minimal distraction when there is impairment in processing information about the environment.

INTERVENTIONS	**R**ATIONALE
Provide a safe environment — free of clutter, well lighted, with consistent visual cues for recognition of schemes. 1. Use mirrors for visual feedback during ADL 2. Keep night light on 3. Keep call light on unaffected side 4. Keep side rails up when in bed 5. Use wheelchair safety belt	Since the client is cognitively impaired and may not recognize the neglect deficits, interventions focusing on maintaining safety are essential.
Provide constant cueing when transporting throughout the hospital, noting landmarks on both sides of the hallway. 1. Place a name card near doorway of room on both sides of the hall 2. Incorporate scanning techniques while transporting	Due to an inability to distinguish stimuli on the neglected side, environmental information is processed incompletely.
Instruct regarding neglect deficits.	Informed significant others can facilitate learning with the client and assist in coping with deficits.
Instruct significant others regarding scanning techniques.	The client may not be able to monitor progress and may always require cueing to enhance awareness of the neglected side.
Community Health/ Home Care Assess extent of neglect and effective use of cues.	The nature of the interventions is based on the presentation of neglect and learned compensatory mechanisms.

INTERVENTIONS	RATIONALE
Provide a safe environment. 1. Remove excess furniture and equipment from main pathways of house 2. Keep house well lighted in areas client may occupy 3. Identify familiar landmarks throughout the home	Familiar landmarks provide a consistent cue for location in the home. A well-lighted environment enhances safety by providing adequate visualization of the environment. Providing a clear pathway for mobility around the environment minimizes the chance of injury.
Arrange household to carryover consistent visual stimulation techniques. 1. Use mirrors for all activities appropriate for client (feeding, dressing, hygiene) 2. Hang full-length mirrors in areas client may ambulate	Providing consistent visual stimulation techniques facilitates carry-over of learned behaviors.
Reinforce system of cueing previously learned.	Building on a system already learned facilitates carry-over of techniques.
Continue to educate care givers in the home about the nature of the neglect.	Reinforcement of previous learning assists in coping with the unilateral neglect and facilitates carry-over.

•REFERENCES/BIBLIOGRAPHY

Booth, K. (1982). The neglect syndrome. **Journal of Neurosurgical Nursing**, **14**(1), 38–43.

Dittmar, S. (1989). **Rehabilitation Nursing Process and Application** (1st Ed.). St. Louis: Mosby.

Hart, G. Strokes causing left vs. right hemiplegia: Different effects and nursing implications. **Geriatric Nursing**. January/February, 1983.

North American Nursing Diagnosis Association. **Taxonomy I** (Rev. 1990). St. Louis: NANDA.

Siev, E., Freishtat, B., & Zoltan, B. (1986). **Perceptual and cognitive dysfunction in the adult stroke patient**. Thorofare, NJ: Slack.

Urinary Retention, Acute

A state in which an individual experiences a sudden onset of urethral pressure so great that little or no urine is allowed to be expelled.

Anne Marie Voith Sherman, R.N., M.S.N.

. . . .

DEFINING CHARACTERISTICS

Absence of urine output
Bladder distention after voiding
Dribbling
Lower abdominal discomfort

Restlessness
Sensation of bladder fullness
Small (e.g., less than 50 cc), frequent voiding

CONTRIBUTING FACTORS

Pathophysiological

Effects of psychotropic medication, anesthesia, opiates, sedatives, antihistimines
Hypertonic sphincter
Partial or complete obstruction of urethra by pressure of swelling or edema (e.g., fecal impaction, surgical site swelling, postpartum edema, strictures, vaginal or rectal packing, prostatic hypertrophy)

Psychosociobehavioral

Anxiety
Psychosis

EXPECTED OUTCOMES

Client's bladder will not be palpable after voiding.
  Voiding occurs in 150–400 cc amounts.
  Absence of dribbling and dysuria is reported.
  Post-void residual is less than 75 cc.
  Problems with voiding are reported promptly.

INTERVENTIONS · RATIONALE

Universal	
Evaluate medications and work with physician to adjust as necessary.	Many medications may contribute to retention.
Assess pain level before voiding; medicate as necessary.	Pain may interfere with ability to void.
Attempt to initiate voiding reflex (e.g., drink water, stroke lower abdomen or inner thigh, pour water over perineum, run water in sink, tap over symphysis pubis, place spirits of wintergreen in commode or bedpan).	These techniques may overcome a neurological block to micturition by strengthening reflex and/or relaxing sphincters.
Have female client squat over toilet using leg muscles, or sit upright. Have male client stand.	This helps relax pelvic floor muscles and uses gravity to assist in emptying of bladder.
Promote relaxation with deep breathing and calming conversation.	Relaxation facilitates voiding.
Perform straight catheterization.	Straight catheterization bypasses the obstruction, allowing bladder emptying while minimizing risk of infection from indwelling catheter.
Provide privacy.	Privacy increases ability to concentrate on urination and/or relaxation.
Remove obstruction, if possible.	Removal of obstruction, such as fecal impaction, reduces urethral pressure, allowing urine to pass.

INTERVENTIONS	**R**ATIONALE
Teach to report problems immediately.	Renal damage can be prevented and treatment can be instituted promptly when early knowledge of problem is identified.
Inpatient None	
Community Health/ Home Care None	

REFERENCES/BIBLIOGRAPHY

*Bergstrom, N.I. (1969). Ice application to induce voiding. **American Journal of Nursing, 69**(2), 283–285.

*Cardenas, D.D., Kelly, E., & Mayo, M.E. (1985). Manual stimulation of reflex voiding after spinal cord injury. **Archives of Physical Medicine and Rehabilitation, 66**, 459–462.

*Greengold, B.A., & Ouslander, J.G. (1986). Bladder retraining. **Journal of Gerontological Nursing, 12**(6), 31–35.

*Gross, J.C. (1990). Bladder dysfunction after a stroke. **Journal of Gerontological Nursing, 16**(4), 20–25.

Voith, A.M. (1988). Alterations in urinary elimination: Concepts, research, and practice. **Rehabilitation Nursing, 13**(3), 122–131.

Urinary Retention, Chronic

A state in which an individual's bladder emptying is chronically incomplete.

Anne Marie Voith Sherman, R.N., M.S.N.

DEFINING CHARACTERISTICS

Catheter residual more than 150 cc, or 20% of voided urine
Dribbling
Dysuria
Frequency (voiding more often than every two hours)
Hesitancy (i.e., inability to void on command)
Nocturia
Reduced force of stream (void less than 10 ml)
Sensation of bladder fullness
Small (e.g., less than 50 cc, frequent voiding)

CONTRIBUTING FACTORS

Pathophysiological

Chronic overdistention
Dehydration (bladder fills so slowly that sensory impulses are not stimulated)
Detrusor atrophy
Hypertonic sphincter
Partial or complete obstruction of urethra (e.g., strictures, prostatic hypertrophy)

Psychosociobehavioral

None

EXPECTED OUTCOMES

Client's bladder will not be palpable after voiding.
  Understanding of causative factors is verbalized.
  Voiding occurs in 150–400 cc amounts.
  Post-voiding residual is less than 75 cc.
  Absence of dribbling and dysuria is reported.
  Treatment regimen is correctly verbalized and demonstrated.

INTERVENTIONS	RATIONALE
Universal	
Determine bladder's ability to contract by attempting urination. Note size and force of urinary stream.	If voiding is possible, Credé's maneuver or other techniques may be an option for successful urination.
Monitor for bladder distention, inability to void, and bladder spasms.	Complications and discomfort result from overdistention.
Assess for effects of medications (e.g., psychotropics, antihistamines, atropine) and consult with physician regarding possible adjustment.	Various medications can contribute to urinary retention.
Assess pain level before initiating voiding; medicate as necessary.	Pain may interfere with ability to void.
Monitor for signs and symptoms of a urinary tract infection (UTI).	Urinary retention may be a precipitating factor for the development of UTIs.
Monitor for signs and symptoms of hyperreflexia.	These are a syndrome of symptoms caused by bladder distention or a blocked catheter. They include excessively elevated blood pressure, bradycardia, throbbing headache, flushing, diaphoresis, blurred vision, nasal congestion, and nausea. Hyperreflexia can be a life-threatening complication leading to seizures and/or stroke, and is usually more dramatic in the spinal cord injured.

INTERVENTIONS	RATIONALE
After voiding, straight catheterize for residual.	Complete emptying is important to prevent problems resulting from prolonged urine retention (e.g., infection, sepsis, and reflux to the kidneys).
Consult with physician regarding use of an alpha-blocker or cholinergic medication.	These drugs reduce outlet resistance.
Encourage voiding at regular intervals, not to exceed every four hours.	Chronic overdistention leads to retention and its complications. By emptying the bladder on a scheduled basis, overdistention may be prevented.
Have male void while standing; female sit upright to void.	Gravity helps empty bladder in this position.
Promote relaxation with deep breathing and calming conversation.	Relaxation facilitates voiding.
Instruct in causative/contributing factors.	Knowledge about the etiology of urinary retention may prevent its occurence and/or promote early intervention.
Instruct in regimen, its reasons, and complications of incontinence.	Understanding facilitates compliance.
Teach Credé's maneuver (deep massage with fingertips together from iliac crest in to midline and down toward pubic bone).	This assists bladder in overcoming urethral pressure. Note: May increase reflux into ureters. Check with physician.
Teach intermittent self-catheterization.	If bladder emptying by voiding is not possible, catheterization is necessary for passage of urine at predictable times. A clean technique is usually sufficient at home.
Teach rectal stretch (insert forefinger into rectum and gently stimulate, "stretch" the sphincters).	This relaxes the sphincters and, in combination with Valsalva's maneuver, allows emptying of the bladder for some spinal cord injured clients.

INTERVENTIONS	**R**ATIONALE
Teach Valsalva's maneuver (have client bear down by holding a deep breath and pushing against diaphragm from below to increase intraabdominal pressure, as if having a bowel movement).	Note: This maneuver is not recommended in the presence of certain conditions (e.g., glaucoma, myocardial infarction, eye surgery, and aneurysm). When this maneuver can be safely used, it relaxes the sphincters and allows emptying of the bladder.
Refer care giver to support group: The Simon Foundation, Box 815, Wilmette, IL 60091; OR; Help for Incontinent People; PO Box 544, Union, SC 29373.	Caring for an incontinent person can be stressful.
Inpatient None	
Community Health/ Home Care None	

REFERENCES/BIBLIOGRAPHY

Gross, C. (1990). Bladder dysfunction after stroke: It's not always inevitable. **Journal of Gerontological Nursing, 16**(4), 20–25.

Ouslander, J.G. (1988). Practical management of incontinence. **Highlights of a Roundtable Discussion**. Kansas City, MO: Marion Laboratories.

Resnick, N.M., & Yala, S.V. (1985). Management of urinary incontinence in the elderly. **New England Journal of Medicine, 313**(13), 800–805.

Voith, A.M. (1988). Alterations in urinary elimination: Concepts, research, and practice. **Rehabilitation Nursing, 13**(3), 122–131.

Violence: Risk

A state in which an individual experiences behaviors that can be physically harmful to either the self or others (NANDA, 1990, p. 102).

Von Best Whitaker, R.N., Ph.D.

RISK FACTORS

Pathophysiological

Anemia leading to affective disturbances and increased irritability
Anesthesia
Biochemical imbalance
CNS disorders (e.g., tumor, cerebral edema, cerebrovascular disease, degenerative dementia, disorientation, head trauma, temporal epilepsy, hypertensive encephalopathy)
Electrolyte imbalance
Endocrine disorder (e.g., hormonal imbalance, hypoglycemia)
Genetics
High fever
Septic shock

Psychosociobehavioral

Adverse substance/chemical reaction
Age
Altered libido
Altered perceptions of territorial space
Cultural heritage
Demanding of instant gratification
Dysfunctional family
Fear attributed to change of environment (e.g., institutionalization, deinstitutionalization)
Feelings of helplessness or powerlessness due to a frustrating environment
Grief or loss (e.g., of familiar environment, home, vision, hearing, limbs, significant other, job)
High dissatisfaction with others

History of attempted suicide or physical harm to self or others
History of childhood brutality
History of destruction of property
Homosexual panic in an attempt to restore self-esteem
Inability to communicate verbally
Lack of human warmth
Loneliness
Low self-esteem
Misperceived communication—either verbal or behavioral
Paranoia
Perception of others as all powerful and impervious to own wishes
Persistent interpersonal conflict
Poor impulse control
Poor interpersonal and interdependent relationships
Poor work history
Possession of destructive objects (e.g., knives, guns, etc.)
Psychiatric illness (e.g,. hallucination, mania)
Self-hatred
Social isolation

EXPECTED OUTCOMES

Impulsive behavior that has potential to harm self and others will be avoided.
    Factors that precipitate violent behavior are recognized.
    Alternative ways of expressing frustration are identified, e.g., verbalization.
    Alternative objects for anger are identified, e.g., punching bag, walking, jogging.
    Limits placed on behavior are accepted.
Client will establish consistency in daily activities.
    A consistent daily protocol is adhered to.
Client's self-esteem will be enhanced.
    Feelings and concerns are verbalized.
    Self-awareness and mutual trust are increased.
    Negative thoughts are cognitively restructured, and strengths rather than weaknesses
        are emphasized.
Client will translate hostile feelings into words.
    Consequences of behavior are identified.
Client will identify target of anger.
    Aggression is expressed verbally.
    Expression of physical aggression is avoided.
Client will establish honesty and trustworthiness.
    Ways in which behavior affects others, as well as self, are identified.
Client will increase interpersonal skills.
    Verbal communication is increased, e.g., reminiscing, recall.

INTERVENTIONS	**R**ATIONALE
Universal	
Assess for family and supportive others as possible additions to the management team.	Inclusion of supportive others helps to decrease isolation, loneliness, and adjustment to loss of independence.
Assess age and sex.	Most violent subgroup is males between the ages of 15 to 33 years.
Assess cultural heritage and needs for personal space.	Definitions of and acceptance levels for violence and needs for personal space vary within cultures.
Evaluate ethnic affiliation.	Myths and stereotypes about violence abound and have been falsely attributed to certain ethnic groups as fact.
Assess religious affiliation.	Religion may be the only hope to hold on to when feelings of hopelessness are present.
Explore immigration status.	Newly arrived immigrants may have difficulty with acculturation due to loss of cultural norms, prejudice, family, etc.
Observe nonverbal cues.	Behavioral action may be indication of impending violence to self or other (i.e., pacing, wringing hands, extreme diaphoresis).
Assess ability to communicate verbally.	Verbalizing aggression decreases possibility of physical aggression.
Note time of day.	Most serious self-harming attempts (e.g., suicide) occur during early afternoon when numerous activities are taking place.
Assess for signs and symptoms of depression.	Most serious self-harm attempts occur when depressed—in particular, when veil of depression is beginning to lift and lost energy is regained.
Monitor clues for increased pacing, inability to remain stationary, and sudden cessation of motor activity.	These are behavioral clues for risk of violence.

INTERVENTIONS

RATIONALE

INTERVENTIONS	RATIONALE
Monitor threatened verbal or physical behavior toward self or others.	Loud speech, profanity, assaultive behavior toward real or imagined objects are behavioral manifestations for risk of violence.
Assess for chemical or substance reaction.	Toxic reactions enhance the acting out of assaultive behaviors without inhibitions.
Respect personal space.	Invasion of certain spacial areas claimed as personal territory enhances risk for violence.
Avoid quick and sudden movements.	Quick or sudden behavior may cause fear of attack or invasion of personal or territorial space.
Never turn away from client.	Vulnerability is increased when unable to see source of attack.
Interview client alone.	Privacy decreases feelings of being overwhelmed, threatened, or vulnerable and maintains dignity and privacy.
Use semi-structured interview techniques.	Semi-structured interview technique allows the disclosing ability to be directed.
Convey calm and self-assurance when approaching client.	Expressing concern over a situation that is occurring and a desire to change it enhances feelings of alliance with care giver.
Use modulated tone when interviewing.	A soft tone tends to deescalate volatile situations at a mild emotional level; but during a high emotional level, use a louder than normal voice and **slower speech** to prevent auditory clutter.
Give behavioral directions using clear, simple, and specific speech.	An aroused state decreases ability to receive and process organized complex information.
Avoid confrontation.	Increased staff-client emotional level heightens volatile situation.
Do not leave client alone.	Leaving the client alone may be interpreted as rejection or could provide opportunity to inflict harm upon self or others while unobserved.

INTERVENTIONS

RATIONALE

INTERVENTIONS	RATIONALE
Allow for verbal ventilation.	Verbalization may alleviate anxiety by allowing client to feel that someone is going to help and hear emotions and feelings.
Be an active listener.	Use of body language (e.g., facial expressions, etc.) and encouraging words demonstrate active listening and caring.
Mutually plan ways to decrease frustration.	Joint planning formulates the rules for acceptable limits while allowing for compromise.
Take nonassaultive posture when violence is imminent (do not argue, clench fists, place hands on hips, move suddenly, display angry facial expressions, fold arms across chest, etc.).	In a panic state, cognitive reasoning may be fragmented, and an authoritative posture may cause feelings of being pressured or trapped.
Negotiate if weapon is present.	The offering of alternatives for the outlet of aggressive feelings may diffuse the volatile situation.
Teach acceptable methods for violence prevention.	Documented organizational behavioral policy to prevent violence gives support for staff behavior during crisis.
Teach the etiology of anxiety, anger, and aggression.	Anticipation, prevention, and skillful interactions decrease the occurrence of violent behavior during crisis.
Provide education addressing ethnic, cultural, and religious diversity.	Cultural, ethnic, and religious factors are frequently ignored; and judgements about care are not predicated upon presenting data and empirical evidence but upon myth and stereotypical perceptions.

Inpatient

Assess precipitating factors for violence.	Knowledge of factors which promote violence can aid in the prevention of violence (e.g., institutionalization; feelings of dependency, anger and rejection by family and staff; illness; anger at self; grief reaction (loss), etc.

INTERVENTIONS	**R**ATIONALE
Assess previous coping patterns.	Knowledge of previous coping patterns provides a map for the present response to crisis.
Assess environment for over-crowding and understaffing.	Overcrowding leads to low morale and a decrease of territorial space, which decreases personal space for acting out feelings and emotions
Provide recreational and occu-pational activities.	Recreational and occupational activities frequently allow for cathartic outlets for hostile urges.
WHEN DANGER IS IMMINENT Forewarn of bodily touch.	Perceived invasion of territory may heighten feelings of being threatened and the inability to control personal self and prevent attack.
Explain what is going to occur in setting and keep repeating state-ments **slowly**.	Explanation helps to decrease anxiety about activities taking place.
Communicate expectations.	When expected and accepted behavior are clearly and concisely stated, the sense of security and control is increased.
Community Health/ Home Care Assess living arrangements (availability of weapons, crowd-ing, and availability of chemical substances, etc., enhances risk of violence).	A suicidal client may become self-destructive at any time during treatment.
Assess the environment for indi-viduals who will encourage client to comply with therapies and medications.	Adherence to medication schedule and therapy routine offers an opportunity to reduce anxiety as well as discuss feelings and thoughts about adjustments and changes occurring.

INTERVENTIONS	RATIONALE
Assess knowledge concerning the actions and side effects of medications.	Knowledge of medications assists in the observations of typical and atypical drug responses. Also, knowledge enhances compliance.
Solicit support to assist in structuring a home environment that has few violence-producing stimuli.	Continued verbalization after discharge enhances problem solving, e.g., the setting of mutual goals, acceptable behavior.
Make contract for outpatient/ group/family psychotherapy.	In group situations there is less opportunity to be manipulative if others are present to encourage honest behavior. Establishment of a contract helps to prevent creation of conditions which precipitate removal from therapy when unwanted emotions surface.
Share the possible changes in life-style that occur with the reentry of a family member who is at risk for violence.	Knowing what alterations in life-style might occur helps to decide if reentry into the home is the best option.
Assist in developing and using community support systems.	Awareness of support systems such as group therapy, community health nurse, visiting nurse, suicide hotlines, family support groups, crisis centers, police, emergency rooms, ministerial counseling, etc., decreases anxiety by knowing that assistance is available.

REFERENCES/BIBLIOGRAPHY

American Nurses' Association. (1989). **Classification systems for describing nursing practice: working papers** (ANA Pub. NO. NP–74 500 1/89). Kansas City, MO: ANA.

Boettcher, E.G. (1983). Preventing violent behavior: An integrated theoretical model for nursing. **Perspectives in Psychiatric Care, 21**(2), 54–58.

Bornstein, P.E. (1985). The use of restraints on a general psychiatric unit. **Journal of Clinical Psychology, 46**(5), 175–178.

Brant, B.A., & Osgood, N.J. (1990). The suicidal patient in long-term care institutions. **Journal of Gerontological Nursing, 16**(2), 15–18.

Brown, M. (1988). Dealing with actual or threatened violence. Nursing: **The Journal of Clinical Practice, Education and Management, 3**(30), 17–19.

Carpenito, L.J. (1987). **Nursing diagnosis—Application to clinical practice**, (2nd ed.). Philadelphia: Lippincott.

Carmel, H., & Hunter, M. (1989). Staff injuries from inpatient violence. **Hospital and Community Psychiatry, 40**(1), 41–46.

Carney, F.L. (1976). Treatment of the aggressive patient. In D.J. Madden, & J.R. Lion (Eds.). **Rage, hate, assault and other forms of violence** (pp. 223–248). Holliswood, NY: Spectrum.

Casseem, M. (1984). Violence on the wards. **Nursing Mirror, 158**(21), 14–16.

Cox, H.C., et al. (1989). **Clinical applications of nursing diagnosis**. Baltimore: Williams & Wilkins.

Dolan, M. (1990). **Community and home health care plans**. Springhouse, PA: Springhouse.

Drummond, D.J., Sparr, L.F., & Gordon, G.H. (1989). Hospital violence reduction among high risk patients. **Journal of the American Medical Association, 261**(17), 2531–2534.

Dubin, W.R. (1981). Evaluating and managing the violent patient. **Annals of Emergency Medicine, 10**(48), 481–484.

Gallahorn, G. (1976). Suicide and self destructive behavior: Clinical summary of recent research. In D.J. Madden, & J.R. Lion (Eds.). **Rage, hate, assault, and other forms of violence** (pp. 153–168). Holliswood, NY: Spectrum.

Gordon, M. (1989). **Manual of nursing diagnosis 1988–1989**. St. Louis: Mosby.

Gordon, M. (1987). **Nursing diagnosis: Process and application**. New York: McGraw-Hill.

Hyman, S.E. (1988). The violent patient. In S.E. Hyman (Ed.). **Psychiatric emergencies** (pp. 23–31). Boston: Little, Brown.

Jones, M.K. (1985). Patient violence: Report of 200 incidents. **Journal of Psychosocial Nursing, 23**(6), 12–17.

Kelly, E.N. (1987). Patterns of violence. In J. Haber (Ed.). **Comprehensive psychiatric nursing**, (3rd ed.) (pp. 601–617). New York: McGraw-Hill.

Kronberg, M.E. (1983). Nursing interventions in management of the assaultive patient. In J.R. Lion, & W.H. Reid (Eds.). **Assault within psychiatric facilities** (pp.225–240). New York: Grune Stratton.

Kurlowicz, L.H. (1990). Violence in the emergency department. **American Journal of Nursing, 90**(9), 35–39.

* Lanza, M.L. (1988). Factors relevant to patient assault. **Issues in Mental Health nursing, 9**(3), 239–257.

* Lanza, M.L., Milner, J., & Riley, E. (1988). Predictors of patient assault on acute in patient psychiatric units: A pilot study. **Issues in Mental Health Nursing, 9**(3), 259–270.

Lehmann, L.S., Padilla, N., Clark, S., & Loucks, S. (1983). Training personnel in the prevention and management of violent behavior. **Hospital and Community Psychiatry, 34**(1), 40–43.

Lion, J.R. (1972). **Evaluation and management of the violent patient: Guidelines in the hospital and institutions**. Springfield, IL: Charles C. Thomas.

Maagdenberg, A.M. (1983). The violent patient. **The American Journal of Nursing, 83**(3), 402–403.

Madden, D.J. (1983). Recognition and prevention of violence in psychiatric facilities. In J.R. Lion, & W.H. Reid (Eds.). **Assaults within psychiatric facilities** (pp. 213–224). New York: Grune & Stratton.

Madden, D.J., Lion, J., & Penna, M. (1976). Assaults on psychiatrists by patients. **American Journal of Psychiatry, 133**, pp. 422–425.

Miller, D., Walker, M.C., & Friedmen, D. (1989). Use of a holding technique to control the violent behavior of seriously disturbed adolescents. **Hospital and Community Psychiatry**, **40**(5), 520–524.

Morrison, E.F. (1989). Theoretical modeling to prevent violence in hospitalized psychiatric patients. **Research-in-Nursing-and-Health**, **12**(1), 31–40.

Monahan, J. (1982). Clinical prediction of violent behavior. **Psychiatric Annals, 12**(5), 509–513.

Morton, P.G. (1987). Staff roles and responsibilities in incidents of patient violence. **Archives of Psychiatric Nursing**, 1(4), 280–284.

Morton, P.G. (1986). Managing the violent patient. **American Journal of Nursing**, **86**(10), 1114–1116.

* Munns, D.C. (1985). A validation of the defining characteristics of the nursing diagnosis "potential for violence." **Nursing Clinics of North America, 20**(4), 711–721.

Navis, E.S. (1987). Controlling violent patients before they control you. **Nursing 87, 17**(9), 52–54.

Nickens, H.W. (1984). Assessment and management of the violent patient. In W.R. Dubin (Ed.). **Psychiatric Emergencies** (pp. 101–109). New York: Churchill Livingstone.

* Neizo, B.A., & Lanza, M.L. (1984). Post violence dialogue: Perception change through language restructuring. **Issues in Mental Health Nursing**, 6(3/4), 245–254.

North American Nursing Diagnosis Association. **Taxonomy I** (Rev. 1990). St. Louis: NANDA.

Percy, D. (1984). Violence: The drug alcohol patient. In J.T. Turner (Ed.). **Violence in the medical care setting: A survival guide** (pp. 123–151). Rockville, MD: Aspen.

Pisarcik, G. (1981). Violent patient. **Nursing 81**, (11), 63–65.

Rada, R.T. (1981). The violent patient: Rapid assessment and management. **Psychosomatics, 22**(2), 101–109.

Rossi, A.M., Hargreaves, W.A., & Shumway, M. (1989). Dangerous behavior and changes in treatment course. **Community Mental Health Journal, 25**(3), 209–217.

Sarsany, S.L. (1988). Violent behavior. **RN, 51**(9), 64–68.

Sclafani, M. (1986). Violence and violence control. **Journal of Psychosocial Nursing, 24**(11), 8–13.

Slack, P. (1983). Facing up to aggression. **Nursing Times, 79**(20), 10–11.

Steadman, H.J. (1976). Predicting dangerousness. In D.J. Madden, & J.R. Lion (Eds.). **Rage, hate, assault and other forms of violence** (pp. 53–70). Holliswood, NY: Spectrum.

Tardiff, K. (1983). A survey of assault by chronic patients in a state hospital system. In J.R. Lion, & W.H. Reid (Eds.). **Assaults within psychiatric facilities** (pp. 3–20). New York: Grune Stratton.

Wood, K.A., & Khuri, R. (1984). Violence: The emergency room patient. In J.T. Turner (Ed.). **Violence in the medical care setting: A survival guide** (pp. 57–83). Rockville, MD: Aspen.

Index